HUMAN ENDOCRINOLOGY

Obstetrics and Gynecology Series
Edited by Claude E. Heaton, M.D.

CONSULTANT IN ENDOCRINOLOGY: Clara Maass Memorial Hospital (Belleville, N. J.); Methodist Hospital of Brooklyn; Mountainside Hospital (Montclair, N. J.); Community Hospital at Glen Cove (N. Y.); St. Francis Hospital (Bronx, N. Y.); United Hospitals of Newark assigned to Presbyterian Hospital; Lutheran Medical Center (Brooklyn); Elizabeth A. Horton Memorial Hospital (Middletown, N. Y.); Newark Beth Israel Hospital (Newark, N. J.); New York Infirmary (New York City).

ATTENDING ENDOCRINOLOGIST: Knickerbocker Hospital (New York City); St. Barnabas Medical Center (Newark, N. J.); French Hospital (New York City); Booth Memorial Hospital (Flushing, N. Y.); Margaret Sanger Research Bureau (New York City).

RESEARCH ASSOCIATE: Veterans Administration Hospital (New York).

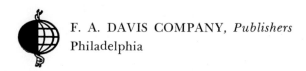

F. A. DAVIS COMPANY, *Publishers*
Philadelphia

HUMAN ENDOCRINOLOGY

1067

ILLUSTRATIONS

29 in color

HERBERT S. KUPPERMAN, Ph.D., M.D.

Associate Professor of Medicine, New York University Medical Center. ☐ Endocrinologist, Kingsbridge Veterans Hospital, Bronx. ☐ In charge of Endocrinology, Obstetrical and Gynecologic Service and Fourth Medical Service at Bellevue Hospital, New York.

Table of Contents
VOLUME 1

Table of Contents
VOLUME 2

Table of Contents
VOLUME 3

volume 2

chapter 11

Nature in her wisdom has so endowed human beings that ovarian failure and incapacity for conception take place at an age when the potential for both fetal abnormalities and complications of pregnancy increases. It appears that the human female is the only one of her gender to live beyond the time that she can bear offspring.[19]

Why the ovary alone is singled out to become the "Achilles' heel"[20] of the glands of internal secretion is not understood. Beneficial as it may appear from the standpoint of eugenics or obstetrics, cessation of ovarian function does create certain disadvantages in many women. The usual age at which women cease to menstruate and are no longer able to bear children is between 45 and 50 years. Barnes[1] has stated that the age at cessation of menses has been extended during the last several hundred years. This comes as no surprise and might even be anticipated, when one considers that human vital statistics in general have shown an increase in life expectancy. In fact, in 1960 the 65-year-old age group was estimated to be about 10 per cent of our population.[21] Thus, menopausal women are encountered in larger numbers, and efforts must be made to make living more pleasant and worth while for them.

The climacteric heralds the beginning of inactivity of ovarian function so that not merely is fertilization impossible but an endocrine dysfunction also ensues. This disturbance may be productive of symptoms constituting the menopausal or climacteric syndrome. These symptoms

Clinical Management of the Climacteric Syndrome*

need not be as sharply demarcated as the sudden cessation of menses, but may be gradual in onset, giving rise imperceptibly to the full-blown clinical picture. On the other hand, the artificial menopause brought on by surgery or irradiation is apt to produce obvious effects more acutely, often in a matter of days, with vasomotor symptoms predominating.

Menopausal Physiology. Griffith[9] has emphasized the extragenital value of the ovarian hormones. It is necessary to consider these physiologic ramifications in formulating any therapeutic regimen to treat the menopause. The basis for this concept is that the ovary cannot be viewed primarily as a reproductive force; by virtue of its internal secretions it plays an important role in metabolic function.

ESTROGEN AND CALCIFICATION. Estrogen, one of the prime sex steroids secreted by the ovary, is essential in protein anabolism and nitrogen retention.[24] This is particularly true in the dynamic processes involved in calcification of bone. When the ovaries cease to function, and especially when they are removed surgically, the stimulus for osteoblastic activity is diminished. As a result, the normal protein bony matrix is reduced and diminished calcification occurs. Osteoporosis may then occur in some women and may be a cause of significant disability. This may progress

---

* This chapter is based in part on a paper on the menopause,[14] portions of which are quoted with permission of the editor of the journal in which it was first published.

to the extent of collapse of a vertebra (Fig. 244). In addition, excessive excretion of calcium may result and be a factor in the formation of renal calculi. The excessive calcium excretion is not attributed to any catabolic process per se but is due to increased amounts of calcium being made available secondary to diminished calcium deposition in bone. Decreased calcification of bone occurs as a result of the diminished protein matrix.

CHOLESTEROL METABOLISM. An intimate relation exists between estrogen and cholesterol metabolism. Hypercholesteremia has been noted after a decrease in estrogen level has occurred. This may account for the fact that patients subjected to bilateral oophorectomy are more vulnerable to hypercholesteremia and its reported adverse effects than are women not so treated. This may well account for the fact that

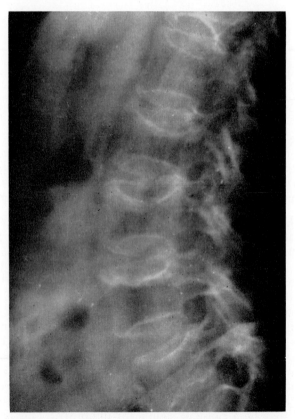

FIG. 244. Patient GA, age 70. Surgical climacteric occurred 25 years ago. Note the marked osteoporosis of the vertebrae with the typical "fish-mouth" appearance of the intervertebral disk. The soft osteoporotic bone is readily compressed by the relatively firm intervertebral disk.

the incidence of coronary heart disease accompanied by hypercholester-emia is comparable in postmenopausal women and in men of a similar age. This is in contrast to the much greater preponderance of athero-sclerotic heart disease in men at the age when active ovarian secretion of estrogens is seen in women. The importance of a functioning ovary in diminishing atherosclerotic coronary disease is inferred by the observation that coronary atherosclerosis is 10 to 40 times more prevalent in men under 40 than in women of a similar age.[28] However, high doses of estrogen can change an abnormal cholesterol pattern in men to a more favorable one and thereby diminish the degree of coronary insufficiency and atherosclerosis.[26] Indeed, it has been said that small doses of estrogen[16-18] which are only minimally feminizing, instead of the larger ones originally used,[2, 6, 15] may also be effective in decreasing blood choles-terol. However, the reported lowering of cholesterol with these dose levels of estrogen did not appear to be outside the range of variation alone.[2, 6, 15]

ADRENOCORTICAL ACTIVITY. Animal experiments have shown that oophorectomy has been associated with adrenal hypertrophy. A similar situation is said to exist in some women in whom an increase in 17-keto-steroid excretion has been reported to occur in the menopause. The in-crease in adrenal cortical secretion of the 17-ketosteroid precursors may account for the increased degree of hirsutism that many women experience during the climacteric (Fig. 245). The increased adrenocortical

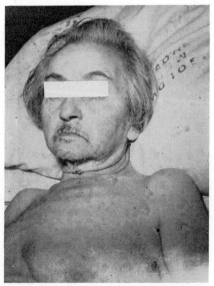

FIG. 245. *Female, age 59, with a diagnosis of idiopathic hirsutism. Her steroid excretion was normal. Her menopause occurred 8 years prior to the time the photograph was taken. She noted an enormous increase in facial hair since her climacteric.*

activity occasionally observed in the menopausal patient may theoretically predispose these patients to cardiovascular disease, as suggested by Selye in his studies on stress.[27] Clinically, the hypertensive phase noted in the climacteric patient probably is associated with the vasomotor instability that these patients exhibit. However, hypertension per se is not likely to appear in a previously normotensive female. Of a group of 200 women in the menopause, including 179 who were surgically castrated, 13 per cent were hypertensive as compared to a 10 per cent incidence of hypertension in the same group of women prior to the onset of the climacteric syndrome.[28]

Diagnosis.   Laboratory Tests.   With the onset of the menopause, follicle-stimulating hormone (FSH) may be excreted in large amounts and the urinary estrogen levels are usually diminished. Assays to determine these changes are costly and cannot be considered as routine procedures. The vaginal smear is helpful, but not absolute. At one time, it was felt that the vaginal smear might be a possible yardstick to use in therapy; at the present time, no definitive relationship has been found to exist between severity of symptoms, clinical response, and degree of cornification shown by the vaginal smear. Randall[23] found that, when the menopause was of from five to 10 years' duration, 44.8 per cent of the women with natural menopause showed estrogen deficiency; with hysterectomy and castration, 30 per cent more had deficient smears than after hysterectomy alone.

Clinical Picture.   Inasmuch as the specific tests used in detecting hormonal insufficiency are too complicated and not precise enough to establish adequately the diagnosis of the climacteric, the clinician must depend on symptoms.

Vasomotor Symptoms.   The principal symptoms noted in the menopause are listed in Table 12. The first four—vasomotor symptoms, paresthesia, insomnia, and nervousness—are the most important, with the

TABLE 12

Menopausal Symptomatology

Vasomotor symptoms	Arthralgia and myalgia
Paresthesia	Headache
Insomnia	Palpitation
Nervousness	Formication
Melancholia	Irritability
Vertigo	Memory loss
Weakness (fatigue)	Inability to concentrate

vasomotor symptoms (hot flashes) exceeding the others in their prominence as far as patient discomfort is concerned. Hot flashes are an interesting and important manifestation of the climacteric. One must stress,
however, that the vasomotor symptoms (flashes or flushes) are a comparatively late manifestation of the climacteric. They do not appear to be
related to the elevated FSH excretion levels but probably are associated
with the decrease in estrogen level. One may administer a dose of estrogen
that will have little if any effect on the patient's FSH excretion but will
adequately control the symptomatology of the climacteric, particularly the
vasomotor symptoms. The precise physiologic mechanism causing the
flashes is not known. Basically, it has been said that the arteriolar changes
of the blush area result from diminution or absence of steroid control.
Reynolds[25] has shown that the loss of this regulator causes hot flushes by
vasomotor instability. Patients with severe flashes may be plagued primarily with abundant perspiration and chilly sensations. One patient
described her difficulty as "like walking out and standing in the rain."
Suddenly her face was covered with sweat, yet no heat was experienced.
These vasomotor complaints may vary from transient feelings of warmth
that are infrequent to objective evidence of reddening. It must also be
borne in mind that exciting factors such as a large meal, joy, anger, or
even the normal vascular changes that occur from relaxation in sleep
may influence the frequency and the severity of the flashes the patient
has been experiencing.

Symptoms Other than Vasomotor. The physician who is aware
of the climacteric syndrome will suspect its presence in a patient
complaining of arthralgia, myalgia, formication, headache, and palpitations, despite the fact that vasomotor symptoms may be minimal or
absent and menses continue. The so-called lesser symptoms, when present
in sufficient numbers, may be equally as distressing as vasomotor complaints and warn the clinician of the impending climacteric syndrome. If
one depends primarily on vasomotor complaints as a guide to determine
the need for therapy, a large group of patients who are suffering with
other manifestations of the menopause, yet who have minimal vasomotor
symptoms, will be neglected. It is necessary, therefore, that the entire
menopausal symptomatology be considered *in toto* both with respect to
the diagnosis and the measurement of the patient's response to drug therapy. It should also be emphasized that the patient may be classified as one
in the climacteric and be treated accordingly if she shows the typical
symptom complex outlined in Table 12, despite the fact that the catamenia is still present, albeit regular or irregular, or consists of staining,
menorrhagia, or hypermenorrhea.

MODE OF INTERROGATION. Before therapy is discussed, several points
should be emphasized with respect to proper interrogation of the patient.
For example, we attach a considerable degree of importance to the symptoms of a patient who claims that vasomotor symptoms, occurring at

night, disturb her sleep. These differ from the vasomotor symptoms seen in the hypertensive patient during the daytime. A hypertensive patient who is not menopausal may experience flashes, but they are not the true vasomotor symptoms of the menopause, inasmuch as when the hypertensive patient sleeps she is not disturbed by the hypertensive flashes or flushing which she had noted previously during the day. The question of palpitations should also be looked into more deeply. The patient should not merely be asked whether or not there is a quickening or acceleration of her heartbeat, but, specifically, whether she observes palpitations in a sitting or a resting position. This is significant palpitation and is not related to physical activity per se. Hence, the physician must be circumspect in his questioning and be aware that certain family and economic problems may enhance or diminish the menopausal symptoms and the need for therapy.

THERAPY

The relief of symptoms and not the change in laboratory data serves the physician best in determining the efficacy of therapy. While we will not take issue with the psychiatric treatment of the menopause, a combined endocrine and psychiatric approach probably will yield infinitely better therapeutic results than either one alone. On the other hand, there is no doubt in our minds that the endocrine management of these patients should be the principal form of therapy resulting in a more reasonable and simpler, yet efficacious, means of treatment.

Placebo Effects.   The principal handicap in determining the effectiveness of endocrine therapy is that in human beings, unlike animals, medication in general exerts a twofold effect—one due to the pharmacologic action of the drug itself and the other to the psychological influence of drug administration. One must be cognizant of the fact that a significant number of patients show an excellent response to a placebo (Table 13). We feel that the dramatic results reported with preparations such as vitamin E and various proprietary "vegetable preparations" on the market at the present time owe their supposed effectiveness to the psychological effects of placebo medication alone.

Who Should Be Treated?   It should be noted that not all women experience menopausal symptoms, when menses cease. It is also difficult to evaluate precisely the number of women who experience vasomotor symptoms as compared to those who do not. A report[8] has shown that, in 1000 cases studied, 50.8 per cent of patients had no symptoms except cessation of menses. Of those who did have symptoms, 89.7 per cent worked as usual without interruption, and only 10.3 per cent were truly incapacitated at intervals. This does not mean that the remaining patients (the 89.7 per cent who worked as usual) did not have menopausal symptoms. A patient may or may not work with vasomotor symptoms, depending on her character and emotional stability. It should be emphasized that drug therapy, psychotherapy, and sedation are reserved only for those patients who request treatment. The fact that the patients are able to perform their household duties and are not completely incapacitated does not preclude the therapeutic use of whatever agent the physician finds helpful. There is no need for stoicism on the part of the patient by refusing appropriate therapy at the time the menopause prevails.

Psychotherapy. If psychotherapy includes kindly treatment of the patient and a truly sympathetic reception of her complaints, it may be offered readily and given frequently. However, psychotherapy may be limited in the minds of certain physicians to the so-called "couch treatment." This type of therapy appears wasteful since the syndrome is readily controlled by organic therapy. However, there is no question that even minimal psychotherapy, when used in conjunction with the drugs mentioned in the next paragraphs, will be synergistic in allaying many of the menopausal symptoms.

ANCILLARY PROCEDURES. Information not easily obtained, yet which may influence a patient's response to therapy, concerns eating habits, especially if the patient is a widow and lives alone. Such patients often do not think that food is important, and dietary deficiencies occur. Also, seven nights a week spent glued to the television set is not relaxing. Clinic patients, notably those who work, would do well with a few suggestions on the allocation of a little time to a few simple diversions. In a large family, the assistance of one of the children or the husband will easily solve problems that the patient herself is apt not to appreciate. This may considerably improve the patient's mental status and thereby prevent an exacerbation of the menopausal syndrome.

Sedation. BARBITURATES. A word of caution should be expressed about the use of phenobarbital continuously and for prolonged periods of time. Usually, more than 24 hours are required before a single dose of phenobarbital may be excreted from the body. Hence, the possibility of cumulative effects due to phenobarbital ingestion must be recognized, with the possibility that barbiturate addiction may take place. One may anticipate that a patient who is so addicted may show symptoms not unlike those noted in the climacteric, despite the fact that barbiturate therapy is continued without cessation. However, with addiction, the need for additional and continuous therapy is evident. As a result, one may create a symptom complex similar to a rolling snowball where, because of habituation, increased doses of the barbiturate are necessary so that eventually the patient may be condemned to the ingestion of increasing doses of phenobarbital. Thus, the repeated use of phenobarbital without restriction may lead, at times, to the undesirable side effect of barbiturate addiction. Such a result would make the treatment worse than the disease.

TABLE 13

EFFECT OF ENDOCRINE AND NONENDOCRINE PREPARATIONS
ON PATIENTS WITH THE MENOPAUSAL SYNDROME

No.	Preparation	Daily Dose in Mg.	No. of Patient Trials	Results		
				Excellent	Moderate	Poor
1.	Placebo	1 tablet	844	203	145	496
2.	Phenobarbital	15.0 t.i.d.	118	26	27	65
3.	Conjugated estrogens equine[1]	1.25	405	308	70	27
4.	Ethinyl estradiol[2]	0.05	312	187	75	50
5.	Estrone	10,000 I.U.	86	36	24	26
		0.5	36	13	11	12
6.	Estradiol	1.0	38	20	13	5
7.	Estradiol linguets	0.25	29	15	11	3
8.	Stilbestrol	0.1 t.i.d.	49	15	15	19
9.	Dienestrol	0.5	91	28	32	31
10.	Hexestrol	3.0	48	14	14	20
11.	Chlorotrianisene	12.0*	124	61	40	23
12.	Methallenestril[3]	3.0	95	38	29	28
13.	Methallenestril	3.0 b.i.d.	33	12	8	13
14.	Ethinyl estradiol & methyltestosterone	0.02 5.0	114	53	38	23
15.	Ethinyl estradiol & methyltestosterone	0.04 10.0	54	24	23	7
16.	Ethinyl estradiol & methyltestosterone & perphenazine	0.04 10.0 4.0	97	57	29	11
17.	Perphenazine[4]	4.0	55	12	12	31
18.	Potassium estrone sulfate ..	1.25	94	47	28	19
19.	Piperazine estrone sulfate[5] .	1.5	75	44	21	10
20.	Estrone sulfate	1.25	82	42	21	19
21.	Estrone sulfate, enteric-coated	1.25	78	35	28	15
22.	Meprobamate	400.0 q.i.d.	51	14	14	23
23.	Hydroxyzine[6]	10.0 t.i.d.	22	2	4	16
24.	Hydroxyzine	25.0 b.i.d.	29	7	7	15
25.	Ectylurea[7]	300.0 t.i.d.	55	7	16	32
26.	Benactyzine hydrochloride[8].	2.5 t.i.d.	14	2	1	11
27.	Benactyzine hydrochloride .	5.0 t.i.d.	11	—	3	8
28.	Chlordiazepoxide[9]	25.0 t.i.d.	16	5	4	7
29.	Chlordiazepoxide	10.0 t.i.d.	44	18	9	17

*Or 24.0 mg. every other day. [1]Premarin; [2]Estinyl; [3]Vallestril; [4]Trilafon; [5]Sulestrex; [6]Atarax; [7]Nostyn; [8]Suavitil; [9]Librium.

TRANQUILIZING PREPARATIONS.   In an attempt to overcome some of the undesirable side effects of phenobarbital administration, particularly those of "hangover" effects and possible addiction, a number of ataractic compounds have been tested in the menopausal patient (Table 13). These have included perphenazine, meprobamate, hydroxyzine, ectylurea, and benactyzine. The data indicated that the use of these compounds in adequate doses did not seem to be therapeutically successful in controlling the climacteric syndrome. As a matter of fact, the response to benactyzine therapy was considerably poorer than that noted after placebo therapy. This was due to the undesirable side effects attributed to the administration of this preparation. In general, the results with the other ataractic drugs indicated that they were no better than those obtained with phenobarbital and slightly better than that obtained with a placebo. More recently, it has been noted that 10.0 mg. of chlordiazepoxide (Librium), t.i.d., offered some relief in a significant number of patients with the climacteric. The results obtained with this preparation were superior to those achieved with phenobarbital (Table 13).

Hormonal Therapy.   In general, the following types of endocrine preparations may be employed in the management of the climacteric: (1) estrogens, (2) estrogens and androgens, (3) androgens alone, and (4) estrogens in conjunction with tranquilizers or sedatives. Hormones may be administered (1) orally, (2) by injection, (3) by pellet implantation, (4) vaginally, or (5) by inunction. In our initial efforts[13] to determine the results of medication in the climacteric, we used both synthetic estrogens and the so-called steroidal groups. The synthetics included diethylstilbestrol (stilbestrol), hexestrol, dienestrol, methallenestril (Vallestril), and chlorotrianisene (TACE). The steroidal estrogens included free estradiol, ethinyl estradiol (Estinyl), conjugated estrogens equine (Premarin, Conestrin), with and without methyltestosterone.

In addition, we employed piperazine estrone sulfate (Sulestrex) potassium estrone sulfate, crystalline estrone sulfate, and crystalline estrone sulfate in an enteric-coated form. Vitamin E preparations, phenobarbital, and placebos were given from time to time with the above estrogenic compounds. In determining the clinical efficacy of the various preparations, particular attention was paid to the appearance of the preparation so that neither the patient nor the physician had any knowledge concerning the nature of the medicament that was being used.

THERAPEUTIC RESPONSE.   The dosages of the various preparations employed are listed in Table 13. Vitamin E was provided in 50.0 to 100.0 mg. capsules or tablets daily. The therapeutic response was judged by the effectiveness of the preparations on the climacteric syndrome as a whole. This is in contrast to attempted evaluation based on the recording of the number of flashes in a 24-hour period, as recommended by Jones.[11] The clinical response was graded as *excellent,* associated with complete relief;

moderate, with minimal residual symptoms; or *poor,* with no relief being noted. The vaginal smear, while taken prior to each patient interview, could not be depended on for true grading of response. The only constant change noted in the vaginal smear was cornification in most patients receiving estrogen therapy.

ESTROGENS. The best results were obtained with ethinyl estradiol and conjugated estrogens equine alone or in combination with androgens. The crystalline estrone sulfate derivatives did not produce results as good as the conjugated estrogens equine, milligram for milligram. Stilbestrol produced nausea in 20 per cent of cases. The frequency of this complaint, plus the darkening of the areolae of the breasts, definitely limited its use. Conjugated estrogens equine were presumed to be the source of two cases of dermatitis. Withdrawal bleeding affected 18 per cent of those receiving combined free and ethinyl estradiol.

The data in Table 13 show that no one preparation could be considered to be 100 per cent effective. Vitamin E, considered a panacea for so many conditions, did no better than a placebo. One other point to be emphasized is that it has been claimed that certain estrogens have less of a bleeding effect on the endometrium than others. We believe that, when a comparable dose of an estrogen is used, it has the same potential hazard of producing endometrial bleeding as any other estrogen. The purported results showing that certain preparations have less bleeding tendency may be explained simply by the fact that a less effective dose of that particular estrogen was being used. When a dose of any estrogen comparable to the clinical effectiveness of 0.05 mg. of ethinyl estradiol was employed, the same bleeding tendency would occur.

ESTROGENS AND ANDROGENS. When androgens, in the form of methyltestosterone, were added to the estrogens, physical vigor and *joie de vivre* became noticeable. Dull personalities seemed to become a bit less so. Occasionally, patients who had been seen for some time modestly whispered about an increase in libido. There were some, however, who did complain of distinct, bothersome clitoral irritation.

The apparent synergism of combined estrogen-androgen therapy permitted us to use smaller doses of each steroid, yet still maintain an equal or greater effect than was accomplished with larger doses of either preparation alone. Vaginal bleeding did not occur. We were constantly alert for masculinizing effects, but there was no evidence of arrhenomimetic phenomena of significance with the doses of methyltestosterone that were employed.

The general degree of improvement in a patient's well being attributable to androgen therapy had a decided effect in ameliorating her anxieties and nervousness which originally were major complaints. Estrogen therapy alone did not seem to be so all-inclusive in effect. The physiologic explanation of the clinical success attributed to the combined steroid medication is perhaps closely related to the enhanced protein anabolism and the maintenance of nitrogen and phosphorus balance that such therapy induced. Osteoporosis of the menopause may thus be better controlled. Although the site of the specific effect of testosterone is unknown, the modus operandi of the estrogens may be ascribed to improved cell permeability.[9] It is reasoned then that, with the basic anabolic property of testosterone and the resultant protein storage, the enhanced cellular activity produced by estrogen increases the potential of the protein anabolic effect of the androgen. The over-all effect of estrogen-androgen combination is to prevent the depletion of body protein substances as age increases. While beyond the scope of this chapter, one must also give serious consideration to long-range steroid therapy in geriatrics, as proposed by Masters.[19] In his hands this regimen effectively influenced 75 per cent of the geriatric persons treated, with notable physical and psychological improvement. We are entirely in accord with Masters' concepts and have confirmed his observations. In addition, it has been noted that such long-continued therapy is not only beneficial from the physical and mental point of view, but also appears to be without danger as far as neoplastic tendencies are concerned.[30]

Advantages of Estrogen-Androgen Medication. It should be mentioned that, in the combined use of estrogens and androgens, we do not mean to imply that estrogens can neutralize the undesirable effects of androgens and vice versa. The advantage of their combined use lies in the fact that smaller doses of each one may be administered, so that undesirable side effects due to either steroid are minimized. On the other hand, the combination of the two steroids results in a synergistic effect, approaching the effectiveness of either one alone when administered in higher doses. In other words, if a patient would bleed when 0.05 mg. of ethinyl estradiol per day was administered, we could not prevent that bleeding by the addition of 10.0 mg. of methyltestosterone. Similarly, if 10.0 mg. of methyltestosterone will produce facial hirsutism in a particularly sensitive patient, we cannot inhibit the iatrogenic hypertrichosis with a dose of 0.05 mg. of ethinyl estradiol. However, one can diminish the dose of ethinyl estradiol to 0.02 mg. and administer 5.0 mg. of methyltestosterone simultaneously and achieve a therapeutic effect comparable to that obtained with either 0.05 mg. of ethinyl estradiol or 10.0 mg. of methyltestosterone alone. In so doing, one diminishes the bleeding propensity which was observed when the 0.05 mg. dose of ethinyl estradiol was employed or the hirsutism noted with the 10.0 mg. dose of methyltestosterone. An interesting possible advantage of therapy with combined estrogens and androgens is that the estrogens at times may promote fluid accumulation and induce increased nervousness, anxiety, and irritability in certain menopausal patients. The value of estrogens and androgens in these patients would be that the tendency for estrogens to produce enhanced nervousness and retention of fluid is diminished with a smaller dose of estrogens, but the clinical efficacy is maintained by the addition of androgens without diminishing the desired clinical effect.

ESTROGENS WITH CENTRAL NERVOUS SYSTEM STIMULANTS OR DEPRES-
SANTS. It has been suggested that the combined use of tranquilizing
drugs or analeptic agents with estrogens and/or androgens would be of
advantage clinically. The simultaneous administration of these preparations might conceivably result in true synergism whereby a more satisfactory therapeutic effect could be achieved with such a combination. Their
use in the management of the climacteric would be obvious.

A bit fearful of the possibilities of accumulation of effect or addiction
to extended barbiturate administration, we did not use the combination
of estrogen and a barbiturate.

Estrogens and/or Androgens with Reserpine.   An attempt was made
to determine clinically the value of combinations of reserpine,[12] the purified alkaloid prepared from *Rauwolfia serpentina,* with different hormones. Women with natural or surgically produced menopause who had
demonstrated their capacities to respond to the preparations mentioned
above were studied. Two clinically proved effective estrogens (ethinyl
estradiol 0.05 mg. per day or conjugated estrogens equine 1.25 mg. per
day) were administered, since a specific clinical response could be anticipated for the prescribed estrogen. Thereby one could ascertain whether
or not a synergistic effect was achieved by the addition of reserpine.
Basically, both of these estrogens generally effected a 70 to 90 per cent
relief of symptoms. Smaller doses of either estrogen when combined with
reserpine were found to be less satisfactory than the steroid alone.

The dose of reserpine was either 0.1 or 0.2 mg. twice daily. Such a
fixed combination of reserpine and an estrogen was found to be somewhat
of a handicap. It was apparent that, when one component is productive
of some untoward response, an attempt at regulation is hindered by an
inflexible combination. Nasal stuffiness and drowsiness, the most bothersome side effects due to the reserpine, caused sufficient discomfort to
exclude the use of this preparation in the management of the climacteric.
Libido was not affected either favorably or unfavorably by reserpine.
Table 14 shows the doses and the types of preparations employed in
combination with reserpine and provides strong evidence for the fact that
no set of combinations superseded the excellent results achieved with
conjugated estrogens or ethinyl estradiol alone (see Table 13). No synergistic action could be demonstrated between reserpine and the estrogens
used, as had been noted when androgens and estrogens were used in
combination. On the other hand, complaints not attributable to the
menopause, but nevertheless apt to accentuate the climacteric symptomatology, took origin in the side effects from the reserpine. As noted above,
with the doses of reserpine employed one encountered nasal stuffiness
and drowsiness, as well as unusual dreams verging on nightmares, and
even Parkinson-like disorders. Therefore, the combination of reserpine
with a steroid in a single tablet is impractical for clinical use in the
climacteric. However, it should be emphasized that, if they are admin-

TABLE 14

EFFECT OF COMBINED THERAPY WITH RESERPINE AND DIFFERENT STEROIDS
ON PATIENTS WITH THE MENOPAUSAL SYNDROME

	Regimen*			Results		
No.	Preparation	Dosage in Mg.	No. of Patients	Excellent	Moderate	Poor
1.	Reserpine ethinyl estradiol	0.1 0.02	43	12	11	20
2.	Reserpine ethinyl estradiol	0.2 0.02	25	12	3	10
3.	Reserpine methyltestosterone	0.2 5.0	35	15	9	11
4.	Reserpine ethinyl estradiol methyltestosterone	0.2 0.02 5.0	57	29	11	17
5.	Reserpine ethinyl estradiol methyltestosterone	0.1 0.01 2.5	50	20	14	16
6.	Reserpine d-amphetamine homatropine methyl bromide	0.25 5.0 5.0	45	7	9	29

* All preparations were administered b.i.d.

istered separately, the simultaneous use of steroids and reserpine may be helpful. A combined tablet did not seem advisable in our patients because of inflexibility of dosage and undesirable effects due to the reserpine itself.

Estrogen-Androgen-Phenothiazine Preparation. On the other hand, a combination of estrogen or estrogen and androgen with a phenothiazine compound seemed to be unusually effective in therapy of the climacteric syndrome. Administration of perphenazine with ethinyl estradiol and methyltestosterone, in the form of a delayed-absorption tablet, appeared to yield a better therapeutic effect than any one of the preparations administered alone (Table 13). No undesirable effects were observed with the doses employed. There was no evidence that perphenazine alone or in combination either induced or accentuated melancholia or depression in the patients studied.

Mode of Administration of Drug Therapy. ORAL. Traditionally, medicaments are most simply and safely administered orally. As a rule, this provided an uncomplicated and convenient mode of treatment in the majority of patients studied. Admittedly, this modality of therapy placed less demand on the physician's time so that less frequent office visits and supervision of therapy were necessary. The frequency of administration depended on the clinical efficacy of the compounds used and their duration of effect. Generally speaking, it was necessary to take steroid medication only once per day. One preparation, chlorotrianisene, had a more prolonged effect, due to possible storage in depot areas in the body, and could be administered once every other day or even less frequently.[7]

PARENTERAL. Intramuscular injections are indicated specifically for those patients who are unreliable and will not or can not remember to take the oral medicaments.

Depo-Preparations. The long-acting parenteral preparations have much to offer by providing a continuous and effective control of the patient's condition. Aqueous suspensions were not satisfactory because they were usually painful. In contrast, esterification of some steroids provided nonirritating, oil-soluble materials that acted over a comparatively long period of time. Two such preparations, estradiol valerate (Delestrogen) and estradiol cyclopentylpropionate (Depo-Estradiol)[10] are very effective and last for a period of two to three weeks.

Table 15 points to the control afforded by these parenterally given steroids as compared to orally taken preparations listed. All of the long-acting preparations were clinically comparable with respect to their ability

TABLE 15

EFFECT OF PARENTERALLY GIVEN STEROIDS ON PATIENTS
WITH THE MENOPAUSAL SYNDROME

No.	Preparation	Dosage in Mg. Given Every 2 Weeks	No. of Patients	Results		
				Excellent	Moderate	Poor
1.	Estradiol cyclopentylpropionate	5.0	51	33	6	12
2.	Estradiol valerate	10.0	110	75	24	11
3.	Estradiol valerate	10.0*	16	6	6	4
4.	Estradiol cyclopentylpropionate Testosterone cyclopentylpropionate	2.0 50.0	29	16	9	4
5.	Estradiol cyclopentylpropionate Testosterone cyclopentylpropionate	2.0 100.0	68	48	13	7
6.	Testosterone cyclopentylpropionate	100.0	28	18	5	5
7.	Polyestradiol phosphate	40.0	43	27	9	7
8.	Placebo	1 cc.	167	51	33	83

* Given every 3 weeks.

to effect relief of menopausal symptoms. Parenterally given placebos, on the other hand, induced a poor effect by comparison. The outstanding result of the long-acting parenteral medicaments was that they achieved adequate relief for 15 to 25 days. These results were encouraging since one could now offer intramuscular administration at two-week to three-week intervals, instead of the tedious two or three times per week administration previously practiced. Estradiol valerate, 10.0 mg., and estradiol cyclopentylpropionate, 5.0 mg., usually given at two-week intervals, were equally as effective as any of the orally given materials that have been used. For those patients in whom oil solutions were poorly tolerated, an aqueous solution of polyestradiol phosphate proved to be an effective substitute. Adequate control of the menopausal syndrome was achieved with 40.0 mg. of this preparation injected every three to four weeks.[3] Oily and aqueous solutions of the long-acting steroids can be used conveniently in patients who cannot swallow pills or tablets. They also provide a method of definitively controlling unreliable patients and make available an additional modality to improve the therapeutic effect of steroid therapy in patients who do not respond well to oral medication.

PELLET IMPLANTATION. Despite the simplicity of oral medication and the availability of the long-acting parenterally given steroids, the menopause induced by surgery may be treated best by pellet implantation. Deanesly and Parkes[5] showed that pellet implantation of steroids resulted in a prolonged release of the material in a manner akin to that observed in the *in vivo* steroid elaboration from the organs of internal secretion. The advantage of this type of therapy was a sustained, continuous, physiologic level of the implanted steroid substance over an extended period of time. Therefore, pellet implantation in the human was seen as a way of offering the patient more constant but physiologic blood levels of the steroid due to the long-continued effect of pellets. Pellets provided the ultimate in replacement therapy, inasmuch as continued maintenance of appropriate levels of the steroids is achieved with little discomfort to the patient. Not only does one get a continuous endocrine effect but also the pellet itself would in substance simulate the secretion of the ablated organ.

To Spare or Not to Spare the Ovaries. The surgically induced menopause frequently may be apparent before the patient leaves the hospital. This is especially true of younger women, particularly those below the age of 35 to 40. It is impossible at this point to proceed without a word about the practice of oophorectomy dependent on age alone. We are in agreement with Randall's[22] strong plea to retain ovaries in the absence of any pelvic disease that makes it imperative to remove these important structures. The present trend does seem to oppose the routine bilateral oophorectomy of normal ovaries, in cases of benign uterine disease, just because of age. This strikes a happy note, since in time the frequency of surgically induced menopause must proportionately lessen.

Method of Pellet Implantation and Preparations. In treating patients who had both ovaries removed at the time of total hysterectomy, we have found it extremely effective to insert pellets of steroid hormone into the rectus muscle beneath the anterior sheath during closure of the abdominal wall (Fig. 246).

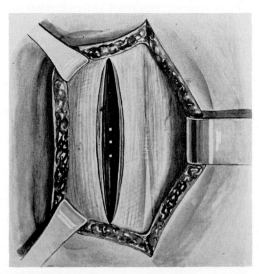

FIG. 246. *Site of pellet implantation. The pellets are placed in the rectus sheath after the total hysterectomy while the abdomen is being closed. Note the spacing of the pellets at the time of their insertion.*

Our earlier studies[4] included at first the implantation of single 25.0 mg. pellets of estradiol. This was quickly increased to three pellets of 25.0 mg. of the same substance.

Initially, we studied a group of surgically castrated women below the age of 40 treated with estradiol pellets alone, and used as controls a corresponding number of castrated women of comparable age who were untreated. The menopausal index means of evaluation[13] showed effective control by the pellets in the majority of patients, with a reduction in severity of complaints up to 15 months. However, not all of the patients receiving pellets were relieved of all symptoms, and not all of the surgically castrated patients in the control series complained of menopausal symptoms despite bilateral oophorectomy. We believe that since a majority of women in the younger age group—i. e., under 40 years of age—who are subjected to castration will usually exhibit profound and incapacitating withdrawal (climacteric) symptoms, implantation of estrogens or estrogens combined with androgens is a propitious and wise form of therapy to be done at the time of surgery before these symptoms can occur.

Thus, estrogen pellets induced a smooth course, free of the postoperative symptoms usually noted in precipitous estrogen withdrawal. The patients in the control series had many minor complaints, notably absent in those treated with estrogen pellet implantation. Accordingly, one may assume that these symptoms were alleviated in the patients treated with pellets. It is possible that the symptoms might not have necessitated medical aid, but still they would have been a burden to the patient.

The vaginal smears provided evidence for the long-continued effects of the pellets, inasmuch as many of the patients showed a normal or increased degree of cornification 12 to 15 months after surgery and implantation. As a rule, the estrogenic response was noted promptly, but occasionally smears did not manifest an effect due to the pellets for the first six weeks.

Estrogen and Testosterone Pellets. In view of the synergistic effect of androgens in the climacteric, we now use three pellets of 25.0 mg. of estradiol plus two pellets of 75.0 mg. each of testosterone propionate. The addition of testosterone pellets to the estrogen was distinctly advantageous in offering the patient a general sense of well being. While the estrogen alone produced a well-controlled and satisfied patient, the combination of androgen and estrogen pellets gave a more effective response; improved spirits were readily apparent, as well as enhanced libido, an important factor in maintaining normal marital relationships. In these cases, we were careful to note any evidence of excessive hair growth. The slow release of androgens from the pellet site in doses of gammas per day could not be considered a factor in hirsutism. However, one must be cognizant of the increased hirsutism that may spontaneously occur in some postmenopausal women. Any hair growth noted is probably a consequence of the natural course of the syndrome and not due to the minute amounts of androgens released from the pellet site.

Post-surgical Pellet Implantation. When, for some reason, pellets were not implanted at operation, we utilized a standard trochar (Kearns injector) for insertion of the pellets. When properly done, this technique is not associated with significant discomfort and should be considered essentially an office procedure. The subscapular or inguinal regions may be used. The same number of pellets are implanted as were used at the time of surgery, and the hiatus created is closed with a single 0000 suture.

Contraindication to Pellet Implantation. It should be emphasized that pellet implantation of estrogens is contraindicated in any patient who has a uterus or ovaries. Estrogen pellets may cause irregular bleeding if the uterus remains *in situ*, as has been reported in 30 to 50 per cent of the cases. Small fibroids in these uteri invariably increase in size. Twombly and Millen[29] advised, and we have reiterated,[4] that an intact uterus is a contraindication to estradiol pellet implantation unless prior destruction of the endometrium by radiation was done. We noted no vaginal spotting (not unexpectedly, as all of our patients had had hysterectomies). Pellet implantation is also contraindicated in patients with breast disease or a history of genital carcinoma. Breast engorgement or tenderness was not noted in any of our patients receiving estrogens alone or in those in whom estradiol and testosterone pellets were implanted.

ESTROGEN SUPPOSITORIES. A relatively infrequent site for the administration of steroids is the vagina. Nevertheless, this mode of therapy may be of tremendous value in the management of patients who have developed senile vaginitis. It is these patients who are especially prone to show loss of tissue elasticity and atrophic local vascular changes conducive to the formation of fissures. Often this results in pain and tenderness, plus the appearance of bleeding areas and a bloody discharge. When this occurs in patients well past the menopause, not only is it a source of physical discomfort, but also the mental anguish because of fear of the presence of anaplastic lesions may cause undue anxiety and apprehension. These lesions responded well to local application of estrogenic creams or suppositories. Of course, adequate testing by smears or biopsy is indicated to rule out the factor of neoplasm. The following creams may be utilized with effectiveness: 0.05 mg. of ethinyl estradiol, 0.1 mg. of diethylstilbestrol, 0.5 mg. of dienestrol, or 1.25 mg. of conjugated estrogens equine per gram of ointment. The local use of these estrogens is associated with prompt relief and usually does not cause any systemic effect. Unfortunately, dyspareunia and pruritus vulvae do not always respond so favorably. The incorporation of 0.1 to 0.25 per cent of 9-alpha-fluoro-hydrocortisone or its equivalent of prednisolone or dichlorisone acetate with the estrogen in these patients has resulted in a better therapeutic response to local application in many patients with atrophic vaginitis and pruritus.

COSMETICS WITH ESTROGENS. A word about the use of estrogen in cosmetics would be appropriate at this time. Startling claims have been made by various manufacturers concerning the induction of youthful effects by estrogens incorporated in facial creams. These advertisements grossly exaggerate the therapeutic efficacy of their products, since the amounts of estrogens which are incorporated are usually considerably below an effective therapeutic level. We believe that estrogens given systemically in adequate doses will have a beneficial effect on the skin by increasing the deposition of elastic tissue. However, if the amount of estrogens for topical application were increased, this would place such creams and lotions in the category of active medicaments with a definite potential of inducing endocrine effects systemically. Consequently, their sale over the counter is prohibited according to our present food and drug laws and regulations. The anticipated therapeutic action of such creams indiscriminately used would be to induce vaginal bleeding and other undesirable effects of hyperestrogenization.

DURATION OF THERAPY. The need for therapy is dependent on the patient herself. If adequate control is achieved, the dose of estrogen used may be diminished gradually after several months of treatment by increasing the interval between steroid administration. Thus, one may give oral medication every second day for several weeks after good control has been accomplished with daily doses. The frequency of administration may then be extended to twice a week, then once per week, and finally no therapy at all. Parenteral medication may also be reduced gradually by giving one half the amount initially injected at appropriate intervals, and finally only one fourth the initial dose. If there is no return of symptoms, the medication may then be discontinued. The gradual weaning of the medication is necessary, since the climacteric symptomatology occurs as a result of precipitous decrease in estrogen levels and may be reinstituted after adequate control if the steroid medication is discontinued abruptly.

GERIATRIC CONTROL. At this time, it would be well to reiterate that long-continued estrogen administration in the postmenopausal or geriatric patient is a wise and appropriate form of therapy, provided that there is some interruption of the continuous estrogen treatment either by stopping the medication or by physiologic interruption of estrogen effects through the use of progestational steroids. The purpose of continuous estrogen therapy is to retard the process of aging. In so doing the skin is maintained in a better state of elasticity. The process of cerebration and recall seems to be improved as does the patient's ability to care for herself and manage her personal hygiene. The daily dose of estrogen should range between one and two times the dose of the standard preparations that provide effective control of the climacteric, which are listed in Table 13. When continuous estrogen therapy is used, one of the following progestational steroids should be administered at five- to six-week intervals:

Norethindrone (Norlutin), 10.0 mg. b.i.d. for seven days,

Norethindrone acetate, 5.0 mg. b.i.d. for seven days,

Norethynodrel (Enovid), 10.0 mg. b.i.d. for seven days,

Medroxyprogesterone (Provera), 5.0 mg. b.i.d. for seven days,

Progesterone (intramuscularly), 100.0 mg. in oil (single injection).

Such therapy would initiate a menstrual flow at these intervals and would thus provide physiologic interruption of estrogenic activity despite its continuous use. This regimen is more appropriate than the one where estrogen therapy is interrupted for one week out of four.

The long-acting parenteral preparations (Delalutin or Depo-Provera) are not suitable for producing a medical curettage because their effects are too prolonged and dissipated too gradually to facilitate adequate endometrial deciduation. The oral agent, dydrogesterone (Duphaston), in doses of 30 mg. per day is also unsatisfactory for this purpose and should not be used.

CONCLUSIONS

The above therapeutic approach to the management of the menopausal and postmenopausal patient has been offered as a means of treating a condition that can be distressing to both the physician and the patient. Wise management by the physician will result in a very grateful patient. The use of placebo therapy in appropriate cases may achieve the same therapeutic response as an estrogen. Placebo therapy in such patients is not a dishonest procedure but a means of treating a patient according to the dictums of our profession. The selective use of sedation, psychotherapy, or estrogens and androgens provides the physician with multiple modes of therapy for a complex problem with the end result of relief for women who ordinarily would have to suffer through a rather unpleasant and possibly dangerous (psychologically and emotionally) period of their lives. There is no need for these patients to suffer and stoically bear their discomfort. Appropriately instituted therapy will create a happier patient from both the psychological and the clinical points of view.

References

1. BARNES, A. C.: In discussion on Masters.[19]

2. BARR, D. P., RUSS, E. M., AND EDER, H. A.: Influence of estrogen on lipoproteins in atherosclerosis. Trans. Assoc. Amer. Physicians 65:102-113, 1952.

3. BRAMBILLA, F., BERCZELLER, P. H., EPSTEIN, J. A., BLATT, M. H. G., AND KUPPERMAN, H. S.: Experiences with the use of polyestradiol phosphate, a long-acting estrogen. Obstet. Gynec. (N. Y.) 17:115-119, 1961.

4. DELAPLAINE, R. W., BOTTOMY, J. R., BLATT, M. H. G., WIESBADER, H., AND KUPPERMAN, H. S.: Effective control of surgical menopause by estradiol pellet implantation at time of surgery. Surg. Gynec. Obstet. 94:323-333, 1952.

5. DEANESLY, R., AND PARKES, A. S.: Factors influencing effectiveness of administered hormones. Proc. Roy. Soc. (Biol.) 124:279-298, 1937.

6. EILERT, M. L.: The effect of estrogens upon the partition of the serum lipids in female patients. Amer. Heart J. 38:472-473, 1949.

7. EPSTEIN, J. A., VOSBURGH, L., VESELL, M., AND KUPPERMAN, H. S.: An oral-depot estrogen. Physiologic demonstration of effect. Obstet. Gynec. (N. Y.) 9:512-516, 1957.

8. FLUHMANN, C. F.: Menstrual Disorders: Pathology, Diagnosis and Treatment. W. B. Saunders Company, Philadelphia, 1939.

9. GRIFFITH, G. C.: Oophorectomy and cardiovascular tissues. Obstet. Gynec. (N. Y.) 7:479-482, 1956.

10. GURTMAN, A. I., ANDRADA, J. A., BLATT, M. H. G., EPSTEIN, J. A., AND KUPPERMAN, H. S.: Long-acting estrogens in amenorrhea and menopause. Obstet. Gynec. (N. Y.) 10:261-265, 1957.

11. JONES, G. S.: Management of endocrine disorders of menstruation and fertility. (American Lectures in Endocrinology.) Charles C Thomas, Springfield, Ill., 1955.

12. KUPPERMAN, H. S., BLATT, M. H. G., VOSBURGH, L. F., CANIS, J., AND WETCHLER, B.: Effect of reserpine, with or without hormonal therapy, upon the female climacteric. J. Amer. Geriat. Soc. 4:160-166, 1956.

13. KUPPERMAN, H. S., BLATT, M. H. G., WIESBADER, H., AND FULLER, W.: Comparative clinical evaluation of estrogenic preparations by menopausal and amenorrheal indices. J. Clin. Endocr. 13:688-703, 1953.

14. KUPPERMAN, H. S., WETCHLER, B. B., AND BLATT, M. H. G.: Contemporary therapy of the menopausal syndrome. J.A.M.A. 171:1627-1637, 1959.

15. LONDON, W. T., ROSENBERG, S. E., DRAPER, J. W., AND ALMY, T. P.: The effect of estrogens on atherosclerosis: A post mortem study. Amer. Intern. Med. 55:63-69, 1961.

16. MARMORSTON, J., MAGIDSON, O., LEWIS, J. J., MEHL, J., MOORE, F. J., AND BERNSTEIN, J.: Effect of small doses of estrogen on serum lipids in female patients with myocardial infarction. New Engl. J. Med. 248:583-586, 1958.

17. MARMORSTON, J., MOORE, F. J., LEWIS, J. J., MAGIDSON, O., AND KUZMA, O.: Estrogen therapy in men with myocardial infarction: Occurrence of lipid changes before feminization. Clin. Pharmacol. Ther. 1:449-453, 1960.

18. MARMORSTON, J., MOORE, F. J., MAGIDSON, L., KUZMA, O., AND LEWIS, J. J.; Effect of long-term estrogen therapy on serum cholesterol and phospholipids in men with myocardial infarction. Ann. Intern. Med. 51:972-982, 1959.

19. MASTERS, W. H.: Sex steroid influence on the aging process. Amer. J. Obstet. Gynec. 74:733-746, 1957.

20. MASTERS, W. H.: Endocrine therapy in the aging individual. Obstet. and Gynec. (N. Y.) 8:61-67, 1956.

21. MASTERS, W. H.: In discussion on Masters.[19]

22. RANDALL, C. L.: Ovarian function and woman after menopause. Amer. J. Obstet. Gynec. 73:1000-1010, 1957.

23. RANDALL, C. L., BIRTCH, P. K., AND HARKINS, J. L.: Ovarian function after the menopause. Amer. J. Obstet. Gynec. 74:719-732, 1957.

24. REIFENSTEIN, E. C., JR.: In Sodeman, W. A. (ed.): Pathologic Physiology: Mechanisms of Disease. W. B. Saunders Company, Philadelphia, 1950.

25. REYNOLDS, S. R. M.: Physiology of Uterus, 2nd ed. Paul B. Hoeber, Inc., New York, 1949.

26. RUSS, E. M., EDER, H. A., AND BARR, D. P.: Influence of gonadal hormones on protein-lipid relationships in human plasma. Amer. J. Med. 19:4-24, 1955.

27. SELYE, H.: Stress of Life. McGraw-Hill Book Company, Inc., New York, 1956.

28. TAYLOR, R. D., CORCORAN, A. C., AND PAGE, I. H.: Menopausal hypertension: Critical study. Amer. J. Med. Sci. 213:475-476, 1947.

29. TWOMBLY, G. H., AND MILLEN, R. S.: Implantation of solid pellets of estrogens in treatment of menopausal symptoms. Surg. Gynec. Obstet 72:605-610, 1941.

30. WALLACH, S., AND HENNEMAN, P. H.: Prolonged estrogen therapy in postmenopausal women. J.A.M.A. 171:1637-1642, 1959.

chapter 12

The growth and development of breast tissue in the female is under endocrine control. Abnormalities of breast growth and physiology, therefore, frequently are due to aberrant endocrine function or abnormal tissue responsiveness to normal hormonal stimulation.

Physiology. The endocrine factors controlling breast growth originate mainly from both the pituitary gland and the ovaries (Fig. 247). Development of breast tissue usually will not occur in the absence of the ovaries. Similarly, it has been demonstrated that, in certain animals, breast tissue will not develop if hypophysectomy has been done despite adequate replacement therapy with estrogen and progesterone.[14, 15, 18, 26, 34] The pituitary factors controlling breast function are probably three in number: *Mammotropin I* is that hormone from the pituitary gland which is concerned with mammary ductal growth. *Mammotropin II* is the principle from the hypophysis which is involved in alveolar maturation and development. *Prolactin,* the third hormone of pituitary origin, probably is concerned with the formation and secretion of milk per se.[28, 29, 32] It has been claimed by some that mammotropin I is released from the pituitary gland under the influence of estrogen, while mammotropin II is released under the stimulus of large doses of progesterone alone or after the combined administration of estrogen and progesterone.[14, 34] The secretion of milk, while controlled to some extent by prolactin, is affected

Clinical Management of Abnormalities of the Breast in the Female

also by factors other than the hormones of anterior pituitary origin. Neurogenic stimuli are of utmost importance in maintaining lactation, and at times even in initiating milk secretion.[11, 12, 19, 21, 22, 25, 30] This effect may be by way of hypothalamic stimuli to the pituitary gland, either directly to the anterior lobe or indirectly via the posterior lobe. However, the action of posterior pituitary hormones appears to be a specific one upon the breast tissue, inducing smooth muscle contraction in the mammary glands to cause milk ejection.[2, 3, 23, 35] Therefore, it seems likely that the stimulatory effect the sex steroids have on breast secretion probably is not mediated via the posterior pituitary gland. Both posterior pituitary hormones, oxytocin and Pitressin, are capable of enhancing the secretion of milk. Either principle, in the chemically pure form, will experimentally increase milk secretion from the appropriately prepared breasts of most mammals. While posterior pituitary hormones do not enhance milk secretion per se, they do induce ejection of milk already formed in the mammary gland.[3, 20, 23, 35]

In the rat, it has been shown that the adrenal cortex and/or ACTH is also necessary for mammary gland development and function.[19, 20, 24, 29] More recently, relaxin, the protein hormone produced by the corpora lutea, has been shown in the same species to play a role in the development and growth of the mammary glands by enhancing the response of breast tissue to pituitary factors, as well as to sex steroids.[13, 36-38] In addi-

449

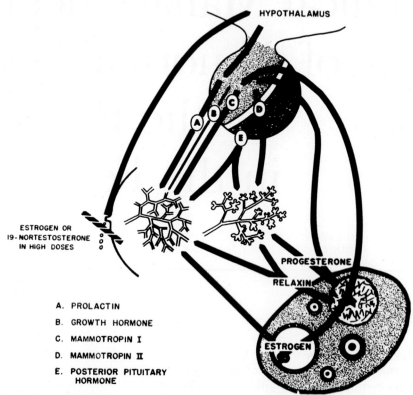

HYPOTHALAMUS

ESTROGEN OR
19-NORTESTOSTERONE
IN HIGH DOSES

PROGESTERONE

RELAXIN

ESTROGEN

A. PROLACTIN

B. GROWTH HORMONE

C. MAMMOTROPIN I

D. MAMMOTROPIN II

E. POSTERIOR PITUITARY
   HORMONE

FIG. 247. *Diagrammatic presentation of the interrelationship between the pituitary and the ovary and the various factors that affect breast growth and secretion. Prolactin (A), mammotropin I (C), and mammotropin II (D) are pituitary factors which have a direct effect on the breast; prolactin causing secretion, mammotropin I causing duct growth, and mammotropin II causing alveolar growth. Growth hormone (B) enhances the effect of prolactin on breast secretion, as does relaxin. Estrogen and progesterone may affect the breast either directly, or indirectly by virtue of their effect in releasing mammotropin I and mammotropin II, respectively. Estrogens or 19-nortestosterone inhibit breast secretion, either by way of the hypothalamus or by direct action upon the breast. Posterior pituitary hormone causes the ejection of milk already present.*

tion, it has been noted that thyroxin may play a permissive role in the response of mammary tissue to appropriate stimulation.[37] Lobule-alveolar growth after estrogen and progesterone was increased by 25 per cent when thyroxin was added.[27]

The role of the pituitary gland in controlling the function of mammary tissue is seen indirectly when inhibition of pituitary secretion is accomplished by sex steroid administration. Inhibition of pituitary function by non-estrogenic steroids results in diminution of mammary growth and secretion. The pituitary inhibitors, such as estrogen and the 19-norsteroids, are potent depressors of breast secretion in both the animal and the human. When estrogens alone are used, however, inhibition of milk secretion occurs with evidence of breast enlargement. The clinical application of these hormones for the control of aberrations of function of the breasts will be discussed later in this chapter.

Embryology. The embryologic development of the breast tissue is rather interesting in that it appears to be related to the origin of the sebaceous glands: both are derived from the ectoderm. Early in the embryologic development of mammary tissue, a bilateral thickening of the ectoderm occurs on each side of the ventral midline, giving rise to the mammary striae or bands. Continued hypertrophy and hyperplasia of the cells in this area result in the mammary line. Centers of proliferation then appear on the mammary line to form the primordial teat or mammary bud. The number of these centers determine the number of mammary glands that will develop. As the breast anlages proliferate, they push the underlying basement membrane into the mesenchymal tissue, which gives rise to the fibro-elastic-muscular tissue of the adult breast.

Columns of cells invaginate from the mammary bud to form the primary sprouts which later give rise to the number of ducts in the mature teat. Man has 16 to 25 of these sprouts in contrast to two for the mare and pig and only one for the rodents, goats, and cattle.

Canalization of the primary sprout takes place, extending down toward the underlying mesenchymal tissue. These plugs of epithelial tissue or sprouts also begin to divide, giving rise to the duct system seen in the adult. During early pubescence, at the time of the thelarche, there is an increase in growth and development of the duct tissue. The secretory components of the breasts known as alveoli develop at the end of the terminal ducts. A group of alveoli, together with their multibranched or divided ducts, comprise a lobule.

Morphology. The ducts are present early in the development of the breast. Only the breast of the adult female and males with gynecomastia will show significant lobulation with alveolar architecture forming the secretory unit referred to as the lobule-alveolar system. The interductal fibrous-like tissue, as well as the glandular portion, will also undergo hypertrophy when beginning development of the breasts occurs. The interductal fibrous tissue consists of eosinophilic elements intermixed with smooth muscle structures. As the thelarche develops, the proliferation of the glandular tissue will lead to lobule-alveolar development in pretty much the same manner as seen in the sebaceous glands. Secretion will also develop at this particular time. The epithelium lining the ducts consists of two rows of epithelial cells while the lobule-alveolar system, the terminal end of the duct, is lined by a single layer of epithelial cells. The cells of the secretory portion are columnar during the active secretory phase and are relatively flat when they are in the quiescent or nonsecretory phase. Myo-epithelial cells lie in close contact with the epithelium of the alveoli and are probably responsible in part for the ejection of milk in response to oxytocin. Marked ductal hyperplasia will usually result in pseudo-striation of the nuclei so that eventual occlusion of the duct may take place.

Cystic Mastalgia.   One of the most common clinical problems concerned with diseases of the breasts is cystic mastalgia. This syndrome is characterized by the presence of cyclic changes in the breast associated with an increase in size, pain, tenderness, and cystic alteration of the tissue itself. These changes usually will occur premenstrually and may start approximately seven to 10 days before the onset of the menstrual period. The changes in breast size during this period of time may be minimal or marked. The degree of discomfort is usually correlated with the increase in breast dimensions as well as with the accompanying severity of the associated premenstrual molimina. The cystic changes may be so marked that they may be demonstrated by transillumination. In addition, x-ray pictures of the breast tissue may also show striking cystic changes in certain selected cases. At times, these cystic structures may reach such proportions that the question of a neoplasm is raised and excisional biopsy must be done to rule out the possibility of malignancy.

The etiology of cystic mastitis is not well delineated although aberrant metabolism of estrogens may be an important factor in initiation of the disease. The discomfort due to the cystic changes is accentuated by the fluid retention that many of these patients may experience. The fluid retention, as well as the breast hypertrophy, has been attributed also to the presence of excessive amounts of unopposed estrogen.

The management of cystic mastalgia may be accomplished by the use of any one of a number of different therapeutic agents. There is one point of agreement recognized by most investigators: estrogens are contraindicated in patients with cystic mastitis because excessive amounts of unopposed endogenous estrogen, particularly that associated with anovulatory cycles, may initiate cystic alterations. The use of progestational and/or androgenic steroids, with or without diuretics, is the procedure of choice and will effectively control many of the patient's complaints. If the patient does not have any associated dysmenorrhea, she may be placed on an oral progestational compound given in sufficient doses to ameliorate the discomfort as well as to prevent or greatly relieve the breast enlargement. The effective doses are of such small quantity that there is usually no interference with the regularity of the catamenia. The following preparations and doses may be used:

Ethisterone (Pranone, Lutocylol), 10.0 mg. t.i.d. for seven to 10 days premenstrually,

Norethindrone (norethisterone) (Norlutin), 10.0 mg. per day for seven to 10 days before the anticipated onset of menses.

Norethindrone acetate (Norlutate) or medroxyprogesterone (Provera), 5.0 mg. per day for seven to 10 days premenstrually.

Norethynodrel should not be used owing to its estrogenic properties. Dydrogesterone (Duphaston) has not proved to be effective in doses of 10 to 20 mg. per day.

Of the steroids with androgenic potential that have been used with some degree of success in premenstrual molimina, methylandrostenediol is a most effective one in diminishing the patient's mastalgia and is the drug of choice if the patient has dysmenorrhea associated with cystic mastalgia. The usual dose is 25.0 mg. b.i.d. for seven to 10 days premenstrually.[17] It should also be noted that relief of the breast symptoms may be accomplished by the pre-ovulatory administration of methyltestosterone in doses of 10.0 mg. t.i.d. for eight days, starting four days before the anticipated day of ovulation. This therapeutic approach is exceedingly effective in controlling both the dysmenorrhea and the associated premenstrual molimina, as well as the mastalgia—provided that adequate timing and doses as suggested above are used.[16, 17]

Any of the chlorothiazide preparations in equivalent dosage may also be employed as ancillary procedures together with the above steroids, or may even be effective in their own right. Following are the preparations that may be used, and their effective doses:

Chlorothiazide, 250.0 mg. once or twice per day,
Hydrochlorothiazide, 25.0 mg. once or twice per day,
Chlorthalidone (Hygroton), 100.0 mg. once per day to once every second day,
Trichlormethiazide (Naqua), 4.0 to 8.0 mg. per day,
Methychlothiazide (Enduron), 4 mg. per day.

Any one of these preparations may be given for the seven to 10 days prior to the onset of menses.

Control of Lactation. POSTPARTUM LACTATION. Another major and common problem facing the clinician, usually requiring hormonal control for the best therapeutic response, is that of postpartum breast engorgement and secretion. Prevention of breast engorgement has been attempted by conservative measures of breast binding, reduction of fluid intake, and the use of cathartics. While such time-honored remedies were those of choice for that period in medicine when the present-day steroid armamentarium was not available, there is no rationale for adhering solely to such archaic procedures now, although they may be used as ancillary measures along with steroid therapy. The relatively simple management of postpartum lactation may be achieved by the use of adequate doses of the synthetic steroidal or nonsteroidal estrogenic preparations or the progestational steroids. These substances will induce a significant degree of relief in the breast pain and discomfort plus the fact that they can shorten considerably the time during which symptoms are prevalent. However, it is obvious that the infant must be withheld from the breast so that the neurogenic stimulus of suckling cannot continue the nervous mechanisms responsible for maintenance of lactation.

The present-day management of postpartum breast engorgement dates from the classic work of Parkes and Bellerby, who showed that lactation could be diminished in the rat by the injection of estrin.[31] Clinically, the older oral estrogens now appear to be primarily of historical interest. The synthetic estrogen stilbestrol was the first one used with any degree of success in the effective management of breast engorgement.[7] The doses of stilbestrol which were capable of inhibiting lactation ranged from 2.0 to 5.0 mg. per day for a period of four to seven days. This was successful in diminishing breast engorgement and secretion. However, there were some undesirable side effects due to the use of stilbestrol. These adverse effects were the associated nausea that was frequently noted, the increase in areolar pigmentation, and the increase of lochia which was a consequence of the estrogenic stimulation of the endometrium. In addition to these maternal undesirable side effects, the infant also showed some somatic changes due to the orally ingested estrogen passing through the mother's milk.

In an attempt to minimize these adverse side reactions, androgens were added to the estrogen so that a lesser amount of the estrogen could be used without decreasing its therapeutic effectiveness. A combination of 2.5 mg. of conjugated estrogens equine plus 10.0 mg. of methyltestosterone t.i.d. for five days has proved to be an effective means of controlling breast engorgement. Here, too, the lochia is occasionally increased.

Estrogens with prolonged effects after oral administration, the so-called "depot estrogens,"[6] also have proved to be effective in controlling postpartum lactation and breast engorgement. Chlorotrianisene, the "oral depot estrogen," in doses of 12.0 mg. q.i.d. for five days successfully controls postpartum breast engorgement. Its therapeutic effects are enhanced when 20.0 to 30.0 mg. of methyltestosterone per day is added.

More recently, the long-acting parenteral steroids, such as estradiol valerate (Delestrogen), together with testosterone enanthate (Delatestryl), in doses of 20.0 and 400.0 mg., respectively, have proved to be effective in controlling postpartum breast engorgement with only a single injection. Similar effects are obtained when estradiol cyclopentylpropionate (Depo-Estradiol), 10.0 mg., is incorporated with 200.0 mg. of testosterone cyclopentylpropionate (Depo-Testosterone). The advantage of the parenteral therapy is that adequate control may be accomplished by only a single injection which may be administered immediately after delivery.

Two of the 19-norsteroids with progestational activity have also proved to be effective in diminishing breast engorgement: 10.0 mg. t.i.d. for seven days of either norethindrone or norethandrolone will be effective in managing postpartum breast engorgement. Norethynodrel in similar doses, while effective in inhibiting pituitary secretion, is not the drug of choice since its estrogen content may lead to the same disadvantages noted for the oral estrogens themselves—a possible increase in breast tenderness and an increase in amount and duration of postpartum endometrial discharge. Medroxyprogesterone, not a 19-norsteroid, when given orally is a relatively poor pituitary inhibitor of lactation. The parenteral form, medroxyprogesterone acetate, has not been evaluated adequately to determine its effectiveness in the treatment of postpartum lactation. Norethindrone acetate has been active in doses of 15.0 to 20.0 mg. per day in controlling breast engorgement in contrast to the 30.0 mg. per day required of the free norethindrone.

There are three other rare clinical states associated with lactation that may be managed by appropriate therapy.

CHIARI-FROMMEL SYNDROME.[4, 10] This syndrome describes those patients who develop persistent postpartum lactation associated with obesity, amenorrhea, castrate vaginal smear, low FSH, and, sometimes, enlargement of the sella turcica. Occasionally, there may even be some aberration of the visual fields. The prognosis in these patients for fertility or the recurrence of spontaneous menses is remote. Cessation of lactation may usually be accomplished by the administration of chlorotrianisene (TACE), 12.0 mg. q.i.d. for four weeks. Following this, the patient is given a progestational steroid in the same doses as listed for the diagnosis and management of the patient with amenorrhea. Menses will usually follow this regimen for one or two months after the progestational steroid administration. However, when menses fail to occur after the course of progestin therapy, the patient is primed once more with chlorotrianisene in the same dose schedule as originally used. The estrogen is then followed by the monthly course of progestational steroid, repeating the entire procedure for as long a time as the patient desires to have menses. In so doing, lactation will be held in abeyance. The estrogen therapy is indicated not only for the purpose of inhibiting lactation, but also as a means of preventing premature aging from occurring due to the lack of endogenous estrogen activity.

FORBES-ALBRIGHT-CASTILLO SYNDROME.[1, 8, 9] This clinical entity, also associated with lactation, has been described by Forbes, *et al.,* and almost simultaneously by Argonz and del Castillo. The clinical picture is characterized by the presence of amenorrhea (usually primary), a low FSH, and an acromegalic-like facies. These patients usually have an enlarged sella turcica but do not show evidence of visual disturbances. They appear to be akin to frank acromegalics (who may also lactate[5]) except that they do not show the organomegaly, increase in soft tissue of the hands, and marked encroachment on the visual fields usually seen with progressive enlargement of the sella. If menses are not desired in the patients with Forbes-Albright-Castillo syndrome, control of lactation may be accomplished readily by the use of 10.0 mg. t.i.d. for ten days of norethindrone, norethandrolone, or norethynodrel. If lactation does not subside, then the course of any of the 19-norsteroids should be continued for a longer period of time—usually for three weeks. The same schedule using chlorotrianisene as that described for the Chiari-Frommel syndrome may also be used with an equal degree of effectiveness where catamenia is desirable.

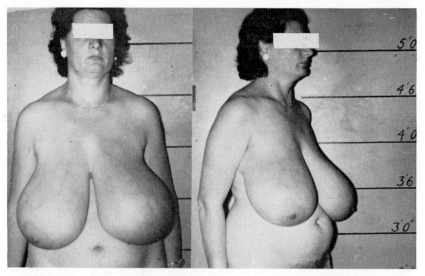

FIGS. 248A and B. Patient AG, age 45 years. Marked enlargement of the breasts had recently occurred without noticeable change in menstrual periods. Their enormous size contributed to the patient's discomfort.

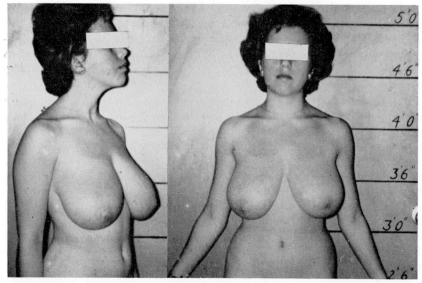

FIG. 249. Patient TD, age 15 years and 10 months. Breasts markedly enlarged. They have increased in size steadily but progressively since the time of her menarche four years ago. The pain and tenderness attributed to the breasts, plus their enormous size, has limited this patient's physical activity.

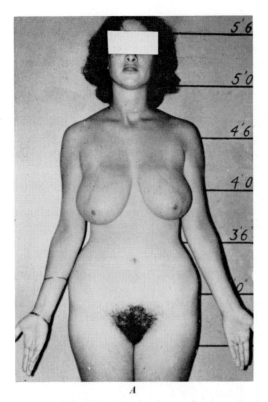
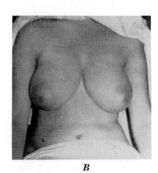

A   B

FIG. 250. Massive breast hypertrophy in young teenage females.

A, Patient MB, age 18 years and 11 months, height 66 inches. Note marked breast hypertrophy; menses are normal. The patient's discomfort and embarrassment were considerable, and in themselves were indications for the need for treatment.

B, Patient KK, age 15 years, exhibiting marked hypertrophy of the breasts which has incapacitated her physical activity and has been associated with excessive engorgement premenstrually. Response to progestational steroids has been excellent. The patient's endocrine work-up showed no abnormality.

POSTSURGICAL LACTATION.   Another unexplained phenomenon associated with lactation occurs in patients after a surgical procedure that may involve removal of the uterus,[33] of the ovaries, or even of viscera not associated with reproduction, such as the gallbladder. Therapeutic control of such lactation may be accomplished readily by the administration of one of the 19-norsteroids in the doses described for the management of the Forbes-Albright-Castillo syndrome. Usually, one course of therapy for ten days will suffice for adequate control of the lactation.

Hyperplasia of Breast Tissue.   The presence of unusually large breasts may present a difficult problem of medical management to the clinician (Figs. 248-250). While such patients are relatively few in number as compared to those with cystic mastitis, the associated discomfort and embarrassment are of far greater magnitude. Excessive breast hypertrophy may occasionally be seen in women in whom normal breast size had been present prior to the enormous enlargement (Fig. 248). On the other hand, marked hypertrophy of the breasts may be due to progressive and excessive growth of breast tissue with the onset of the menarche, the so-called virginal hypertrophy of the breasts (Fig. 249).

Enlargement of the breasts may take place following a number of different types of surgical procedures. For example, it has been reported after hysterectomy, ovariectomy, and even after abdominal surgery for conditions not related to the genitourinary tract. The mechanism of the resultant enlargement or the etiologic factors responsible for the galactorrhea in such cases are not known. It has been suggested that such hypertrophy may be an outcome of elaboration of a hypothalamic factor causing release of mammotropin principles from the hypophysis with breast enlargement resulting.

The management of bilateral breast hypertrophy, regardless of the cause or type, may be achieved readily by the use of gonadotropic suppressive doses of medroxyprogesterone acetate, thereby bringing about abeyance of the menstrual periods with a resultant decrease in the enormously enlarged breasts. Usually, the patient will have to be maintained on this parenteral steroid for a period of several months to years, during which time she will be amenorrheic. The dose employed is 100.0 to 150.0 mg. of the preparation, given intramuscularly every seven to 10 days. The breasts usually will diminish in size very rapidly. It is recommended that the patient be kept on such therapy for a number of months so that more normal proportions may be attained. After the medication is discontinued, hypertrophy may recur in over half of the patients so treated, but it will be rather slow in onset and may never attain the original engorged state.

Oral therapy with norethindrone may also be used in doses of 10.0 mg. t.i.d. However, this dose may produce some evidence of increased hair growth, acne, and seborrhea. Cessation of menses usually will be achieved, and there will be an associated diminution in breast size. The duration of therapy should be the same as that suggested for the medroxyprogesterone acetate.

Obviously, the use of plastic surgery may be recommended for those individuals in whom cessation of menses may be a source of concern. However, one must consider the fact that, after the plastic surgery, there may be difficulty in duct drainage and lactation if pregnancy takes place subsequently.

Hypoplasia of the Breasts. A most distressing syndrome which faces the young adolescent and adult is failure of breast development or marked mammary hypoplasia (Figs. 251-256). While such a clinical state is not

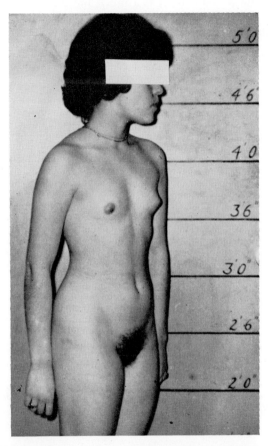

FIG. 251. Patient BH, age 18 years, having marked hypoplasia of the breasts despite the fact that she has normal menstrual periods and no abnormal findings on pelvic examination. Patient is emotionally upset by failure of breast development.

associated with physical discomfort, breast hypoplasia may cause such emotional difficulties in the patient that, if she be told that there is little or no hope for her breasts to increase in size, deep depressive states may occur; indeed, in one patient this was associated with suicidal tendencies. As a rule, if these patients menstruate regularly, while the problem is not an impossible one to manage, it is a much more difficult one to treat in contrast with the excellent therapeutic response that is achieved with replacement therapy in one with ovarian failure.

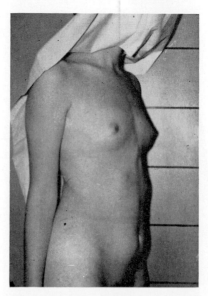

FIG. 252. Patient SA, age 15½ years, height 61½ inches. Normal menstrual periods. Note the marked hypoplasia of both breasts. This has been a source of concern and anguish to the patient, who otherwise is endocrinologically normal. She was placed upon the therapeutic regimen recommended with oral estrogen and showed an adequate response.

The treatment of these patients, while not hopeless, should not be offered with any profound degree of optimism since only 20 to 30 per cent of the patients show a response that can be considered adequate. The following regimen has been employed and will usually not be associated with significant alteration of the regularity of the menstrual cycle: ethinyl estradiol, 0.05 mg. per day for the first 14 days of the menstrual cycle, followed by 0.05 mg. b.i.d. for the next 10 days. The patient then stops her medication, and resumes with the first day of her next menstrual period. This procedure has proved to be effective in increasing breast

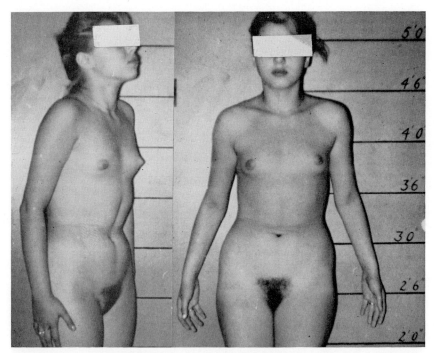

FIG. 253. *Patient EG, age 16½ years. Normal menstrual periods. Moderate breast hypoplasia. Due to the patient's unhappiness concerning the failure of her breasts to develop, she has avoided all social contacts.*

size in approximately one fifth of our patients without evidence of disturbing the regularity of the previously established cyclic catamenia.

If the above procedure is without effect, a more intensive course of therapy with estrogen may be used, which will invariably be associated with cessation of menses during the time the patient is on therapy. The fact that the menses are held in abeyance during hormonal administration does not mitigate against the use of such therapy, for, whenever the estrogen is discontinued, the catamenia will take place again with the same degree of regularity as prior to the institution of these high doses of estrogen. The following dose regimen may be used: ethinyl estradiol, 0.05 mg., two tablets b.i.d. to t.i.d. continuously. An increase in breast size usually will be noted in most of the women so treated. In order to induce physiologic interruption of the continuous estrogen therapy, periodic menses are induced in these patients by the administration of norethynodrel in doses of 10.0 mg. b.i.d. for seven days at four-week intervals. This progestational steroid will produce menses without adversely affecting the growth of the breast that had been achieved by

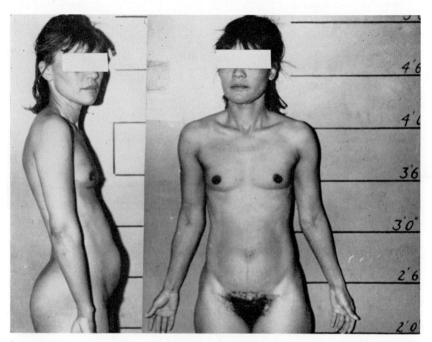

FIG. 254.   Patient LM, age 22 years, married female with two children. Breast hypoplasia has persisted despite two pregnancies and lactation. Menstrual periods are normal.

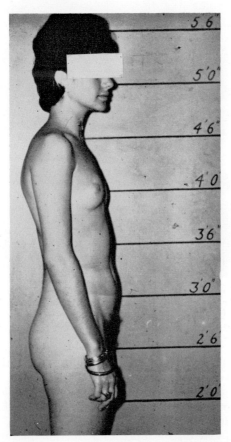

FIG. 255.   Patient LK, age 19 years. Marked hypoplasia of the breasts which has caused the patient to adopt an antisocial behavior. She refuses to go swimming because of self-consciousness over the hypoplastic breasts. Menstrual periods are normal.

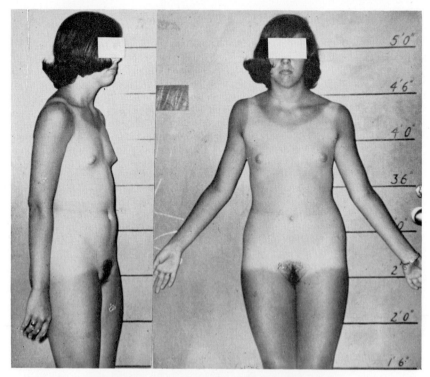

FIG. 256. Patient LS, age 16 years, 11 months, with regular menses. Note marked breast hypoplasia. This has caused a great deal of mental anguish, and the patient consequently has limited her social life and activity. The need for therapy is obvious. Patient's endocrine work-up showed no abnormality.

the continuous estrogen treatment. The purpose of the progestational steroid is to prevent cystic hyperplastic changes from occurring in the endometrium, as well as to ward off the possibility of abnormal nuclear changes in the female reproductive tract as a result of the continuous use of the estrogenic substance.

When therapy is discontinued, a reduction in breast size may be noted. However, the gain that had been achieved may be maintained at its peak level by reinstituting the therapy initially recommended above, where there is no interruption of the regularity of the menstrual cycle. Both forms of therapy have been helpful in dissipating the anxiety and depression that many of these young girls may show as a result of their hypoplasia of the breasts.

Unilateral Breast Hypoplasia. An almost insurmountable clinical problem of aberrant breast development is the young female with asymmetrical breast development (Figs. 257-259). The hypoplastic breast is usually

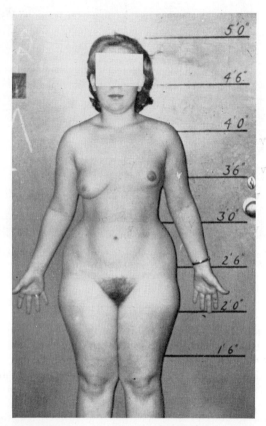

FIG. 257. *Patient MKJ, age 15 1/3 years, height 59½ inches, with a normal menstrual history. However, note the marked asymmetry of the breasts where the left breast is markedly underdeveloped and the right breast is adequately developed. Patient has been placed upon topical estrogen and progesterone therapy to be applied to her left breast area.*

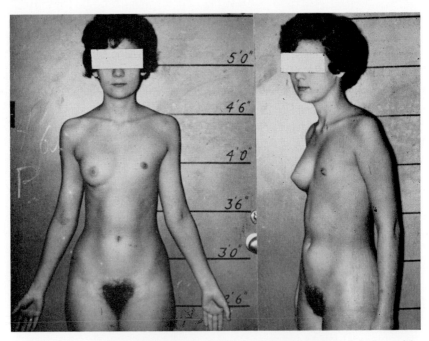

FIG. 258. *Patient CP, age 16 years, with normal menstrual periods but with breast asymmetry. No surgical procedure had been performed on the atrophic breast. The asymmetry of her breasts has caused mental anguish and has resulted in her refusing to appear in a bathing suit.*

resistant to treatment, so that the institution of estrogen therapy will bring about further stimulation of the normally developed breast despite the fact that the hypoplastic breast may or may not show some growth.

A minimal degree of success has been accomplished by the topical application of estrogenic cream or lotion to the hypoplastic breast tissue. It should be emphasized again that none of the products sold over-the-counter is worthy of trial since the dose of estrogen per gram of ointment is homeopathic and will be without significant activity when used for this purpose. The following lotion may be of some benefit:

$$\left.\begin{array}{c}\text{Ethinyl estradiol, 0.05 mg.}\\ \text{and}\\ \text{Progesterone, 5.0 mg.}\end{array}\right\}\begin{array}{l}\text{per cc. of 50\%}\\ \text{ethyl or denatured alcohol}\end{array}$$

The use of 2 to 3 cc. of this preparation on the hypoplastic breast may be associated with some minimal degree of effectiveness and may be worth while.

In discussing asymmetrical breast development, one should emphasize

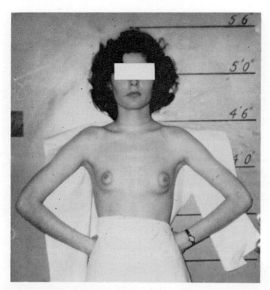

FIG. 259.   Patient KB, age 15½ years, with secondary amenorrhea with hypo-plasia of the breasts and moderate asymmetry.   It is felt that her secondary amenorrhea, when treated, will result in more normal breast development.

the use of restraint before breast biopsy is attempted in an infant or a pre-adolescent female with some evidence of nodular formation in the breast. Ordinarily, at this age, one would not expect to find anything except beginning development of breast tissue. Breast hypertrophy may occur for many different reasons, so that the apparent neoplastic nodule may merely represent precocious development of normal breast tissue. However, if this area is biopsied, it may well be that the anlage for future breast development is removed so that further growth is impossible. As a result, permanent aplasia on that side would prevail with hopeless asymmetry occurring. This tragic iatrogenic cosmetic defect can be avoided if judgment is exercised earlier.

Precocious Thelarche.   This may occur at any age up to puberty. It is characterized only by the precocious development of breast tissue not accompanied by any evidence of precocious or excessive estrogen secretion. The normal vaginal smear and bone age would indicate the non-endocrine nature of the disease. A patient with significant enlargement of the breast is depicted in Fig. 260. Endocrine work-up revealed no abnormal findings.

Summary.   Disturbed breast function or physiology may be managed by appropriate endocrine and/or supportive therapy. Breast discomfort rates

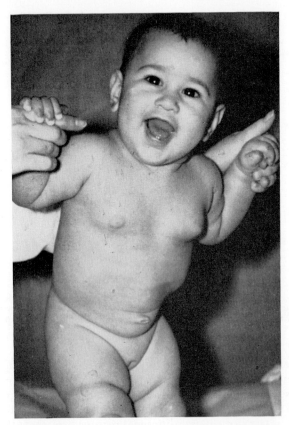

FIG. 260. Patient ER, age 5 months. Thelarche occurred at about age of 3-4 months. Note definite development of breast tissue associated with true glandular growth. Vaginal smear castrate. Bone age within normal limits.

high on the list of common complaints seen in many female patients. The therapy recommended has been most effective and is associated with a minimum degree of undesirable side effects.

References

1. ARGONZ, J., AND DEL CASTILLO, E. B.: A syndrome characterized by estrogenic insufficiency, galactorrhea and decreased urinary gonadotropins. J. Clin. Endocr. 13:79-87, 1953.

2. BELLER, F. K., KRUMHOLZ, K. H., AND ZEININGER, K.: Vergleichende oxytocin-Bestimmungen gemessen durch den lactagogen effect der milchdrüse (milk-ejection). Acta Endocr. (Kbh) 29:1-8, 1958.

3. BERDE, B., AND CERLETTI, A.: Über die workung pharmakologischer oxytocindosen auf die milchdrüse. Acta Endocr. (Kbh) 34:543-557, 1960.

4. CHIARI, J., BRAUN, C., AND SPAETH, J.: Klinic der Geburtshilfe und Gynäkologie. F. Enke, Erlangen, 1855, pp. 371-372.

5. DAVIDOFF, L. M.: Studies in acromegaly. III. The anamnesis and symptomatology in one hundred cases. Endocrinology 10:461-483, 1926.

6. EPSTEIN, J. A., VOSBURGH, L., VESEL, M., AND KUPPERMAN, H. S.: An oral-depot estrogen. Physiologic demonstration of effect. Obstet. Gynec. (N. Y.) 9:512-516, 1957.

7. FIELDS, F.: The influence of stilbestrol upon lactation. Amer. J. Obstet. Gynec. 49:385-390, 1945.

8. FORBES, A. P., HENNEMAN, P. H., GRISWOLD, G. C., AND ALBRIGHT, F.: A syndrome distinct from acromegaly, characterized by spontaneous lactation, amenorrhea and low follicle-stimulating hormone excretion. (Abstract.) J. Clin. Endocr. 11:749, 1951.

9. FORBES, A. P., HENNEMAN, P. H., GRISWOLD, G. C., AND ALBRIGHT, F.: Syndrome characterized by galactorrhea, amenorrhea, and low urinary FSH: Comparison with acromegaly and normal lactation. J. Clin. Endocr. 14:265-271, 1954.

10. FROMMEL, R.: Ueber puerperale atrophie des uterus. Zeitschrift fur. Geburtsh. v. Gynäk. 7:305-315, 1882.

11. GAINES, W. L.: A contribution to the physiology of lactation. Amer. J. Physiol. 38:285-312, 1915.

12. GAINES, W. L., AND DAVIDSON, F. A.: Rate of milk secretion as affected by advance in lactation and gestation. Illinois Agr. Exp. Stat. Bull. 272:1-24, 1926.

13. GARRETT, F. A., AND TALMAGE, R. V.: The influence of relaxin on mammary gland development in guinea pigs and rabbits. J. Endocr. 8:336-40, 1952.

14. GOMEZ, E. T., AND TURNER, C. W.: Further evidence for a mammogenic hormone in the anterior pituitary. Proc. Soc. Exp. Biol. Med. 37:607-609, 1938.

15. GOMEZ, E. T.: Mammary gland growth in hypophysectomized castrated guinea pigs. Endocrinology 31:613-618, 1942.

16. KUPPERMAN, H. S., AND GOODMAN, S. J.: Effective treatment of dysmenorrhea and menstrual molimina by the preovulatory administration of methyltestosterone or methylandrostenediol. Amer. J. Obstet. Gynec. 65:141-149, 1953.

17. KUPPERMAN, H. S., AND STUDDIFORD, W. E.: Endocrine therapy in gynecologic disorders. Postgrad. Med. 14:410-424, 1953.

18. LEWIS, A. A., GOMEZ, E. T., AND TURNER, C. W.: Mammary gland development with mammogen I in the castrate and hypophysectomized rat. Endocrinology 30:37-47, 1942.

19. MAQSOOD, M., AND MEITES, J.: Induction of mammary secretion in rats by electrical stimulation. Proc. Soc. Exp. Biol. Med. 106:104-106, 1961.

20. MEITES, J., AND NICOLL, C. S.: Hormonal prolongation of lactation for 75 days after litter withdrawal in postpartum rats. Endocrinology 65:572-579, 1959.

21. MEITES, J., TALWALKER, P. K., AND NICOLL, C. S.: Initiation of lactation in rats with hypothalamic or cerebral tissue. Proc. Soc. Exp. Biol. Med. 103:298-300, 1960.

22. MEITES, J., TALWALKER, P. K., AND NICOLL, C. S.: Induction of mammary growth and lactation in rabbits with epinephrine, acetylcholine and serotonin. Proc. Soc. Exp. Biol. Med. 104:192-194, 1960.

23. MEITES, J., TALWALKER, P. K., AND NICOLL, C. S.: Failure of oxytocin to initiate mammary secretion in rabbits or rats. Proc. Soc. Exp. Biol. Med. 105:467-469, 1960.

24. MEITES, J., TRENTIN, J. J., AND TURNER, C. W.: Effect of adrenalectomy on the lactogenic hormone and initiation of lactation. Endocrinology 31:607-612, 1942.

25. MEITES, J., AND TURNER, C. W.: Studies concerning mechanism controlling initiation of lactation at parturition. Endocrinology 31:340-344, 1942.

26. MIXNER, J. P., BERGMAN, A. J., AND TURNER, C. W.: Relation of mammogenic lobule-alveolor growth factor of the anterior pituitary to other anterior pituitary hormones. Endocrinology 31:461-466, 1942.

27. MIXNER, J. P., AND TURNER, C. W.: Influence of thyroxin upon mammary lobule-alveolar growth. Endocrinology 31:345-348, 1942.

28. NELSON, W. O.: Studies on the physiology of lactation. IV. The assay of the lactogenic hormone of the anterior hypophysis. Anat. Rec. 60:69-76, 1934.

29. NICOLL, C. S., TALWALKER, P. K., AND MEITES, J.: Initiation of lactation in rats by nonspecific stresses. Amer. J. Physiol. 198:1103-1106, 1960.

30. OTT, I., AND SCOTT, J. C.: The action of infundibulum upon mammary secretion. Proc. Soc. Exp. Biol. Med. 8:48-49, 1910.

31. PARKES, A. S., AND BELLERBY, C.: Studies on the internal secretions of the ovary. III. The effects of injection of estrin during lactation. J. Physiol. 62:301-314, 1927.

32. RIDDLE, O., BATES, R. W., AND DYKSHORN, S. W.: A new hormone of the anterior pituitary. Proc. Soc. Exp. Biol. Med. 29:1211-1212, 1932.

33. SACHS, H. B.: Lactation after hysterectomy in a nulliparous woman. Amer. J. Obstet. Gynec. 78: 204-207, 1959.

34. SELYE, H.: Effect of chronic progesterone overdosage on the female accessory sex organs of normal, ovariectomized and hypophysectomized rats. Anat. Rec. 78: 253-271, 1940.

35. STEWART, R. H., AND NELSON, R. N.: Synthetic oxytocin: I. Comparison of effect with alkaloids of ergot in the third and fourth stages of labor. II. Evaluation of its results on milk let down. Obstet. Gynec. 13:204-212, 1959.

36. TRENTIN, J. J.: Relaxin and mammary growth in the mouse. Proc. Soc. Exp. Biol. Med. 78:9-11, 1951.

37. WADA, H., AND TURNER, C. W.: Role of relaxin in stimulating mammary growth in mice. Proc. Soc. Exp. Biol. Med. 99:194-197, 1958.

38. WADA, H., AND TURNER, C. W.: Effect of relaxin on mammary gland growth in female mice. Proc. Soc. Exp. Biol. Med. 101:707-709, 1959.

chapter 13

The endocrinologist, despite the protestations of the psychiatrist, firmly believes that, in addition to any neurologic and supertentorial influences, the endocrine glands play a major role in the mechanism of libido.[4] The biochemical factors responsible for increasing libido are the steroid hormones elaborated by the gonads with a common denominator being responsible for augmenting sexual desire in both the male and female. Paradoxically, androgens in the female[1, 2, 4-6] and, as to be expected, androgens in the male are unique in their role in enhancing libido in both sexes. Despite our support of the role androgens play in increasing libido in both the female and male, the importance of psychosomatic factors cannot be overlooked.

The role of androgens in enhancing libido in the female received emphasis when they were administered for purposes other than increasing libido. The androgen-treated females volunteered the information that the androgens, in addition to accomplishing an effect entirely unrelated to libido, actually increased their libido. For example, the preovulatory administration of methyltestosterone in doses of 30 mg. a day for eight days to control dysmenorrhea not infrequently has been accompanied by an increase in libido. This was attested to by the enthusiastic comments of husbands who frequently state, "I don't know what you are giving my wife, but keep on giving it to her." Similarly, the administration

Endocrine Management of Disorders of Libido

of androgens in high doses to control the metastatic spread of breast carcinoma has resulted in an inordinate increase in libido in many of these patients. This takes place much to the distress of the husband, whose sexual desires are disrupted by his anxiety concerning his wife's life expectancy. The unexpected effectiveness of androgens in potentiating libido in the female may be due to the role the clitoris probably plays as the center for eroticism in the female.

While it is apparent that androgens increase libido in the female, such specific hormonal therapy would be valueless in those females who have never experienced libido: that is, where frigidity has existed through the entire sex life of the individual (Fig. 261). On the other hand, where libido had been present but has since been lost, and where orgasms, previously achieved, can no longer be reached there is little question that such a patient will be benefited if appropriate hormonal therapy is used.

The human female stands alone in the feminine animal world in that sexual receptivity may be present throughout the year without relationship to time, season, or climate. In the animal kingdom, males are acceptable to the female only during certain times of the year when adequate levels of estrogen and progesterone are present in the female. The use of androgens in female animals has never been known to be of value in

473

Type of Patient	Extent of Libido Before Therapy		Extent of Libido After Therapy	Result
Patient with no libido at present, but who had experienced libido in the past	Lack of sex desire	Androgen	♂♂♀	Increase in libido noted
Patient who had never experienced libido	None	Androgen	None	All organic therapy is ineffective – Psychotherapy is indicated
Nymphomania associated with marked increase in libido	♂♂♂♂♂♂♀	Progesterone (Pellet or I. M.)	♂♂♀	Nymphomanic tendencies decreased by suppressing libido
Normal sexual desire	♂♂♂♀	Progesterone	◌ or ♂♀	Normal desire for sexual intercourse partially suppressed by progesterone

Lack of sex desire ◌   Normal sex desire ♂♂♀

FIG. 261. Diagrammatic presentation of the comparative effects of androgen and progesterone on libido in the human female.

promoting sexual receptivity, in contrast to the human female in whom the process of libido can be significantly augmented by the addition of androgens and diminished by the use of progestational steroids.

The usual dose of androgens that is necessary and the preparations that may be used for the management of libido deficiencies in the female are as follows:

1. Methyltestosterone (Oreton M), 10 mg. a day for the first 20 days, followed by 5 mg. per day thereafter. This latter dose may be diminished to once every second day and finally stopped when the pattern has been established. There may, of course, be a need to reinstitute therapy if the effects are completely dissipated.

2. Fluoxymesterone (Halotestin, Ultandren), 5 mg. once per day for 20 days, followed by 2.5 mg. per day thereafter.

3. Testosterone cyclopentylpropionate (Depo-Testosterone), 50 to 75 mg. intramuscularly (IM) every four weeks.

4. Testosterone phenylacetate (Perandren Phenylacetate), 50 to 75 mg. IM every four weeks.

5. Testosterone enanthate (Delatestryl), 100 mg. IM every four weeks.

The dose of the parenteral preparations may be reduced to one-half the amount suggested above after an appropriate response has been established.

Topical application of androgenic creams to the clitoris may be of value in the treatment of diminished libido in the female. The advantage of such treatment would be that there would be little possibility for a generalized systemic arrhenomimetic phenomenon to occur. Preparations containing 10 mg. of testosterone per gram of vanishing cream base have been of help in augmenting libido in the female. Daily application of 1.0 Gm. of the ointment is usually sufficient. Obviously, when such therapy is used, the possibility is always raised that the mode of application alone might be sufficient to provide clitoral stimulation and thereby enhance libido. This is a moot question; but despite the obvious effect that mechanical stimulation may have, it does appear that the addition of androgen to the cream has been helpful in reestablishing the desire for coitus in the unresponsive female.

The use of androgenic preparations, despite the apparent paradox, has also been found to be helpful in some patients with nymphomania. However, the excessive sex drive in these patients appears to be due to repeated sexual contact being sought because of an inability of the patient to achieve a climax. Androgens in these patients may release a trigger mechanism whereby an orgasm can be accomplished, thus diminishing the need for repeated sexual gratification. On the other hand, the nymphomaniac who readily achieves an orgasm and desires such repeated episodes because of the associated pleasure may best be treated by the administration of progesterone in an attempt to decrease her libidinous drive (Fig. 261). Progesterone may also be used for the treatment of those females in whom erotic or libidinous dreams occur which are disturbing to the patient's mores. In addition, this steroid may be employed to suppress the desire for coitus in women whose husbands are incapable of satisfying their sexual needs. The dose of progesterone and related steroids that may be employed for its antilibidinous effects is as follows:

1. Progesterone suppositories, 50 mg. per evening for several weeks, followed by 25 mg. per evening, and then the amount received further diminished by intermittent therapy.

2. The various progestational agents which are available for oral use are of some help in these patients provided the steroid lacks androgenic potential. Medroxyprogesterone (Provera), 5 mg. a day, would be helpful in this respect, as would 5 mg. per day of norethynodrel (Enovid).

The treatment of libido deficiencies in the male is a much more difficult problem than in the female and many times has been fraught with failure. The use of androgens orally or parenterally is usually ineffective since the psychiatric component in men as far as libido goes is of tremendous importance. As discussed in previous chapters, one may anticipate an increase in libido in the male with androgen therapy if the patient shows a low 17-ketosteroid excretion for his age, or if an elevated follicle-stimulating hormone (FSH) excretion level is present. In the male with normal FSH and 17-ketosteroids, the likelihood of an adequate therapeutic response to androgens is poor. Where the FSH excretion is elevated and the 17-ketosteroids are low, the following therapeutic regimen may be used with some degree of success being assured, particularly if there is poor beard development and the body hair growth is below normal:

1. Methyltestosterone, 20 mg. b.i.d. to t.i.d. with the dose being diminished if an adequate therapeutic effect is accomplished.

2. Fluoxymesterone, 10 mg. b.i.d. to t.i.d. Here, too, the patient is to adjust his dose according to the success of the treatment.

The following parenteral preparations may be administered at two-week intervals:

1. Testosterone cyclopentylpropionate (Depo-Testosterone) or testosterone phenylacetate (Perandren Phenylacetate), 150 to 200 mg. every two weeks.

2. Testosterone enanthate (Delatestryl), 300 to 400 mg. every two weeks.

There is another vital question that must always be considered when androgens are administered chronically in the male: whether or not a neoplastic lesion of the prostate is present. In individuals with prostatic neoplasms, androgenic treatment may be conducive to bringing about accelerated progress of growth of the neoplasms. If anaplasia is present, metastasis may be enhanced. This, however, is a calculated risk and can only be controlled by adequate and frequent prostatic examination. The likelihood of androgen therapy initiating a neoplastic process is remote.

Excessive libido in the male may be managed by suppression of gonadotropic hormone through the use of progestational agents of the 19-norsteroid group. These preparations will suppress endogenous testosterone secretion by inhibition of gonadotropin secretion. Obviously, only those steroids which are not androgenic should be used for this purpose. Medroxyprogesterone acetate (Depo-Provera) intramuscularly, 100 to 200 mg. every 10 days, would be effective, as would oral administration of 10 mg. of norethynodrel (Enovid) b.i.d. The need for such therapy is meager, but it should be considered and used where indicated. The use of estrogens would also be of value in the male as a pituitary gonadotropin suppressant. However, the undesirable side effects of these steroids in inducing feminization would markedly limit their usefulness.

Priapism. There is one clinical entity, priapism, which at times has been allied with problems of libido. Its presence does not necessarily mean that there is an augmented libidinous drive. Not infrequently priapism may be due to a neurologic disorder or to some urologic disease involving the genitourinary tract. The use of hormones for its management is invariably of little value. However, before any extensive neurologic or surgical procedure is advised, and obviously before any detrimental effects (gangrene of the glands, etc.) due to priapism occur, it would be wise to attempt a course of therapy with estrogens, using a preparation such as ethinyl estradiol, 0.1 mg. t.i.d., or conjugated estrogens equine, 2.5 mg. t.i.d., for several days. The use of norethynodrel in doses of 10 mg. three to four times a day may also be helpful. However, if success is not accomplished with these steroids within a relatively short period of time, their continued use is probably ill-advised.

Summary. Libido deficiencies and their management have been discussed. The therapeutic control of these defects by androgens in the appropriately selected patient has been more than adequate.

References

1. GREENBLATT, R. B., MORTARA, F., AND TORPIN, R.: Sexual libido in the female. Amer. J. Obstet. Gynec. 44:658-663, 1942.
2. KUPPERMAN, H. S.: Modern concepts of endocrine therapy in gynecic disorders. Exhibit at A.M.A. Meeting, 1951.
3. KUPPERMAN, H. S.: Hormonal aspects of frigidity. Quart. Rev. Surg. 16:254-257, 1959.
4. KUPPERMAN, H. S.: Hormones, Sex. *In* Ellis, A., and Abarbanel, A. (eds.): The Encyclopedia of Sexual Behavior, Hawthorn Books, Inc., New York, 1961, pp. 494-502.
5. KUPPERMAN, H. S., AND STUDDIFORD, W. E.: Endocrine therapy in gynecologic disorders. Postgrad. Med. 14:410-424, 1953.
6. SALMON, U. J.: Rationale for androgen therapy in gynecology. J. Clin. Endocr. 1:162-179, 1941.

chapter 14

The vaginal mucosa mirrors the endocrine status of the ovary and serves as an excellent measure of physiologic activity of either endogenous or exogenous ovarian hormones. The mucosal layer of the vagina continuously regenerates from the basal cell layer with maturation of the cells occurring in their migration towards the mucosal surface. In the progressive maturation of the cells from the basal germinal cell layers to the superficial portion of the mucosa, there are specific forces at work which influence the histologic picture of the spread made from the vaginal pool containing the desquamated cells. While there are other factors which influence the rate of growth and desquamation of the vaginal cells, there is no doubt that the major influences governing these processes are the physiologically active levels of estrogen and progesterone that are present.

Estrogen Effects. Estrogen has a cohesive action as far as the vaginal epithelium is concerned: it prevents the cells from being sloughed off and will keep them firmly adhered to the underlying cells of the mucosal layers until complete maturation of the cytoplasm and nucleus has occurred (Fig. 262[6]). In the process of cell maturation, estrogen and progesterone influence the developmental changes of both the nucleus and cytoplasm, as well as the biochemical nature of the vaginal mucosa.

The nuclei of the young immature cells of the basal cell layer are large and vesicular. They become less vesicular and diminish in size until

478

Use of the Vaginal Smear as a Diagnostic Test in Endocrinopathies

they eventually assume a pyknotic appearance as the cell migrates towards the surface and matures. In contrast to the nuclear changes, the cytoplasm is sparse and is approximately equal to the nucleus in size in the basal cell or immature stage. However, as the cell matures, under the influence of estrogen, the cytoplasm increases in magnitude and eventually far exceeds the nucleus in size both as far as relative and actual measurements are concerned. As the estrogenic effect continues, the large cornified cell with pyknotic nucleus may eventually be devoid of nuclear structures to enter a keratotic stage. Keratosis is even more prone to occur when there are associated vitamin deficiencies in addition to the continuous uninterrupted action of estrogen.

Progesterone Effects. Progesterone, on the other hand, is a desquamative hormone as far as the vaginal epithelium is concerned. Inasmuch as it promotes early desquamation of the cells, complete maturation of the cell cannot take place in the presence of adequate levels of progesterone. The cohesive force of estrogen is nullified and the cells are shed before their nuclei reach the pyknotic stage or before the cytoplasm attains its maximal proportions. As a result, under progestational activity, the nuclei of the cells in the vaginal smear made from the desquamated cells are in the intermediate or pre-intermediate cell stage (Fig. 262[6]). In general, they retain their vesicular normochromic appearance. In addi-

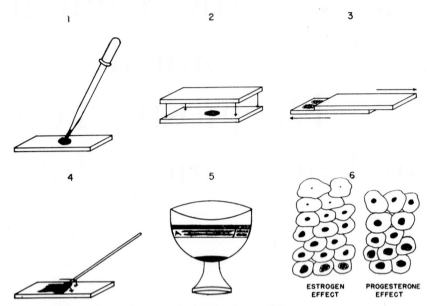

FIG. 262.   *1, Expression of vaginal aspiration on slide.*

2, The secretion obtained from the cul-de-sac area is covered with another slide.

3, The two slides are pulled apart so that an even spread is obtained.

4, Vaginal smear evenly prepared by rolling a cotton swab containing the vaginal cells on a clean glass slide.

5, Lugol's solution in a cup over which a slide containing the dried vaginal smear is suspended face down, thus permitting the iodine fumes to stain the glycogen cells brown (see Fig. 267).

6, The effect of estrogen and progesterone upon the vaginal mucosa. Estrogen prevents desquamation of the cells, while progesterone enhances desquamation so that cornification of any extent is usually not seen.

tion to these nuclear alterations, there are other changes that are invariably noted during the progestational phase which enable the cytologist to distinguish between the proliferative and secretory phases of ovarian activity. Changes during the progestational phase include the following:

1. An increased number of cells are desquamated so that the number of cells in the vaginal smear usually exceeds by far that noted during the proliferative or estrogenic phase.

2. There is an increased degree of cellular folding. Instead of the flattened appearance of the cells noted prior to ovulation, the post-ovulatory (secretory) phase is associated with a folding or rolling of the cells.

3. An increased number of oval or elongated nuclei is evident.

4. There is infiltration of the smear with polymorphonuclear neutrophils. One should note that specific vaginal infections, such as Trichomonas or Candida, or non-specific infections may alter the general

appearance of the vaginal smear so that the typical cyclic changes may be absent. For example, the presence of Döderlein bacilli may cause marked cellular lysis resulting in the presence of bare nuclei devoid of formed cytoplasmic structures. These changes are seen more frequently in states of deficient estrogenic activity or in the secretory phase.

Technique of Obtaining the Smear. ASPIRATION. When there is an adequate amount of vaginal secretion a satisfactory specimen may be taken by the use of a long (8 inch) glass pipette, attached to a rubber bulb. The tip of the pipette should be elongated (1 cm.) and be one third to one fourth the diameter of the shaft of the pipette. This will permit forceful expulsion of the vaginal secretions, which are obtained by aspiration of the posterior cul-de-sac area, onto a slide (Fig. 263). Such a pipette, whose widest diameter is 4 to 5 mm., is easily inserted even in a patient with a virginal introitus. The aspirated material is then expressed on the glass slide and evenly spread by placing another slide on top of the vaginal secretion (Fig. 262 [1-3]). The two slides are then pulled apart and placed back-to-back in the special Mylex fixative or a fixative containing 50 per cent of ether and 50 per cent of 95 per cent ethyl alcohol.

COTTON SWAB. If the vaginal mucosa is atrophic or if there is little vaginal secretion available for aspiration, the pipette method may not be satisfactory since a sufficient amount of material cannot be obtained to prepare a satisfactory slide. In such patients a cotton swab may be inserted into the vaginal introitus and twirled in the area of the posterior vaginal vault (Fig. 264). The material on the swab is then applied to the slide with a rolling motion (Fig. 262[4]). The slide is then fixed in the wet state as described above.

NO DOUCHE PRIOR TO SMEAR. The patients should be instructed never to take a douche prior to vaginal examination. While a douche may be hygienically desirable, it creates an area rather barren of cells so that an inadequate smear is obtained when a slide is made of the vaginal pool.

Staining the Smear. There are several staining procedures that may be employed to prepare the smear for examination.

POLYCHROME TECHNIQUES. These include the methods of Papanicolaou and of Shorr.

Papanicolaou Method.[4-6] The Papanicolaou technique (Fig. 265) is the standard one for the detection of nuclear pathologic change—particularly for the determination of anaplastic changes. Obviously this technique is also ideal for ascertaining the endocrine status of the patient.

Shorr technique.[8] The Shorr technique (Fig. 266) is more rapid and yields the same information as the Papanicolaou procedure as far as the endocrine status of the patient is concerned. However, it is not as desirable for the detection of anaplastic changes and should not be used

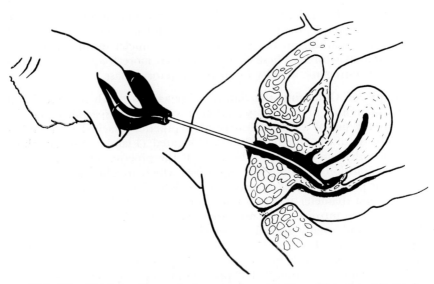

FIG. 263. Obtaining the vaginal smear by aspiration. The glass pipette is inserted into the posterior cul-de-sac, and the contents are aspirated and placed upon the slide as shown in Figure 262 [1].

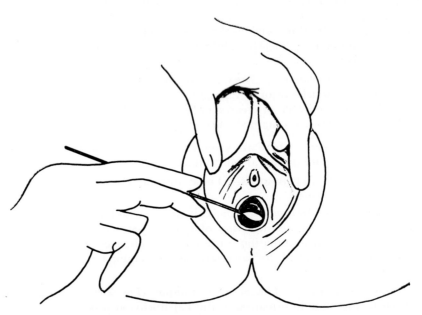

FIG. 264. Obtaining the vaginal smear with the aid of a cotton swab. This is necessary only in patients with diminished vaginal secretion. The smear is transferred to the slide as depicted in Figure 262 [4].

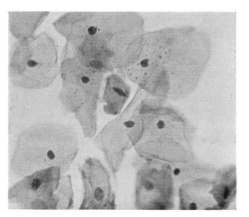 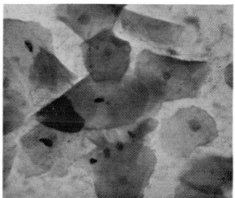

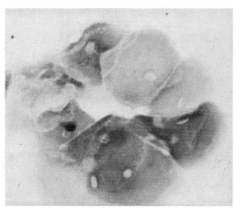 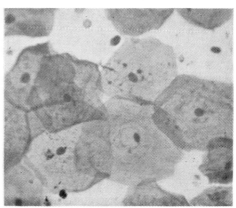

265 (top)   266 (top)

267 (bottom)   268 (bottom)

FIG. 265. *Papanicolaou stained vaginal smear. Note the excellent nuclear and cytologic differentiation.*

FIG. 266. *Vaginal smear stained with Shorr's polychrome stain. Note the excellent cytologic differentiation but poor nuclear characteristics. This technique is excellent for endocrine evaluation.*

FIG. 267. *Mack's iodine stain. Note that the glycogen cells are stained brown. Glycogen deposition is increased with enhanced estrogenic activity. The smear is stained as shown in Figure 262 [5].*

FIG. 268. *Fuchsin stain. Note the excellent cytologic staining qualities but poor nuclear differentiation.*

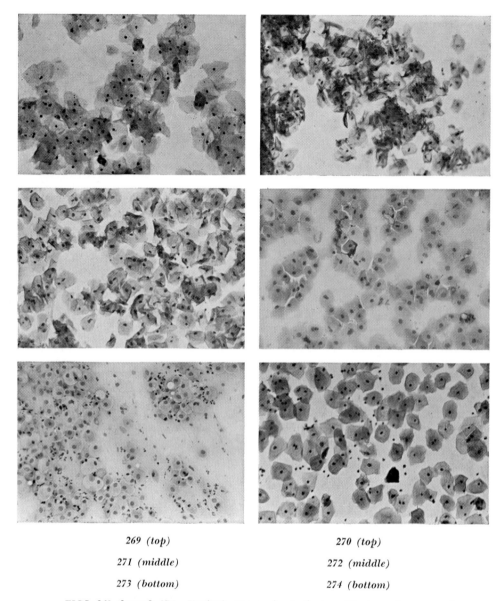

269 (top)
271 (middle)
273 (bottom)

270 (top)
272 (middle)
274 (bottom)

FIGS. 269 through 274. *Vaginal smears in patients with precocious sexual development showing the effect of different therapeutic regimens that were employed to obtain a correct diagnosis.*

FIG. 269. *Vaginal smear obtained from a patient with sexual precocity. Note the excellent cornification.*

FIG. 270. *Vaginal smear from same patient shown in Figure 269 after intramuscular administration of 100 mg. of depot-medroxyprogesterone (Depo-Provera) every seven days for three weeks. Note the excellent secretory change without evidence of decreased estrogenic activity. Diagnosis was that of a neoplastic process causing the sexual precocity. This was confirmed by finding a granulosa cell tumor.*

FIG. 271. *Vaginal smear in a young female child, PR, age 15 months, with sexual precocity and menstruation.*

FIG. 272. *Vaginal smear taken from same patient as shown in Figure 271 after receiving Depo-Provera, 100 mg. every seven days. The vaginal smear showed marked estrogenic deficiency. Constitutional sexual precocity was established on this basis and confirmed by laparotomy.*

FIG. 273. *Decreased estrogenic activity in vaginal smear noted in patient with significant breast development. The diminished estrogenic function in this patient would point towards the diagnosis of the thelarche rather than sexual precocity.*

FIG. 274. *Vaginal smear from patient with sexual precocity showing increased degree of cornification and excellent breast development. The precocious development of the breasts would rule out the thelarche in this patient since the vaginal cornification would point towards an endogenous source of estrogens, either neoplastic or constitutional in origin.*

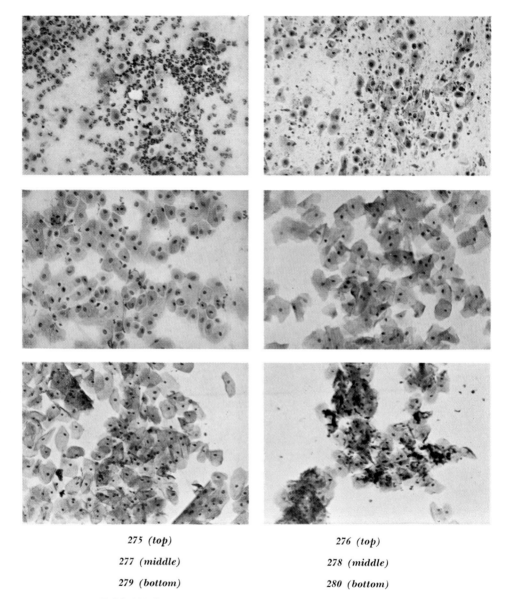

275 (top)

277 (middle)

279 (bottom)

276 (top)

278 (middle)

280 (bottom)

FIGS. 275 through 280.   The diagnostic usefulness of the vaginal
smear in patients with amenorrhea.

FIG. 275. *Vaginal smear obtained from patient with primary amenorrhea showing evidence of lack of estrogenic activity.*

FIG. 276. *Vaginal smear from the same patient as shown in Figure 275 after a 3-week course of gonadotropin therapy (Equinex). Note the persistence of diminished estrogenic activity associated with typical castrate-like changes. This failure of ovarian stimulation to occur would support the diagnosis of ovarian agenesis or primary ovarian failure.*

FIG. 277. *Vaginal smear obtained from patient with primary amenorrhea. Note the typical changes commensurate with estrogenic deficiency.*

FIG. 278. *Vaginal smear from same patient as in Figure 277 after a 3-week course of PMS gonadotropin. Note the excellent degree of maturation of the vaginal spread, indicating that the patient has ovaries capable of responding. This would rule out ovarian agenesis or gonadal dysgenesis, and would indicate the diagnosis of decreased pituitary secretion of gonadotropins.*

FIGS. 279 and 280. *Vaginal smears obtained from patient with primary amenorrhea with excellent secondary sex development, normal breasts and pubic and axillary hair. Figure 279 shows excellent vaginal cornification. Figure 280 demonstrates the typical changes seen during the secretory phase. Failure of menses in this patient, plus the finding of cyclic changes in the vaginal smear, would indicate the diagnosis of uterine agenesis. This was confirmed by laparotomy.*

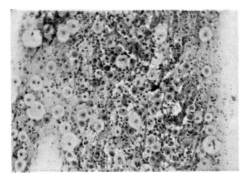 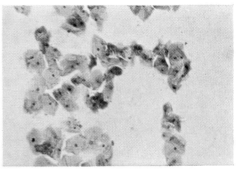

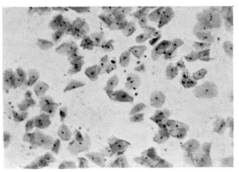

281 (left)   282 (right)

283 (center)

FIGS. 281 through 283. *The diagnostic value of an atrophic smear as well as those with marked cornification in patients with amenorrhea or oligomenorrhea.*

FIG. 281. *Vaginal smear taken from patient with excellent breast development but who showed an absence of pubic and axillary hair. The decreased estrogenic activity in the vaginal smear, together with the above clinical picture, would support the diagnosis of testicular feminization. This was confirmed by laparotomy, and the finding of a negative chromatin pattern and increased FSH excretion.*

FIG. 282. *Vaginal smear from patient with oligomenorrhea and vaginal cornification noted throughout her menstrual cycle. Menses readily followed administration of progesterone. This would indicate anovulatory function in this patient.*

FIG. 283. *Vaginal smear from another patient with irregular menses in whom vaginal cornification was noted before and after the onset of her spontaneous menses. Such findings would indicate that the patient has anovulatory cycles.*

when examination of the smear for neoplastic disease is the prime pre-requisite.

OTHER TECHNIQUES.   There are two other simple but valuable pro-cedures that are adaptable for endocrine survey. These are the Mack's iodine technique and the fuschin stain.

Mack's Iodine Technique.[2, 3]   Mack's iodine stain is a simple one and is based upon the fact that the glycogen deposited in the epithelial cells under the influence of estrogen and progesterone will be stained brown by the iodine fumes emanating from Lugol's solution. The method may be performed as follows: A dried vaginal smear is obtained by the methods described earlier. The slide is then placed face down over a small amount of Lugol's solution so that the fumes will strike the cells in the vaginal spread (Fig. 262 [5]). The slide is kept over the fumes for a period of two to three minutes. The number of cells with glycogen (stained brown) in contrast to the cells free of glycogen (yellow stain) is propor-tional to the degree of estrogenic activity that is present (Fig. 267). Complete glycopenia is noted in marked estrogenic deficiency. Excellent estrogenic activity would be characterized by the presence of glycogen in 75 to 80 per cent of the cells which will be stained brown. These slides will fade with age but may be readily re-stained by replacing them over Lugol's solution whenever desired. Regardless of how long the slide had been stored in a dried state, the glycogen stain will reappear in the same percentage of cells as previously noted.

Fuchsin Stain.[1, 7]   Aqueous carbolfuchsin may be used as a 1 to 2 per cent solution, or, as suggested by Salmon and Frank,[7] a 3 per cent alcoholic solution of fuchsin diluted 1:8 with water may be employed. Either stain provides the physician with a relatively simple and economic technique. The dried vaginal smear, obtained as described above, is flooded with the fuchsin solution of choice for two to three minutes. The slide is then washed and examined (Fig. 268). The basal, intermediate and cornified cells are readily distinguished from one another by nuclear and cytoplas-mic ratios. The cytoplasm is well outlined, as is the nucleus which may be adequately characterized. The nucleus takes a darker stain than does the cytoplasm (Fig. 268). However, the vesicular, hyperchromic or ana-plastic nature of the nucleus is difficult to judge with this stain. The relative proportion of nuclear and cellular size is an index of relative estrogenic function, i. e., a large nucleus in a small cell indicates low or absent estrogenic function; a small pyknotic nucleus in a large squamous cell points toward adequate estrogenic function.

Clinical Application of the Vaginal Smear Procedure.   The clinical importance of the vaginal smear as a diagnostic procedure in the different endocrinopathies must never be overlooked. A study of the vaginal smear at periodic intervals or after certain therapeutic procedures may offer the clinician a relatively simple method to solve many difficult clinical pro-

blems. Since most of the applications of the vaginal smear have been discussed in the pertinent chapters in which the specific endocrinopathy was being considered, only a brief outline of the clinical usefulness of the vaginal smear will be reviewed here.

SEXUAL PRECOCITY (ISOSEXUAL). If repeated vaginal cytologic studies show evidence of a persistent degree of marked cornification over a period of several months, the possibility of an estrogen-producing neoplasm as the principal causative factor in the sexual precocity must be considered. However, if cyclic changes are noted in the study of the vaginal smears obtained at intervals of every five days, one can assume that the patient either has constitutional sexual precocity or precocious development due to some intracranial disorder or disease that has resulted in premature but cyclic secretion of pituitary gonadotropins.

On the other hand, if there is still some indecision as to the exact nature of the disturbance causing the sexual precocity, one may then determine the child's response to norethisterone (10 mg. t.i.d.) or depot-medroxyprogesterone (100 to 150 mg. given intramuscularly every seven to ten days). If the administration of these steroids over a period of four to six weeks causes persistent secretory changes in the vaginal smear, then the possibility of a neoplastic cause is most likely (Figs. 269, 270). If, on the other hand, a castrate-type smear is obtained with such treatment, this must be considered as good evidence for the diagnosis of constitutional sexual precocity (Figs. 271, 272). The rationale behind this differential point is that in patients with constitutional sexual precocity, the recommended dose of the progestational hormone inhibits endogenous gonadotropic secretion so that ovarian function is held in abeyance. The castrate smear then reflects cessation of ovarian function. On the other hand, since a neoplasm is not dependent upon pituitary tropic hormones for its activity, it will continuously secrete its hormone responsible for the sex precocity, and the progestational steroid will merely alter the morphologic expression of the neoplasm's estrogenic activity by inducing changes in the vaginal smear commensurate with the secretory phase. Hence a castrate-like picture will not be seen since the tumor will be continuously secreting estrogen.

THELARCHE. Premature development of the breasts is noted at times in infants and children and may or may not be associated with progressive sexual precocity. Since the premature thelarche (development of the breasts not associated with increased ovarian activity) may take place at all ages during infancy and early childhood, it is important to establish the presence or absence of ovarian activity. A castrate vaginal smear (normally seen in children prior to the onset of ovarian activity) would point towards the diagnosis of premature thelarche alone (Fig. 273), and would rule out the possibility of increased estrogenic secretion due to constitutional sexual precocity or neoplasm (Fig. 274).

PRIMARY AMENORRHEA (WITHOUT DEVELOPMENT OF BREASTS AND PUBARCHE). In patients with primary amenorrhea without sexual maturation, one may determine the presence or absence of ovaries capable of functioning by studying the vaginal changes in a patient given a gonadotropin rich in FSH. If the administration of 500 to 1000 I.U. of pregnant mare's serum (Equinex) three times per week for three weeks is not associated with any vaginal maturation, one can then conclude that there is probably ovarian failure or agenesis, or gonadal dysgenesis (Figs. 275 and 276). On the other hand, some degree of vaginal maturation occurring in response to a course of exogenous gonadotropins would indicate the presence of ovaries capable of functioning and would rule out the possibility of the above diagnoses (Figs. 277 and 278). In such a patient the prognosis would not be hopeless, as it would have to be in those patients showing no evidence of increased estrogen activity after exogenous gonadotropic stimulation.

PRIMARY AMENORRHEA WITH ADEQUATE SEXUAL MATURATION. Primary amenorrhea associated with good development of secondary sexual characteristics and normal cyclic changes in the vaginal smear would point towards the diagnosis of uterine agenesis or endometrial failure (Figs. 279 and 280). This would be particularly so if large doses of estrogen and progesterone fail to bring about a catamenia. If one is unable to obtain a vaginal smear and notes a bulging perineum and/or hematosalpinx or uterine enlargement, these findings would support the diagnosis of gynatresia, imperforate hymen, or cervical stenosis.

If there is evidence of an atrophic smear (Fig. 281) in a patient with well-developed breasts and diminished or absent pubic or axillary hair, the diagnosis of testicular feminization is likely and will be confirmed by the presence of a negative chromatin pattern. This can be further ascertained by noting a failure of menses to follow cyclic therapy with estrogen and progesterone (same dose regimen recommended in Chapter 6, Amenorrhea).

MENSTRUAL IRREGULARITIES. Excessive, prolonged and irregular catamenia associated with increased cornification in the vaginal smear (Fig. 282) obtained when the patient is not menstruating would point towards anovulatory cycles and persistent estrogenic secretion. This diagnosis is all the more definite if the heavily cornified smears are obtained just before the onset or just after cessation of menses. Persistent and marked vaginal cornification in a patient with oligomenorrhea would also support the diagnosis of unopposed estrogenic secretion seen in the anovulatory female (Fig. 283).

Conclusion. In conclusion it may be said that accurate interpretation of the vaginal smear and the response to therapy serves as an excellent diagnostic modality for the physician. It offers the examiner a simple, rapid, and yet highly instructive means of unraveling some perplexing endocrinopathies in gynecology.

References

1. Greenblatt, R. B.: Office Endocrinology. Charles C Thomas, Springfield, Ill., 1947.

2. Mack, H. C.: A new and rapid method of staining vaginal smears based upon a specific color reaction for glycogen. Harper Hosp. Bull. 1:54-56, 1942.

3. Mack, H. C., and Ale, T.: Appraisal of estrogenic activity by the vaginal glycogen index. J. Clin. Endocr. 2:361-364, 1942.

4. Papanicolaou, G. N.: A new procedure for staining vaginal smears. Science 95: 438-439, 1942.

5. Papanicolaou, G. N., and Traut, H. F.: Diagnosis of uterine cancer by the vaginal smear. The Commonwealth Fund, New York, 1943.

6. Papanicolaou, G. N., Traut, H. F., and Marchetti, A. A.: The epithelia of woman's reproductive organs. A correlative study of cyclic changes. The Commonwealth Fund, New York, 1948.

7. Salmon, U. J., and Frank, R. T.: Hormonal factors affecting vaginal smears in castrates and after menopause. Proc. Soc. Exp. Biol. Med. 33:612-614, 1936.

8. Shorr, E.: New technic for staining vaginal smears. Science 91:321-322, 1940; 91: 579-580, 1940.

chapter 15

Microscopic study of samples of the endometrium will often provide the clinician with information concerning the endocrine function of the ovary which cannot be as easily obtained by other chemical tests or biologic procedures. The endometrium, like the vagina, mirrors the hormonal activity of the ovary.[4] In general, there are two characteristic, hormonal-dependent phases of the endometrium which are histologically and chemically different from one another and have been designated as the phase of proliferation and the phase of secretion.

Proliferative Phase. The proliferative phase is one in which the endometrium is primarily under the influence of the estrogens secreted by the developing follicle prior to ovulation. This phase starts with the first day of menstruation, i.e., the first day of the menstrual flow, and continues, in the normal cycle, to ovulation. The primary effect of estrogen on the endometrium is one of growth, hence the term "proliferative phase." The glands at this time are straight and show little or no coiling.

Morphologic Appearance. Pseudostratification of the nuclei of the endometrial glands is noted early in the proliferative phase (Fig. 284). As the patient approaches her ovulatory phase, the glands become larger and the lining mucosal cells show a greater degree of pseudostratification. The stroma becomes more densely cellular as compared (Figs. 285 and

Diagnostic Value of the Endometrium in Menstrual Abnormalities

286) to the stromal edema (of the late proliferative phase) which reaches a peak effect in the midportion of the estrogenic or proliferative phase (Fig. 287). There is a considerable increase at this time in the number of mitoses in both the glands and stroma. The pseudostratification of the glandular cells and their nuclei becomes less marked and eventually disappears entirely. Subnuclear vacuolization begins to appear and, when noted, implies that the proliferative phase is at an end, plus the fact that the secretory phase is being ushered in (Figs. 288 and 289). The pseudo-stratification is replaced by glandular cells present as a single layer of cuboidal to columnar mucosal cells. These changes are diagrammatically listed in Figure 290, which is based in part upon the earlier description of Hertig and Rock.[3]

Secretory Phase. MORPHOLOGIC APPEARANCE. Vacuolization appears beneath the nucleus just after ovulation occurs, causing the nucleus to be pushed from the basal area towards the periphery so that it becomes located in the midportion of the cell. This process may start in the late proliferative phase and is seen characteristically on days 15 to 17 of a normal 28-day cycle. As the secretory phase progresses, there is an increasing amount of secretion from the cells. Maximal secretory activity occurs at days 22 to 24, which is the midportion of the secretory phase (Figs. 292-294). Edema of the stroma is also maximal at day 22 (Fig.

489

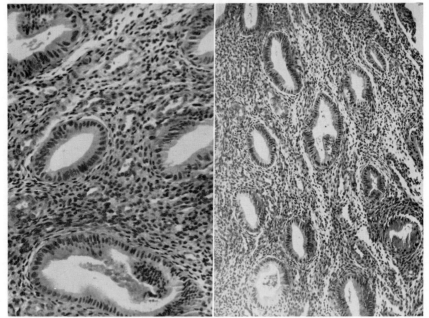

FIG. 284   FIG. 285

FIG. 284.   Early proliferative phase. Note the moderate density of the stroma and beginning striation of nuclei of the endometrial gland. Specimen obtained from infertile patient with anovulatory periods.

FIG. 285.   Mid-proliferative phase. Note compactness of the stroma plus nuclear stratification. Beginning stromal edema is noted.

293). It should be noted, however, that while stromal edema also is accentuated at about day 9 to 10 of the proliferative phase, it is much more intense and pronounced on the seventh postovulatory day (Figs. 295, 296). Pseudo-decidual formation in the stroma is never seen in the proliferative phase but occurs only during the latter portion of the secretory phase (Fig. 297). There is an increased number of stromal mitoses about day 23 to 24. The number of cells with mitotic activity is comparable to that noted during the preovulatory phase. Prior to menstruation, beginning approximately on day 25, there is an increase in polymorphonuclear neutrophil infiltration of the stroma (Figs. 290 and 298). This will persist during the early portion of the proliferative phase at the time of the catamenia, which ushers in the beginning of estrogenic activity for the subsequent cycle. These changes are also presented in schematic form in Figure 290.

Menstrual Phase. When menstruation does take place, proliferative phase activity has already begun again so that there is significant regrowth

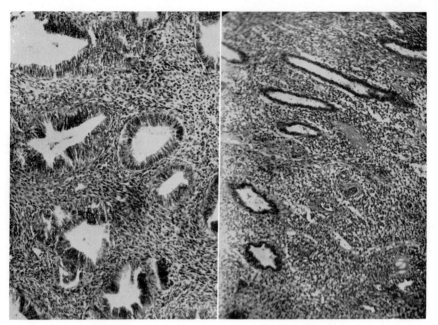

FIG. 286   FIG. 287

FIG. 286.   Mid-proliferative phase. The striation of the glands is more extensive.
The stroma is compact yet shows evidence of beginning edema.

FIG. 287.   Edema of the stroma with decreased striation of the nuclei in the
glands. There is no evidence of secretion.

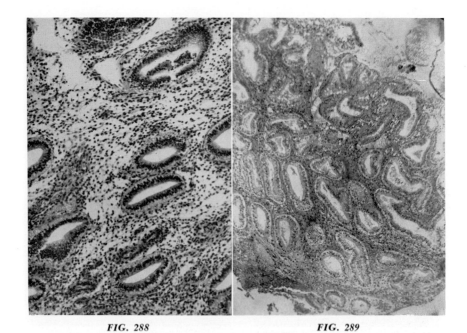

FIG. 288   FIG. 289

FIG. 288. Endometrium at the sixteenth day of the menstrual cycle. Note the subnuclear vacuolization without evidence of secretory activity at the periphery of the cells. Stromal edema is diminished.

FIG. 289. Endometrium obtained on day 16 to 17. Note the subnuclear vacuolization as seen in Figure 288. No evidence of secretory activity. The stroma is more compact than that in Figure 288.

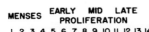

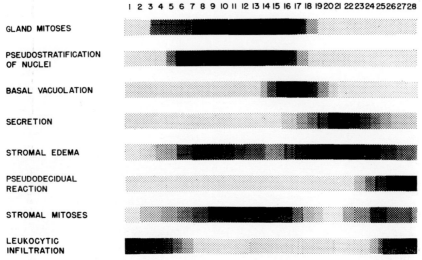

FIG. 290. A diagrammatic presentation of the changes seen in the endometrium. The intensity and variation of the changes noted are characterized by differences in shading. The darker the bar, the higher the intensity of the characteristic that this bar portrays.

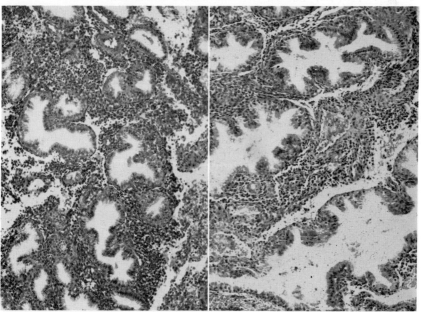

FIG. 291   FIG. 292

FIG. 291. Day 21. Note the secretory activity of the glands with a fairly compact stroma. Edema of the stroma is minimal and is commensurate with the histologic picture normally anticipated for this phase of the cycle.

FIG. 292. Day 22. Note increased secretory activity with beginning of stromal edema.

493

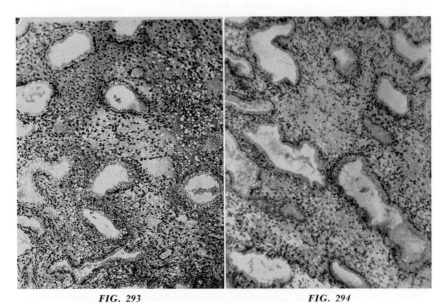

FIG. 293   FIG. 294

FIG. 293. Day 22 to 23. Note the unusual degree of stromal edema
associated with endometrial hyperplasia.

FIG. 294. Day 24. Note the marked edema with excellent
secretory activity of the glandular epithelium.

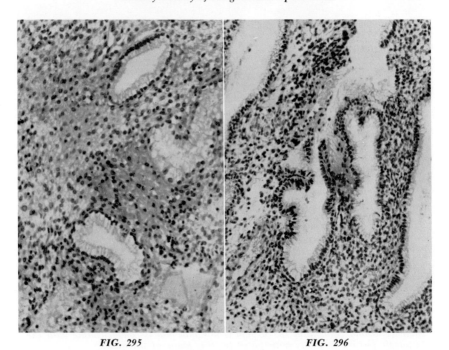

FIG. 295   FIG. 296

FIGS. 295 and 296. Day 23, high-power view of endometrium. Stromal edema
well demonstrated plus active secretion depicted by the glandular epithelium.

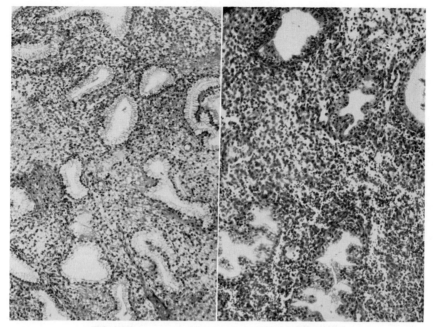

FIG. 297   FIG. 298

*FIG. 297.   Pseudodecidua reaction noted in the stroma of the endometrium
taken on the twenty-fourth day of the menstrual cycle.*

*FIG. 298.   Day 26 to 27.   Polymorphonuclear neutrophil infiltration of the
stroma. Secretory activity of the glands is still high.*

of the endometrial glands, despite the fact that the secretory endometrium is being almost completely shed. At the time of menstruation, the endometrial glands begin to show pseudostratification of the nuclei. Hence, while one would anticipate that menstruation would normally be associated with degradation, glandular development and growth are actively in progress at this time.

Clinical Importance of Endometrial Biopsy.   The physiology of menstruation has been discussed in a previous chapter and will not again be elaborated upon here. However, emphasis will be placed on the role and the importance of the endometrium in evaluating the endocrine status of the patient as a whole, or of the ovary in particular. The following pertinent facts should be noted.

USEFULNESS OF BIOPSY IN DETERMINING OVULATION.   Endometrial biopsy specimens taken on the first day of menstruation are of inestimable value in establishing the adequacy of the secretory activity of the corpora lutea. An adequate, mature, secretory endometrium implies that ovulation has taken place. If the endometrial specimen shows poor secretory changes

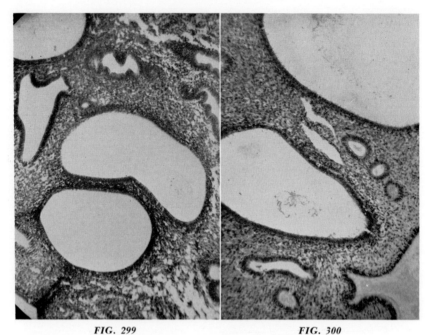

FIG. 299   FIG. 300

FIGS. 299 and 300. Cystic glandular hyperplasia of two endometrial specimens obtained from patients with anovulatory cycles. Note the marked change in the glands of the endometrium characterized by dilation of the glands with cystic changes. The stroma is compact. Nuclear striation is evident.

with little decidua-like alteration of the stroma, this points towards the possibility of inadequate production of progesterone by the corpus luteum. Such a finding leads one to the diagnosis of an inadequate secretory phase, which may occur when the synergistic effects that normally exist between progesterone and estrogen are probably not functioning at their maximal capacity at this time.

"BLEEDING BIOPSY." The biopsy specimen obtained as soon after the onset of menses as possible has been designated as a "bleeding biopsy." The advantage of the bleeding biopsy is that when the specimen is obtained via instrumentation at this time, the physician is reasonably safe in assuming that there is little chance of disturbing a viable pregnancy. Moreover, it is at this time that one would anticipate the maximum histologic response to endogenous ovarian hormone secretions.

Significance of Proliferative Activity. If the endometrium obtained at "bleeding biopsy" shows only a proliferative phase type of response, one may then conclude that the patient was anovulatory in the preceding menstrual cycle.

Significance of Cystic and/or Hyperplastic Changes. If an endometrial biopsy reveals a proliferative phase associated with hyperplastic and cystic changes in the endometrium (Figs. 299, 300), one can safely assume that there has been unopposed continuous estrogenic activity, and thus the possibility of ovulation having occurred in the preceding four to six weeks is remote. In other words, the finding of cystic, hyperplastic changes of the endometrial glands would imply that there has been a lack of secretory activity for some time, plus the fact that adequate or more than adequate estrogenic activity was present during this same period of time.

Endometrial Hypoplasia. An endometrial biopsy showing proliferative phase activity but one characterized by atrophy would point towards diminished proliferative phase function or decreased estrogenic secretion by the ovary.

Diagnosis of Infection. The presence of amenorrhea in a patient in whom the endometrial biopsy reveals marked round cell infiltration with multinucleated giant cells would point to the diagnosis of an acid-fast infection involving the endometrium. In such an individual, culture or guinea pig inoculation of the menstruating endometrium could confirm the diagnosis of tuberculous endometritis. In the event that the patient does not menstruate, scrapings obtained by the suction curette can be used for diagnostic purposes and can be subjected to both culture and guinea-pig inoculation.

Usefulness of Biopsy in Characterizing the Activity of Newer Progestational Steroids. The endometrium study also serves as a biologic assay method in establishing the progestational potential of new steroids. The possible progestational effects of steroids under investigation may be studied either in patients with persistently anovulatory cycles or in those in whom ovarian function is absent and in whom the endometrium has been adequately primed with estrogen. The presence of minimal secretory changes in the endometrial glands of such a biopsy specimen, associated with decidua-like alterations in the stroma, would indicate that the steroid being investigated is similar in effects to the 19-norsteroid compounds (Figs. 301-305). The endometrial biopsy specimen in these cases serves well to characterize the biologic activity of the unknown steroid in the human being, and this information obviously supersedes any biologic information obtained from animal studies.

The endometrial pattern will also help to characterize the possible ovulatory-inducing effects of certain analogues of chlorotrianisene, such as clomiphene (MRL 41). The tissues obtained by biopsy shown in Figures 307 and 308 are anovulatory, but were taken from patients with an ovulatory biphasic basal body temperature curve. The biopsies proved beyond doubt that normal ovulation did not take place.

FIG. 301   *FIG. 302*

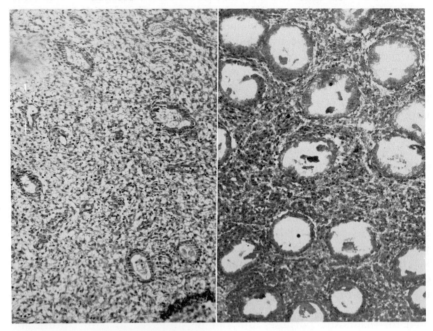

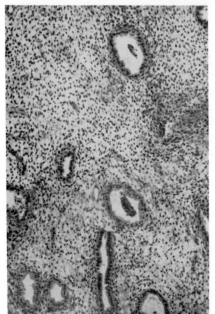

FIGS. 301-305. *Different endometrial specimens obtained from patients treated with the 19-norsteroids. Note the apparent dichotomy between the development of the glands and the stroma. Marked decidua-like changes are noted in Figures 302 through 305, while glandular development is poorly developed and only slightly secretory. Figure 301 shows only minimal decidua change with adequate glandular development.*

FIG. 303

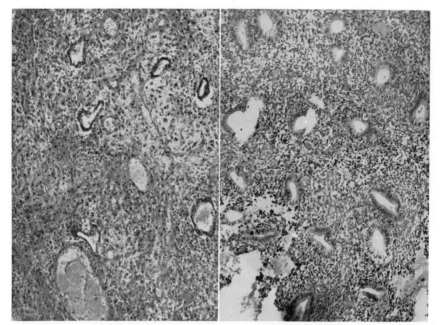

FIG. 304   FIG. 305

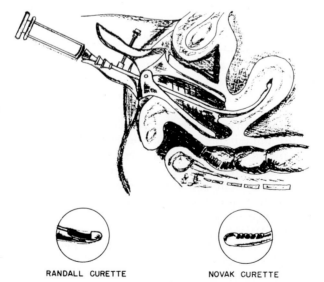

RANDALL CURETTE   NOVAK CURETTE

FIG. 306. *Diagrammatic sagittal section showing the attachment of the curette to a syringe and insertion into the uterine cavity. The Randall curette is non-serrated and is to be compared with the serrated Novak curette.*

Obtaining the Endometrial Biopsy Specimen.   There are several techniques that one may use to obtain an endometrial biopsy specimen.

SUCTION CURETTE.   The optimum method in my experience and that
of my colleagues entails the use of a suction curette[2]—either the Novak
(serrated) or Randall (non-serrated) curette is the instrument of choice
(Fig. 306). The curette is inserted into the uterine cavity and is attached
to a 10 cc. Luer-lock syringe. This procedure provides ease of manipula-
tion of the curette and sufficient negative pressure by pulling back on the
plunger of the syringe.

Use of Preoperative Analgesia.   Prior to obtaining an endometrial
biopsy specimen it behooves the physician to premedicate the patient with
32 mg. of codeine plus 65 mg. of dextro-propoxyphene and acetylsalicylic
acid (Darvon Compound 65). This combination usually provides satisfactory analgesia for most patients so that the procedure is a tolerable
one and the physician achieves the advantage of minimizing patient
resistance to the technique. Parenteral administration of 50 mg. of
meperidine may also be used to prevent pain and allay the fears of the
patient for the procedure. It appears to be wantonly sadistic to deny the
patient analgesic medication prior to the procedure. Moreover, since the
use of appropriate analgesia will change an unwilling, apprehensive
patient to a most cooperative one, the physician also benefits from the
premedication. This is particularly true if biopsy specimens must be
obtained repeatedly for diagnostic or investigative purposes.

Sounding the Uterus.   Prior to the insertion of the curette, the
cervical os should be treated with an antiseptic solution after adequate
exposure provided by use of a bivalve speculum. The uterus may be
sounded to determine its size, shape, and position prior to the insertion
of the curette. This would also tend to ease the way for the insertion of
the curette, which has a somewhat larger diameter than the sound.

Necessity for Tenaculum.   As a rule, there is little need to use a
cervical tenaculum to immobilize the cervix since the curette may be easily
introduced into the uterine cavity after the uterine sound has been passed.
The pain associated with application of the tenaculum to the cervix makes
such a procedure undesirable since the benefit it achieves is not worth
the discomfort to which the patient is subjected.

Performing the Suction Biopsy.   The actual technique necessary in
order to obtain a sufficient amount of endometrial tissue involves the
application of negative pressure on the curette by pulling back on the
plunger of the syringe and then gently moving the curette up and down
in the fundus until tissue from all four quadrants has been obtained.
The tissue in the curette is then expressed into a Petri dish containing
saline solution. All the tissue is washed out of the curette and syringe
barrel by aspiration and then the fluid with the contained endometrial
material is expelled into the dish. The pink-white tissue is removed
from the saline wash and placed into an appropriate fixative, usually 10
per cent formalin.

COLLECTION OF MENSTRUAL ENDOMETRIUM. Another method for obtaining samples of the endometrium for study is that of actually collecting menstrual blood in an appropriate container. This collected sample may then be centrifuged and the sediment fixed. Sections of this material will provide the physician with the same information as that given by the suction curette technique and will help to establish data on the functional and cyclic activity of the endometrium and the ovaries. The advantage of this method is its painlessness. On the other hand, it is not the most aesthetic procedure in which the patient may be asked to participate.

Value of Endometrial Biopsy in the Diagnosis of Neoplastic Disease. While the use of the endometrial biopsy is of unquestionable value in characterizing the functional state of the endometrium and the ovaries, the diagnostic use of the suction curette biopsy technique for the detection of neoplastic or anaplastic lesions is probably not as reliable as the more thorough dilatation and curettage procedure. Theoretically, one could well miss the areas containing the neoplastic changes in the endometrium with the suction curette, so that a false negative histologic picture may be obtained. The suction curette technique and the endometrial fragments obtained thereby should not be used primarily for the diagnosis of pathologic changes but should be employed basically as a method for obtaining specimens of the endometrium in order to establish the correct diagnosis as to the functional endocrine status of the ovary.

Relation between Endometrial Response and Basal Body Temperature (BBT). In characterizing the effect of endogenous progesterone or of other exogenous steroids upon the endometrium of the human being there are several points that should be stressed concerning the minimal dose of a progestational steroid which is necessary to bring about secretory changes as compared to the amount of progesterone required to induce a hyperthermic effect.

INCREASE IN BBT CHART WITHOUT SECRETORY CHANGES. Ten milligrams of progesterone in oil per day for five days will usually not induce an adequate secretory effect on the endometrium, but will cause a definite hyperthermic rise in basal body temperature. Five milligrams of norethindrone acetate or norethynodrel given twice a day will cause a hyperthermic response, but will also provide an adequate secretory effect with decidua-like changes in the stroma. Five milligrams of medroxyprogesterone twice a day will also produce a hyperthermic response and endometrial secretory changes, but will not cause a decidua-like reaction in the stroma. This dichotomy between the hyperthermic response to progesterone and its failure to induce a secretory effect in the aforementioned dose level should raise some doubt concerning the reliability of the basal body temperature chart as an absolute method for demonstrating the adequacy of corpus luteum function, and that ovulation has taken place at all (Figs. 307, 308). In other words, the amount of progesterone

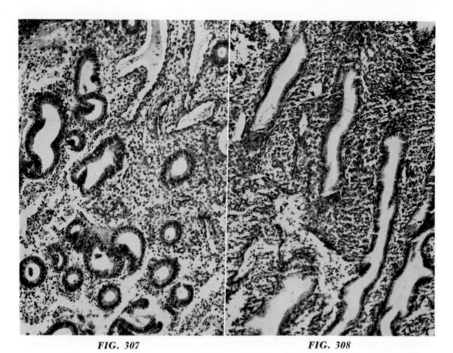

FIG. 307   FIG. 308

FIG. 307. Tissue from patient MM, anovulatory, treated with clomiphene (MRL 41). The patient's temperature chart showed biphasic changes. The endometrial biopsy specimen showed evidence of stromal edema but essentially a proliferative phase activity as far as the glands were concerned.

FIG. 308. Tissue from patient with history of infertility and anovulatory cycles. Clomiphene (MRL 41) induced biphasic temperature changes. Endometrial biopsy revealed poor if any secretory activity with some evidence of stromal edema.

necessary to produce the same degree of hyperthermia noted in the biphasic basal body temperature graph is less than that necessary to bring about adequate secretory changes in the endometrium. Usually a total dose of 100 mg. of parenteral progesterone or 250 mg. of 17-hydroxy-progesterone caproate will bring about good secretory changes in the endometrium.

Chemical Changes. While the morphologic picture is one of prime importance in establishing ovulation or an adequate progestational effect, there are also certain specific chemical changes in the endometrium that are measures of ovulatory or progestational effects. Chemical findings in the endometrium which are characteristic of the pre- and postovulatory phase are an increase in glycogen deposition and alkaline phosphatase activity. Glycogen, while present in minimal quantities during the proliferative phase, increases to a maximum level five to seven days postovulatory (when nidation takes place). The relationship between glycogen and adenosine triphosphatase (ATP) is interesting in that when glycogen is high, ATP is low, and vice versa. Alkaline phosphatase increases during the proliferative phase and reaches its peak at the time of ovulation. Following this, it then decreases in amount. These two chemical constituents (glycogen and ATP) occur in greatest amounts when estrogen and progesterone are both present. Estrogen alone, however, will induce glycogen deposition in a female with absent ovarian function. This cannot be accomplished when progesterone is given to a female castrate without preceding estrogen priming. The same is probably true for alkaline phosphatase activity.

Is Progesterone a Desquamative Hormone?   In studying the effect of progesterone upon the endometrium and vaginal mucosa, it appears that, unlike its effect upon the vagina, progesterone is not a desquamative hormone as far as the endometrium is concerned. In other words, when progesterone is administered exogenously, or secreted endogenously, it actively induces desquamation of vaginal epithelium during its peak activity. On the other hand, the administration of effective doses of progesterone is not associated with any deciduation of the endometrium (deciduation is a more correct term than desquamation since the endometrial lining is not made up of stratified squamous epithelium). As long as the progestational steroid is being administered, there will be no catamenia or shedding of endometrial tissue. However, when progesterone administration is discontinued or its endogenous production brought to a halt, one then obtains a progesterone withdrawal catamenia associated with complete deciduation of the endometrium. It is for this reason that it is incorrect to designate progesterone as a desquamative hormone as far as the endometrium is concerned. Not only is there an absence of desquamative changes, but the progesterone level must fall before there will be any evidence of deciduation.

The endometrium has been, and will continue to be, an excellent diagnostic structure, not only for detecting neoplastic changes but also to ascertain the endocrine status of the patient. In addition, its study in characterizing the new progestational hormones is paramount in the human being and should supersede all other clinical methods to determine the clinical activity of progestational agents.[1]

References

1. GREENBLATT, R. B., AND ROSE, F. D.: Delay of menses: Test of progestational efficacy in indication of pseudo-pregnancy. Obstet. Gynec. 19:730-735, 1961.
2. KLINGLER, H. H., AND BURCH, J. C.: Suction in obtaining endometrial biopsies. J.A.M.A. 99:559-560, 1932.
3. NOYES, R. W., HERTIG, A. T., AND ROCK, J.: Dating the endometrial biopsy. Steril. Fertil 1:3-25, 1950.
4. PHELPS, D.: Menstruation (pp. 55-87). In Essentials of Human Reproduction; clinical aspects. New York, Oxford University Press, 1958.

chapter 16

Knowledge of the interrelationship existing between the pituitary and the testes is paramount to appropriately diagnose and manage aberrations of gonadal function in the male. However, in order to understand these interrelationships, it would be well to review the embryologic development and the anatomy of the testes and related secondary sex organs.

EMBRYOLOGY

Indifferent Stage. The testes and the ovaries have a common origin—the gonadal anlage located in the germinal ridge.

GERMINAL RIDGE. The germinal ridge is first recognizable at the fifth week of gestation as a minute projection on the ventral medial border of the mesonephros (Fig. 309). The early stages of differentiation beginning in the germinal ridge are the same for both male and female gonads. The germinal ridge may be formed by either the covering mesothelium or by germ cells migrating from the yolk-sac. There are those who believe that the germ cells are derived in their entirety from the migrating yolk-sac cells and others who feel that the germinal epithelium may proliferate as needed to replenish dying or dead germ cells and thereby maintain the necessary biologic factors required for procreation. Be that as it may, the male gonadal anlage becomes recognizable as such by the seventh to eighth week of gestation.

Male Endocrinology: Hypogonadism in Adolescent Male and Cryptorchism

Medullary Cords. Unlike the ovarian anlage, the medullary components of the germinal ridge become accentuated to form the cord-like elements seen in the embryonic testes. These cord-like structures migrate toward the mesorchium and will eventually give rise to the seminiferous tubules.

Tunica Albuginea. The tunica albuginea, which is derived from fibrous, connective-tissue-like cells, is recognized early in the embryologic development of the testes. It unites with the underlying septula which have radiated from the mediastinum testis. The tunica separates the primary sex cords from the overlying layer of germinal epithelium. The connective tissue septula lie between the cord-like elements of the testis. They join with the tunica to divide the testis into functional components.

Rete Testis and Collecting Ducts. These cord-like structures, representing the beginning development of seminiferous tubules, are initially solid columns of cells. They develop central lumina at about the seventh month of gestation similar to the tubules of the postnatal testes and join in the region of the mesorchium to form the rete testis. The rete testis connects with the cephalid mesonephric tubules known as the ductuli efferentes. Thus, while the mesonephros degenerates, its duct system and principal collecting duct, the Wolffian duct, remain to form the spermatogenic duct collecting system necessary to transfer the sperm from the

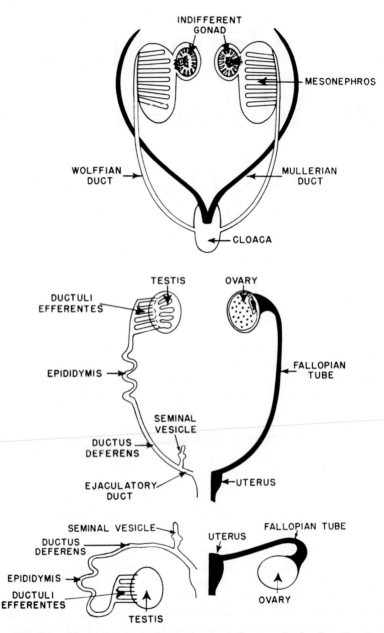

FIG. 309. *The embryologic development of the gonads showing the similarity in origin of the ovaries and the testes. The duct systems involved in both the male and the female are delineated.*

seminiferous tubules to the urethra. In order to accomplish this, the ductuli efferentes then join with the proximal end of the Wolffian duct (mesonephric duct). This portion of the Wolffian duct is termed the epididymis. The remaining portion of the mesonephric duct gives rise to the ductus deferens with the distal portion terminating in the urethra.

Male Gonad and Male Accessories.   At about the fourth month of gestation, the seminal vesicles form as outpouchings of the vas deferens just before it joins the urethra. The segment of the vas between the seminal vesicle and the urethra becomes known as the ejaculatory duct. The prostate and Cowper's glands differentiate from the urethra before the formation of the seminal vesicles at about the third month. The male gonadal anlage, when recognized as such, consists of the cords of cells, which are the source of the gamete in adulthood, and the interstitial cells or the endocrine secreting elements.

Leydig or Interstitial Cells.   Interstitial cells can be recognized by the tenth week of gestation and are present in large numbers as early as the twelfth to fourteenth week of gestation. These cells increase in number until about the seventh month of gestation, following which their numbers actually decrease. The diminution in interstitial cells continues after birth so that there are relatively small numbers of these cells present until puberty occurs. The increase in size and number of the interstitial cells may correlate well with the secretion of chorionic gonadotropin by the placenta itself. Since there is a marked decrease in chronic gonadotropin level at the third trimester, the decrease in size and number of Leydig cells at this time points toward the importance of chorionic gonadotropin in the early proliferation of the Leydig cells during the embryonic development of the testis. The regression of both the size and the number of the interstitial cells is also associated with the regression of the fetal zone layer of the adrenal cortex. The decrease in fetal zone layer appears to correlate with the decrease in size of the adrenal cortex. The question also arises as to whether or not the interstitial cells, which appear to increase in size and number at the peak of chorionic gonadotropin, might well play a role in the marked hypertrophy of the fetal adrenal, as has been suggested by Lanman in his studies of the immature male rat.[32, 33]

Tissue Organizers.   The development of the male duct system appears to be related to some intrinsic component in the testicular anlage itself. Evidence presented by Jost has indicated that such a factor actually exists in the testes of the fetal rabbit, for when the gonadal anlage of the male is removed prior to the eighteenth to nineteenth day of pregnancy, feminization of the reproductive system occurs.[21, 22] This feminization is believed to be due to a tendency by the maternal organism to feminize its offspring and will occur when the testicular influence is removed despite the negative chromatin nature of the fetus.

Position of Embryonic Testes. The embryonic testes are located initially high in the abdominal cavity in a position comparable to that of the adrenals and the kidneys. As the embryo develops, the testes tend to migrate toward a more caudal position. The entire development and migration of the testes take place retroperitoneally.

DESCENT OF THE TESTES. *Anatomic Factors.* The testes in their migration seem to follow the pathway of the folding of the coelomic epithelium (known as the processus vaginalis) which extends down into the scrotum. The factors responsible for the descent of the testes are not known; however, the descent does not appear to be directly related to the gubernaculum testes.[3, 57, 60] Shortening of the gubernaculum probably plays little or no role in the testicular descent but merely serves as a guide for the path of the caudad migration of the testis from its original abdominal position to the scrotum. Experimentally, it has been noted that, when the gubernaculum is removed early in the development of the fetus, descent of the testes will still proceed in an orderly manner in most of the animals so treated.

Endocrine Factors—Prenatal. No doubt endocrine factors are also involved in promoting the descent of the testes.[3, 8] The hyperplasia of the interstitial cells of the fetal testes may be an indication of endogenous androgen production. If so, these fetal androgens may play a role in the migration of the testes to the scrotum. However, it must be admitted that all of this is conjecture since the precise factor responsible for the lodging of the testes in the scrotum is still one of the mysteries of medicine.

Endocrine Factors—Postnatal. The role of hormones in the descent of the testes in the postnatal period in the human being will be discussed further in the therapy of cryptorchism. However, it should be stated that the removal of the pituitary in immature animals will prevent the descent of the testes when they are not normally located in the scrotum in the neonatal period of life. These findings emphasize the role of hormonal factors in the postnatal period which are necessary for maintaining the scrotal position of the testes. Similarly, in the human being, not infrequently spontaneous cure of cryptorchism may occur at the time of puberty due to the increase in androgenic secretion during this period of life.

ANATOMY OF THE TESTES

Testes and Scrotum. The adult testes lie in the scrotum, with the left testis tending to be positioned therein somewhat lower than the right. The distance of the testes from the body is dependent on the redundancy of the scrotum. The redundancy of the scrotum appears to be related to the temperature of the scrotum and is influenced by both the environmental and endogenous body temperatures. Neurogenic stimuli (fright, cremasteric reflexes) and the androgenicity of the individual will also influence the dependent nature of the scrotum. The size or the weight of the testes plays no role in determining the degree of redundancy of the scrotum.

GROWTH OF THE TESTES.   At the time of birth, the testes are very small but firm. They show no significant growth until the child is five or six years of age. At that time, a minimal increase in growth of the gonads occurs until the individual is approximately eight to 10 years of age. Then, with the onset of puberty, there is a relatively rapid growth of the testes until they reach adult size by the time the boy is 17 or 18 years of age.

Connective Tissue.   The testes are covered by a layer of connective tissue, the tunica vaginalis propria, beneath which there is a dense, white, fibrous capsule known as the tunica albuginea. The tunica vaginalis propria represents the fold of coelomic tissue or peritoneum which is invaginated extraperitoneally during the process of descent of the testes. As noted in the embryologic development of the testes, septula arise from the tunica albuginea and radiate toward the mesorchium. The connective tissue lobules converge toward the posterior surface of the testes to form the mediastinum testis which is present near the upper pole. Blood vessels and nerves enter and leave the testis through the mediastinum. The mediastinum also contains the rete testis which communicates proximally with the seminiferous tubules and distally with the ductules of the epididymis. Connective tissue in the form of septa radiate peripherally from the mediastinum, to subdivide the testicular substance into numerous pyramidal lobules. There are approximately 200 to 300 of these lobules in the testes, each containing several long, curled, markedly convoluted structures—the seminiferous tubules.

Seminiferous Tubules.   The tubules may be about 30 to 70 cm. long and approximately 150.0 to 250.0 microns in diameter. Canalization of these seminiferous tubules, as previously noted, occurs approximately in the seventh month of gestation, much later than the canalization of the lower collecting system.

TUBULI RECTI AND ANASTOMOSING DUCTS.   At the apex of each pyramidal lobule the tubules become less tortuous and abruptly lose their convolutions to form the tubuli recti. These structures represent the first portion of the excretory duct system necessary to convey the sperm from their origin, the germinal epithelium, to the ejaculatory duct. The tubuli recti anastomose to form the rete testis. These then divide into 12 to 15 ductuli efferentes, which open into the ductus epididymis. The epididymis empties into the vas deferens, which connects to the urethra.

Blood Supply.   ARTERIAL VESSELS.   The blood vessels responsible for the major source of supply to the testes are derived principally from the internal spermatic artery, which is a direct branch of the dorsal aorta. To a lesser extent, blood is also supplied to the testes by the cremasteric arteries as well as by the deferential arteries, both branches of the inferior vesicular and the deep epigastric arteries. Occasionally, the superior vesicular arteries also supply blood to the testes. As a rule, there are anastomoses between the various arteries listed above. However, regardless of the interconnecting network of arterioles and arteries, the internal spermatic artery is still the prime artery supplying the testes. If this artery were severed, the network of anastomoses made up of the other arteries would usually be insufficient to maintain the integrity of the testicular tissue for normal spermatogenesis.

VENOUS AND LYMPH DRAINAGE. The distribution of the venous drainage parallels that of the arterial network. The spermatic vein leaves the gonads via the mediastinum, to form an extensive plexus known as the pampiniform plexus. This plexus forms a single trunk near the internal inguinal ring to give rise to the spermatic vein. The left spermatic vein drains into the renal vein, the right into the vena cava. The left spermatic vein obviously is considerably longer than the right and consequently is more prone to develop varicosities or varicoceles so that these vascular abnormalities are noted more frequently in the region of the left gonad.

Lymphatic drainage of the testes is believed to take place via the pre-aortic lumbar lymph nodes. These nodes drain that area of the body which was responsible for the embryologic origin of the testes—i. e., the region of formation of the testicular anlage prior to their descent.

Nerve Supply. The nerve supply to the testes is derived from three sources:

1. The external spermatic branch of the genitofemoral nerve which supplies the anterior and lateral portion of the testes.

2. Perineal branches of the pudendal nerves innervating the posterior portion of the testes.

3. Posterior femoral cutaneous nerves supplying the inferior portion of the testes.

SYMPATHETIC SUPPLY. The renal, the aortic, and the hypogastric plexuses are the source of sympathetic fibers to the testes. It should be stated that very little is known as to the precise terminal innervation of the testes. However, connections between the neurons and the epithelial cells of the testes have been described as being comparable to the picture seen for the cells of the adrenal medulla with the neuron fibrils terminating directly in the cells themselves.

HISTOLOGY OF THE TESTES

Since the morphologic appearance of the testes varies with their developmental stage, it becomes necessary to describe the histologic variations noted in the different stages of development and maturation.

Seminiferous Tubules.   The seminiferous tubules, the basic morphologic components of the testes, are covered by a basement membrane, which, in turn, is capped by the tunica propria. The tunica propria consists of dense, fibrous connective tissue which offers a protective outer covering for the seminiferous tubule. The tubules during embryonic life and the early postnatal period contain primarily two types of cells—undifferentiated cells and spermatogonia.

SERTOLI CELLS.   The undifferentiated cells are excessive in number and appear to give rise to the Sertoli cells, which are present in lesser numbers in the adult tubule. In the adult, the Sertoli cells are tall and extend from the basement membrane (tunica propria) toward the lumen of the tube. The borders of the cells are adjacent to germ cells in all stages of development and are irregular, with the cell taking the shape of an imperfect pyramid. The nucleus of the cell is relatively hypochromic and vesicular, and may lie at the base or middle portion of the cell. Division of these cells is rarely noted.

SPERMATOGONIA.   The spermatogonia, of course, represent the parent cells of the sperm itself. These cells are spherical or cuboidal in shape, with a hyperchromic nucleus. The spermatogonia continually show evidence of active division. The cytoplasm contains a fair amount of lipid material.

LEYDIG OR INTERSTITIAL CELLS.   The Leydig or interstitial cells lie in the area between the tubules and are usually adjacent to the tunica propria or may be positioned in the mesenchymal-like matrix. The Leydig cells appear early in the embryologic development of the testes. During fetal development they do not contain a significant amount of lipid material, nor are they vacuolated to indicate active hormonal production. Increasing lipid deposition and evidence of steroid production occur shortly before the end of the first decade of life.

In vitro techniques as well as vital staining methods have suggested that the Leydig cells in their endocrine active state, despite their fibro-blastic-like appearance, contain lipids, steroids, alkaline phosphatase, lipase, and ascorbic acid. The fibroblastic nature of the Leydig cells has led some authorities to believe that these cells may revert to connective tissue cells. The connective tissue cells arising from the Leydig cells take up a pyrrole blue or trypan blue stain, whereas the Leydig cells themselves remain unstained. The Leydig cells have sparse cytoplasm and contain relatively large vesicular, spherical nuclei.

Spermatogenesis.   Although canalization of the tubules is usually noted at about the seventh month of gestation, this process may not become very definite until after the first or second year of postnatal life. With the onset of puberty, spermatogenesis begins.

Spermatogenesis takes place in several stages of development: the first is one of proliferation, where the spermatogonia divide by the usual method of mitotic division, so that in their division each cell has the full quota of 46 chromosomes; after an adequate degree of proliferation has occurred, the spermatogonia grow and mature into primary spermatocytes. The primary spermatocyte is about 17.0 to 20.0 microns in diameter and is by far the largest cell seen in the tubule. As is to be expected, it contains the full number of chromosomes—that is, 46.

The nuclei of the spermatocyte are vesicular, with the chromatin material showing a variable picture depending on the state of division. With the formation of the primary spermatocyte, further division by the method of meiosis occurs very promptly.

Meiosis is a method of cell division by which the daughter cells contain only one half the number of chromosomes of the parent cell. There are two meiotic divisions—the first one is reductional and is concerned with the transition from the primary to the secondary spermatocyte. The chromosome divides longitudinally to form two chromatids. Prior to cell division, these may cross one or several times to provide an interchange of chromatin material. The second meiotic division is noted when the secondary spermatocyte changes into the spermatid. This method of division corresponds to mitosis in that each chromatid splits longitudinally to form a chromosome, with each half being identical in all respects.

Thus, the secondary spermatocytes contain only 23 chromosomes. The cell is consequently smaller than the primary spermatocytes and is about 15.0 microns in diameter. However, in the formation of the spermatids, 23 chromosomes are also present, indicating that the division of the secondary spermatocytes is actually a form of mitosis. This must be so since a spermatid contains the same number of chromosomes as its parent cell, the secondary spermatocyte.

The spermatids are smaller in size than the secondary spermatocytes and measure about 9.0 to 10.0 microns in diameter. The spermatozoa are derived from the spermatids by the process of maturation or growth of the spermatids. Normally, the spermatids or spermatozoa contain 22 somatic chromosomes, and either an X or a Y sex chromosome to make up the total number of 23 chromosomes.

The sperm cell itself, a potentially motile cell, is first stored in the seminiferous tubule, and then migrates down the tubules to the epididymis or vas deferens. The seminiferous tubules are believed to be the principal source of nutrient for the sperm cells after they have developed from the spermatids. The Sertoli cells may be the major site of nourishment for the spermatozoa.

Chemical Constituents of Cells.   Generally speaking, it may be said that vital staining procedures fail to demonstrate the presence of steroid substances in the Sertoli cells. However, they do contain lipid material other than steroidal substances, as well as glycogen and alkaline phosphatase. Lipid-like material as well as glycogen has also been demonstrated in spermatogonia and primary spermatocytes but not in the secondary spermatocytes, spermatids, or spermatozoa. Alkaline phosphatase activity is present in all of the cells of the spermatic series. Steroid-like substances have been found in the germinal epithelium by some workers, while their presence has been denied by others.[1, 54, 55] Steroidal-like substances have invariably been identified in the Leydig cells as well as evidence of phosphatase and glycogen activity.

PHYSIOLOGY

Pituitary-Testicular Interrelationship. TROPIC HORMONES. The endocrine function of the testes, as is true of the other pituitary-dependent glands previously studied, is maintained by pituitary tropic hormones. The pituitary gland also maintains and promotes gametogenic activity. In the male there are only two specific active gonadotropic principles: one is the gametogenic hormone, which is similar to the follicle-stimulating hormone (FSH) in the female; the second is the interstitial cell-stimulating hormone (ICSH), which has been allied to the luteinizing hormone (LH) in the female (Fig. 310).

Gametogenic Hormone (FSH). The gametogenic hormone is responsible for stimulating the growth and maturation of the cells of the germinal epithelium of the seminiferous tubules. The gametogenic hormone apparently has the single and specific function in the male of maturing the gamete. It does not appear to have any male hormone or androgenic stimulating activity.

Interstitial Cell-Stimulating Hormone (ICSH). In contrast, the ICSH principle is necessary for stimulating the interstitial cells. Inasmuch as these cells secrete androgens, testosterone production by the testes is maintained by ICSH stimulation. It has been suggested by some investigators that pure FSH would be ineffective in producing adequate spermatogenesis inasmuch as some ICSH is necessary in order to bring about an adequate degree of sperm maturation. It may well be that the testosterone secretion under the influence of ICSH[18, 51, 56] is the substance necessary for FSH to appropriately stimulate spermatogenesis.[18, 36, 51, 56, 59]

Estrogenic Secretion. The interstitial cells, in addition to their elaboration of testosterone, may secrete estrogen. The data to support the findings that estrogen is produced by the interstitial cells have been based on certain experimental work. It has been shown in the human that stimulation of the interstitial cells of the testes by chorionic gonadotropin prepared from human pregnancy urine has been associated with increased estrogen excretion in the urine of these patients.[37, 38] Whether this is due to a direct elaboration of estrogenic substances per se or may be ascribed, secondarily, to a breakdown of testosterone into estrogen[43] is not known at the present time (see Fig. 2, p. 6).

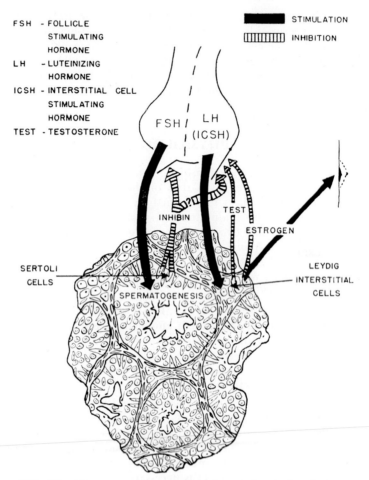

FIG. 310. *Diagrammatic presentation of normal testicular-pituitary interrelationship.*

Metabolism of Testosterone. In addition to a possible conversion of testosterone into estrogen, testosterone is also metabolized into androsterone and etiocholanolone, which apparently have little if any androgenic effects in their own right.[5, 12] Indeed, it has been reported that, unlike testosterone, androsterone may actually lower blood cholesterol in humans with hypercholesterolemia as well as in patients with normal blood cholesterol levels.[19] High doses of etiocholanolone, on the other hand, while not exhibiting any known metabolic activity, have been shown to induce hyperpyrexia in the human being.[4, 23, 24]

17-Ketosteroid Excretion. The androgens produced by the testes are excreted in the urine as neutral 17-ketosteroids. One should note that the major portion of the urinary 17-ketosteroid substances excreted in the male is derived from the adrenal cortex.[5, 53] Hence, of the total amount excreted in the urine in the male, about two thirds come from adrenal androgens and one third is from testosterone of testicular origin.

CHEMICAL DERIVATION AND SIGNIFICANCE OF 17-KETOSTEROID EXCRETION. A word about 17-ketosteroids and the derivation of the term would be appropriate at this time. Testosterone itself is not a 17-ketosteroid, inasmuch as there is a hydroxy-group at the 17 carbon atom. However, when testosterone is metabolized by the liver, it is broken down into a neutral 17-ketosteroid and is excreted as such in the urine. It should be noted that all 17-ketosteroid precursors are not androgenic in effect. Estrogens are also 17-ketosteroid substances and are excreted as such. The excretory products of estrogenic origin, however, do not contribute to the chemical assay for 17-ketosteroids inasmuch as the parent compound is a phenolic substance and as such is removed in the chemical procedure for 17-ketosteroid determination by the addition of alkaline substances such as potassium or sodium hydroxide. The phenolic derivatives are removed after the urine has been extracted with the organic solvent necessary to extract the various steroids or lipid-soluble substances from the hydrolized urine. The steroid metabolites which are present after alkaline extraction are referred to as total neutral 17-ketosteroids and, as noted above, are derived from androgenic precursors produced by either the adrenal or the testes. While some of the androgenic progenitors arising from the ovary are not excreted as 17-ketosteroids, occasionally elevated 17-ketosteroid levels may occur in abnormal states as Leydig or adrenal rest cell tumors and in arrhenoblastomas.

ROLE OF THE LIVER IN 17-KETOSTEROID EXCRETION. In considering the excretion of 17-ketosteroids in the urine, it is important to emphasize the role of the liver in the metabolic breakdown of testosterone or testicular and adrenal androgens into 17-ketosteroids. The liver is vital in the conversion of both endogenously secreted and exogenously administered testosterone into 17-ketosteroid substances.[5, 45, 46]

17-Ketosteroid Excretion After Oral or Parenteral Testosterone. In addition, it should be emphasized that, as far as exogenously administered steroids are concerned, the route of administration plays little part in their metabolic breakdown into 17-ketosteroids. If one were to give the patient 50.0 mg. of testosterone orally or intramuscularly, the total amount of 17-ketosteroid excretion in the urine would probably be higher after the oral dose than after the parenteral one, despite the fact that, biologically, the parenteral route is considerably more effective (Fig. 311).[46]

Conjugation of Steroids in the Liver. The liver is essential in the conjugation and inactivation of androgens. Rapid inactivation and thereby decreased physiologic activity are more prone to occur after ingestion because of rapid uptake by the liver of the orally administered material. Nevertheless, despite its rapid inactivation, conjugation also

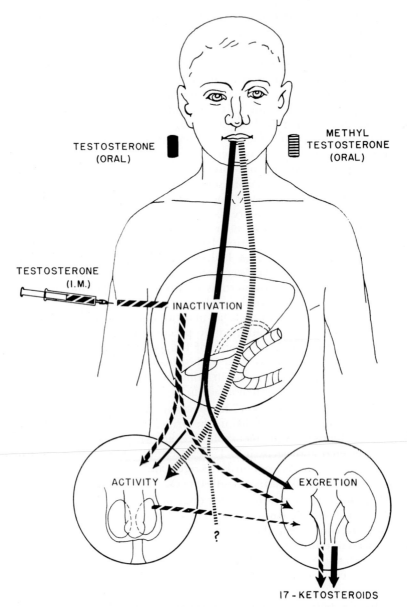

FIG. 311. *The effect of different androgens on 17-ketosteroid excretion. Note that oral administration of testosterone results in an elevated 17-keto-steroid but poor physiologic activity. Parenterally, testosterone is also partially inactivated by the liver but has definite physiologic effects. The metabolic excretory product of methyltestosterone is unknown, designated as "?" in the illustration. However, it does influence total endogenous 17-ketosteroid excretion by diminishing endogenous androgen production.*

occurs in the liver so that relatively elevated excretion of 17-ketosteroids takes place after oral therapy.[5, 29] Conjugation in the liver so alters the steroid molecule that a soluble complex is formed, thereby permitting higher levels of soluble circulating androgens with their prompt excretion into the urine. As a rule, in the process of conjugation, a sulfate radical is added to the steroid molecule. This permits a chemical union with protein, to form a steroid-protein complex.

Effect of Methyltestosterone on 17-Ketosteroid Excretion. The role of the liver in steroid metabolism is emphasized further when one gives methyltestosterone, a synthetic androgen, which is as effective after oral administration as it is after parenteral injection. However, methylation prevents rapid destruction of the steroid by the liver, and also prevents the liver from converting the steroid into a 17-ketosteroid metabolite. Consequently, despite its androgenicity, methyltestosterone is not excreted as a 17-ketosteroid.[11, 47] As a matter of fact, if a high enough dose of this steroid is administered, a depression of total neutral 17-ketosteroids may occur in the male. The decreased 17-ketosteroid excretion is attributed to the fact that the exogenous steroid inhibits endogenous gonadotropic secretion which, in turn, is associated with diminution in the endogenous androgenic secretion by the interstitial cells of the testis itself. Consequently, suppression of the secretion of the testicular precursors of the endogenous 17-ketosteroids occurs with the resultant diminution of total 17-ketosteroid excretion.[47] Ethinyl testosterone, as well as the ethyl and ethinyl derivatives of 19-nortestosterone, also act like methyltestosterone in that they are effective oral androgens, but are not excreted as 17-ketosteroids, and will, in fact, suppress 17-ketosteroid excretion by the same mechanism as described for methyltestosterone.

17-Ketosteroid Excretion in Gout and Hepatic Disease. Peculiarly enough, there are other conditions associated with diminished 17-ketosteroid excretion despite the absence of any evidence of diminution of androgenic or adrenal cortical function. These aberrations are noted in patients with gout as well as those with hepatic disease. The patient with gout, for some unknown reason, does not excrete normal levels of 17-ketosteroid despite the fact that males so affected show no stigmata of testicular or adrenal insufficiency.[84] Their low levels of 17-ketosteroid excretion may approximate those of patients with panhypopituitary insufficiency. Hepatic disease is also accompanied by diminished 17-ketosteroid excretion, probably because of an inability of the liver to metabolize and conjugate the androgen into 17-ketosteroid derivatives.[35, 66]

BILIARY EXCRETION OF 17-KETOSTEROIDS. In addition to its role in the metabolism of testosterone, it should be noted that the liver excretes a considerable portion of the androgens as well as the other gonadal steroids into the bile and thence into the intestinal tract. Some of the steroidal material excreted via the bile into the intestinal tract is partially reabsorbed from the gut, carried by the circulatory system to the kidney, and re-excreted via the urine as a 17-ketosteroid.[45, 46] Thus, the entero-hepatic system in dogs, with respect to ingested and to a lesser extent parenterally administered material, plays an important role in the level of 17-ketosteroids excreted into the urine. Consequently, the presence of a biliary fistula may mitigate against an increase in urine 17-ketosteroid excretion usually anticipated after administration of a standard dose of testosterone. The reason is that much of the steroid material which is conjugated by the liver and secreted into the bile tract, because of the fistulae, is excreted, and hence not made available to the intestinal tract for reabsorption and excretion by the urinary tract.[45, 46] However, studies done in the human being have failed to confirm these findings.[48] It may well be that the dichotomy in these studies lies in the fact that the biliary fistula studies in the human were done in patients with diseased livers in contrast to the healthy animals used by Paschkis and associates.

IN VIVO SYNTHESIS OF TESTOSTERONE. Testosterone is synthesized in both the testis and the adrenal. As a result of studies with radioactive-carbon labeled acetate and cholesterol, it was shown that testosterone of adrenal or testicular origin may arise from either acetate or cholesterol. Either precursor can be converted into testosterone by incubation with testicular or adrenal tissue *in vitro*.[5, 10] Since acetate itself can be converted via cholesterol into testosterone by either the testis or the adrenal, it is apparent that cholesterol is not a necessary intermediary product for the biosynthesis of androgens.[5] Androgens may be produced by either organ directly from dietary cholesterol, or from cholesterol derived endogenously from acetate.

Testosterone and Estrogenic Excretion. The close relationship existing between testosterone and estrogen is evident by the fact that, when testosterone itself is administered, an increased amount of estrogenic substances may be obtained in the urine of animals or patients so treated.[5, 43, 66] Therapeutically, this is important, as will be pointed out later, since certain feminizing characteristics noted in the male (gynecomastia) cannot be treated effectively by administering androgens. While it might appear logical to administer androgens to offset clinical manifestations of femininity in the male, the addition of this hormone does not alter the effect of endogenous estrogen production. As a matter of fact, androgens (methyltestosterone in particular) may be more prone to cause gynecomastia than they are to counteract its development.

The gynecomastia seen in males at puberty has been taken as clinical evidence of estrogenic secretion by the testes at this time. While it has been suggested that estrogen may be secreted by the Leydig cells of the testes, it may well be that the increased estrogen levels noted after testicular stimulation with human chorionic gonadotropin merely represents the formation of estrogenic material from the metabolic breakdown of the increased endogenous secretion of testosterone. This is not peculiar to the human since it has been known for some time that the stallion, the epitome of maleness in the animal kingdom, puts out more estrogen per liter of urine than any other animal.[34, 65] That the source of estrogen appears to lie in the testes is evidenced by the fact that castration of the stallion, to produce a gelding, causes the high estrogen levels in the urine to fall to barely detectable activity.

Inhibin. In addition to the steroids noted above, a third hormone has been said to be elaborated by the testes. This hormone, originally referred to as inhibin by the McCullaghs, is an aqueous-soluble substance with strong pituitary gonadotropic inhibitory properties.[39-41] Inhibin lacks steroidal hormone activity of its own. It is believed to be secreted by the Sertoli cells and is elaborated in adequate amounts to regulate pituitary gonadotropic secretion through its inhibitory properties.[25, 39-41, 58] The concept of inhibin has been denied by some workers. Testosterone, on the other hand, is a relatively poor pituitary gonadotropin inhibitor unless fairly large amounts of the steroid are administered. One must postulate the presence of a more potent pituitary gonadotropin inhibitor; hence, the concept of inhibin is an attractive one from the clinical point of view.[49] The gonadotropic inhibiting effects of testosterone are far inferior to those of estrogens; this has been demonstrated by the parabiotic technique. On a weight basis, approximately 50 to 75 times as much testosterone, as compared to estrogen, is required to achieve equivalent gonadotropic inhibitory effects.[20, 42]

Androgens and Spermatogenesis. The role of androgens in spermatogenesis is an interesting one. It appears that, while there are two distinct functions of the testes (i. e., gametogenic and hormonal), gametogenic activity cannot exist without androgenic production. On the other hand, testosterone secretion from the Leydig cells can take place in the absence of spermatogenesis or in the absence of tubular development or function. While FSH is the prime hormone necessary for the stimulation of the seminiferous tubules, its effect is dependent, in part, on the presence of an androgen[20] or ICSH.[1, 18, 51, 54, 55]

STUDIES IN HYPOPHYSECTOMIZED RATS. While spermatogenesis primarily is dependent on FSH, in hypophysectomized animals there is a concomitant need for ICSH (LH) to permit the gametogenic effect of FSH to be expressed. ICSH acts on the interstitial cells to secrete the necessary androgens. The synergism existing between FSH and testosterone is demonstrated by the fact that enhanced spermatogenesis occurs only when both are administered to the hypophysectomized rat. This effect of androgens on spermatogenesis appears to be paradoxical since ordinarily one would expect testosterone or related steroids to have an inhibitory or suppressive effect on sperm production.

  Direct Effect of Androgens on Testicular Tissue. The role of androgens in spermatogenesis is indicated further by the experimental data of

Nelson, Smith, and Dvoskin, who showed individually that, if one administers testosterone to the hypophysectomized animal (either rat or monkey) immediately after surgery, then spermatogenesis will be maintained.[6, 7, 44, 52] It was also noted that, if a pellet of testosterone was placed in one testis and not in the other testis at the time of hypophysectomy, the testis containing the pellet would show maintenance of spermatogenesis in contrast to the azoospermia and tubular atrophy in the contralateral organ.[7, 52]

Mechanism of Action.   The mechanism of action of testosterone in maintaining spermatogenesis in the hypophysectomized animal or in enhancing the spermatogenic response of the rat to FSH is not understood. Nevertheless, this principle has been used with some success clinically as a means of promoting a better spermatogenic response to exogenously administered gonadotropic substances, as well as by increasing sperm production and motility when testosterone is administered alone.

Biologic Activity of the Undescended Testes.   In the discussion of the embryologic development of the testes, it was noted that the testes originate as abdominal organs so that their position early in embryonic life is cephalad as compared to their final adult dependent location.

SPERMATOGENIC FUNCTION.   The scrotal position of the testes is an important factor in sperm production inasmuch as failure of spermatogenesis is noted when a testis stays in the abdomen.[3, 10] The reason for this is that the temperature of the abdomen is sufficiently high to prevent normal spermatogenic development. Normal spermatogenesis can take place only when the testis is brought down into the scrotum from its original abdominal position.

HORMONAL SECRETION.   It is interesting to note that, despite the failure of spermatogenesis to take place in the abdominally located testis, androgenic function and secretion will still persist due to continued function of the Leydig cells. Stimulation of the interstitial cells by LH apparently goes on unimpeded despite the fact that the tubular elements undergo atrophy.

ANAPLASTIC CHANGES.   The abdominal position of a testis, however, will eventually be harmful to all testicular function, not only because of the failure of the abdominal testis to develop sperm but also because the longer the testis stays in the abdomen the greater the possibility that certain neoplastic changes may take place.[3] It has been shown statistically that the incidence of neoplasia in the abdominal testis is significantly higher than that in the scrotal gonad. Hence, it is necessary to consider any testis which has shown a failure of descent to have a greater malignant potential than a scrotal testis. Hormone therapy or orchiopexy should be attempted in order to bring the abdominal testis down to its normal scrotal position. It should be noted that, once the abdominal testis is fixed in the scrotum, the high incidence of malignancy still persists. The testis can be more directly examined in the scrotum, however, and abnormal growth can be detected with greater ease.

FIBROTIC DEGENERATION. In addition to the propensity for neoplasia, the longer the testis stays in the abdomen, the greater is the possibility that irreparable damage to the tubular structures will then occur. When the testis is finally fixed in the scrotum, only poor, inefficient, or incomplete spermatogenesis may be noted. If the testis remains in the abdomen after the age of 30 or 35, not only is spermatogenesis permanently absent but also hormonal secretion will be significantly diminished. This is due to the fact that total degeneration of the testis may occur as a result of complete testicular fibrosis, and this can be so extensive that premature failure of androgenic function takes place when both gonads are involved. Androgenic production by the testes is likely to persist normally if the abdominally positioned testis is relocated in the scrotum before puberty.

Biologic Properties of Androgens. GENITAL EFFECTS. The biologic effects of androgenic steroids are complex and extensive. The anticipated effects of androgens on the secondary sexual characteristics of the male are well known when appropriate doses of the androgens are administered. Androgens will cause an increase in size of the underdeveloped phallus of the hypogonadal male. They will accentuate the redundancy of the scrotum and cause an increase in both size and secretion of the prostate and the seminal vesicles and any other structures associated with the reproductive tract in the male.

EXTRAGENITAL EFFECTS. There are other phenomena attributed to androgens which may be noted during the administration of physiologically effective doses or when sexual maturation occurs.[5]

Muscle Development. Androgens will cause an increase in muscle mass, resulting in a broadening of the shoulder girdle. There is usually an associated loss of fat in the pelvic girdle area, causing a decrease in the hip measurements.

Hair Growth and Distribution. Facial and body hair growth are initiated or intensified under the influence of male hormone. The increase in growth of hair on the body is fairly characteristic and is manifested by an increase in growth of axillary and pubic hair with an extension of the latter toward the umbilicus.[53, 65] The pattern of hair growth on the body in response to androgenic activity is also specific and is manifested by increased hair growth on the chest, peri-areolar areas, arms, legs, back, and intercrural regions, as well as in the presacral region. Sacral hair growth may become very marked. The quantitative aspects of hair growth under the influence of androgens are also dependent on the racial heritage of the patient. The Nordic individual may show less response as far as body hair growth is concerned; on the other hand, the southern European will show an inordinate amount of hair growth following even relatively small doses of androgens. There are certain other racial differences—the Negro and the Oriental show a diminished hair growth response to androgens as compared to the Caucasian. If androgen therapy is continued, some decrease in cephalic hair growth will usually be noted. This will be discussed in Chapter 23, Hirsutism.

Skin and Androgens. There are other effects of androgens on the integument which frequently occur during adolescence at the time when androgens are first materially increased. Androgens will cause an increase in sebaceous secretion. This is responsible, in turn, for an accentuation or initiation of acneiform eruption.[17] It has been suggested that the excessive sebaceous secretion is prone to cause a greater degree of inspissation of sebum. Inspissated sebum promotes a foreign body reaction which produces an infiltration of polymorphonuclear neutrophils, associated with an inflammatory reaction, bringing about the typical acneiform dermatitis. This explains the increased incidence of acne in the adolescent boy who is exposed to increased endogenous androgen production at the time of puberty. Similarly in the female, androgen secretion may precipitate the advent of acneiform eruption. Many times, acne is accentuated prior to the onset of menses. It is at this time that the excretion of 17-ketosteroids is at its peak. This would point to elevated endogenous androgenic levels.[9, 17, 27]

Nitrogen Retention. There are other specific biologic effects which may be attributed to androgenic activity. For example, androgens in adequate amounts can induce nitrogen retention and bring about anabolic effects resulting in decreased creatine excretion. While anabolic activity is anticipated with all androgenic preparations, these steroids may differ in their ability to retain nitrogen. For example, methyltestosterone has a much less definitive effect on creatine retention than testosterone. As a matter of fact, methyltestosterone may actually cause increased creatine excretion. However, despite this, methyltestosterone is anabolic as far as both muscle mass and protein anabolism are concerned.[5]

Electrolyte and Water Metabolism. Androgens will influence electrolyte metabolism to a degree. Under certain conditions, testosterone in high doses will cause a mild to moderate degree of sodium retention. The effect of androgens on potassium excretion, on the other hand, may be inconsistent. The anabolic effect of androgens may cause potassium retention rather than loss. The potassium retention following testosterone therapy is due to the need for potassium by the tissue when protein is stored or being formed. Indeed, in patients with some measure of renal failure, testosterone may significantly lower elevated potassium levels by virtue of its effect on nitrogen retention and in preventing protein catabolism.

Renal Effects. Testosterone has also been shown to have a renotropic effect, so that it can cause an increase in size and function of the kidneys.[5, 26] As a matter of fact, in some of his early studies Selye showed that testosterone could definitely nullify the nephrotoxic effect of mercurials on the cyto-architecture of the renal tubules.[50] This sparing action of testosterone in reversing the toxic manifestation of mercurials on the kidney has been said to be due to the renotropic activity of androgens in general.

Gynecologic Properties. Testosterone has physiologic effects which make it valuable in the treatment of certain gynecologic disorders in the female. It will induce some measure of hemostasis as far as uterine hemorrhage is concerned.[16] Cessation of uterine bleeding after administration of testosterone may be attributed to the effect of the steroid on the myometrium in producing vasoconstriction merely by increasing muscle mass.[16, 31] It may also cause some alteration of endometrial activity—not directly, but rather indirectly—by diminishing ovarian activity via gonadotropic inhibitory effects when sufficiently large doses of androgens are used. Testosterone may also cause a decrease in size of the breasts, not by competing with the action of estrogen per se, but rather by pituitary tropic inhibition of either the gonadotropic complex or mammotropic principles, or both. In adequate doses, testosterone will increase the size of the clitoris and will usually cause enhancement of libido in female patients.[28] Androgens may decrease the size, or slow down the growth rate, of bony metastases from carcinoma of the breast in the female. All of these phenomena are reviewed in other chapters concerned with gynecologic endocrinology.

Growth Stimulating Effects. Androgens will induce some acceleration of growth in children,[62, 63] but, when given in *excessive dosage,* may cause premature epiphyseal closure, so that while an increase in growth may be achieved initially, eventually the final stature of the individual will be short.

Need for Accurate Diagnosis and Appropriate Therapy. The External Genitalia. The external position of the male genitalia provides the physician with a fairly accurate means of estimating the relative physiologic potential of the patient's genital function by inspection alone. These clinical criteria are most important in establishing the need for further evaluation and provide the basic standards that the physician may use in determining the physiologic capabilities of the genitalia. In contrast to the female, the easy accessibility of the genitalia of the male for clinical evaluation is of advantage in determining the presence of any gross anatomic defects. Consequently, the need for further investigation or therapy in the obviously hypogonadal male is readily apparent.

Psychologic Effects. However, the advantage that inspection of the genitalia has for the physician is of equal disadvantage to the patient with small genitalia that are grossly deviated from normal, for the patient's deficiencies are apparent to his fellow confreres whenever he steps into a gymnasium, a public pool, or a shower. The hypoplastic nature of his genitalia may be of such degree as to provoke certain psychological aberrations of overcompensation or feelings of inferiority.

Ridicule of the Hypogonadal Male. Such adverse psychological effects can be accentuated still further if there are added the derision and the ridicule so frequently offered by the normally endowed male. This is particularly true in the hypogonadal adolescent, where the cruelty of youth not only may force these youngsters to withdraw from physical activity requiring disrobing, but also may create abnormal psychological patterns. As a result, the hypogonadal boy will usually find all sorts of excuses for not attending gymnasium or other physical activities, inasmuch as he knows that he will have to expose himself to the critical vision of his peers and be subjected to their cruel ridicule. The adverse effects of such criticism are accentuated further by the fact that the self-induced limitation of adequate physical activity, usually required for adequate muscular development, may lead to obesity and a tendency toward an even more grotesque physical build; a delay in normal muscular maturation may follow. Poor muscular development is also apparent in the young boy where frank hypogonadism is associated with decreased androgenic secretion. The lack of myotropic effects of adequate amounts of testosterone in these youths causes the "baby body fat distribution" to persist for a much longer period of time than is normal.

THERAPEUTIC APPROACH. Obviously, appropriate gonadotropic or androgenic therapy would appear to be the treatment of choice in these youths. The question arises, however, as to when such therapy should be started and what goal is to be achieved. Similar queries may be raised concerning the appropriate management of the hypogonadal adult male. In both the adult and the adolescent there is also the question as to whether or not the prescribed therapy may be dangerous or could be associated with potential harm to either adolescent or adult testes. An attempt will be made to elaborate upon these aspects in the clinical management of male hypogonadism.

HYPOGONADISM IN THE ADOLESCENT MALE

Classification. Testosterone deficiency will give rise to the multiple manifestations of hypogonadism. Gonadal insufficiency in the male may be characterized as being either primary or secondary in nature.

Primary Versus Secondary Hypogonadism. Primary hypogonadism refers to primary testicular failure; secondary hypogonadism occurs where testicular failure is secondary to factors other than the testes, particularly to pituitary gonadotropic hyposecretion.

CLINICAL HISTORY. In obtaining the history, the following facts will usually be noted: (1) Potentia is absent, poor, or markedly reduced;

(2) the patient is unable to achieve an orgasm; there is little or no stimulus toward masturbation; and if an erection is achieved, it is poorly maintained; (3) the patient usually notes that he is incapable of the usual physical activities which are expected from a normal male; he lacks physical stamina and usually is not only unable but also disinclined to partake in contact or competitive sports requiring some measure of muscular coordination and development.

CLINICAL FEATURES.   Physically, and from the point of view of the history, primary or secondary hypogonadism may be indistinguishable and present clinical features which are similar. However, if the patient with secondary hypogonadism also has panhypopituitarism, the stigmata due to hypofunction of the pituitary-dependent endocrine glands also would be present. In such a case, one could definitely delineate this type of patient from one with primary testicular failure by the composite picture of the pluriglandular deficiency.

Hair.   All patients with hypogonadism show a tendency toward poor secondary sex hair growth (Figs. 312-315). However, in primary hypogonadism, axillary and pubic hair will be present, albeit in feminine distribution, in contrast to its absence in patients with secondary hypogonadism associated with panhypopituitarism. While stigmata of hair distribution will be obvious in the post-pubertal hypogonadal male, they are more difficult to recognize in the prepubertal male.

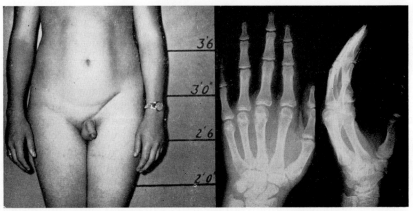

FIG. 312   FIG. 313

FIG. 312.   Patient JC, age 18 years, height 68¼ inches. Complete absence of secondary sex hair development. Genitalia are hypoplastic. 17-Ketosteroids 10.8 mg. per 24 hours; protein-bound iodine 4.7 gamma per cent; chromatin pattern negative.

FIG. 313.   X-ray picture of hand and wrist of patient in Fig. 312 revealed open epiphyses of the phalanges, the metacarpals, and the distal part of both ulna and radius. Significant retardation of bone age. Patient had excellent response to HCG therapy, which was anticipated in view of the open epiphyses.

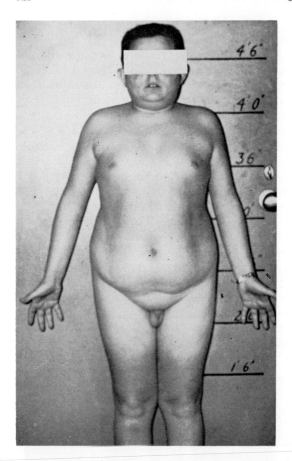

FIG. 314. Patient AC, age
19 years, height 57 inches.
Note complete absence of
secondary sex hair development, immature facies, and
marked hypogonadism. FSH
= 6 mouse units per 24
hours; 17-ketosteroids 9.9 mg.
per 24 hours; protein-bound
iodine 6.1 gamma per cent;
chromatin negative; epiphyses practically closed. Poor
response to therapy.

Testes and Phallus. In both types of hypogonadism, the primary
sex glands, the testes, as well as the phallus are usually poorly developed
(Figs. 316, 317). The hypoplasia may vary from moderate to marked.
The testes are usually small, and the scrotum is poorly redundant.
If the hypogonadal state has been present prior to puberty the testes are
firm to hard. Conversely, the testes in the patient where hypogonadism
is acquired, post-pubertally or during adulthood, will usually be larger
than in the prepubertal group but the testes will be soft and flabby instead
of firm. The penis will be small in both the flaccid and the erect states
(Fig. 315). The overall length of the penis in the untreated adult hypogonadal patient will be less than 6 to 7 cm. One should note that, when
hypogonadism does occur after adequate penile development has been
accomplished, in all probability only the testes, and not the penis or
the scrotum, will be sufficiently affected to reflect the hypogonadal state
(Fig. 318).

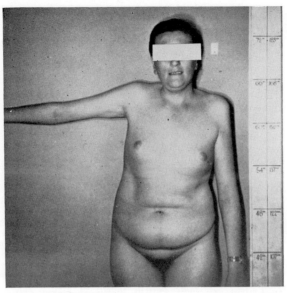

FIG. 315. Patient SR, age 32 years, height 72 inches. FSH greater than 211 mouse units per 24 hours; 17-ketosteroids 12.4 mg. per 24 hours. Epiphyses closed; chromatin pattern negative. Patient had bilateral cryptorchism with testes incapable of responding. Note female fat and hair distribution. Therapy withheld as teenager because of therapeutic nihilism and watchful waiting.

FIG. 316. Patient SK, age 33 years, height 79 inches. Low 17-ketosteroid, elevated FSH, chromatin negative. Note marked hypoplasia of genitalia, particularly of the phallus. The testes were small, firm and hard, but in the scrotum.

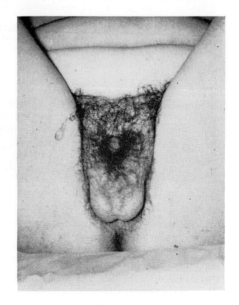

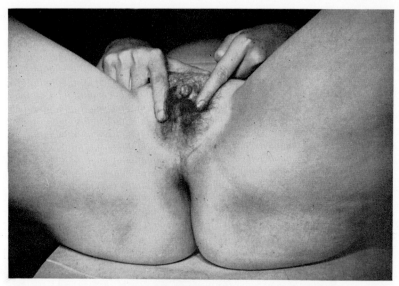

FIG. 317. Patient SR, same patient shown in Figure 315. Note small phallus, no testes. Patient had closed epiphyses. His phallus never increased in size despite massive doses of androgen.

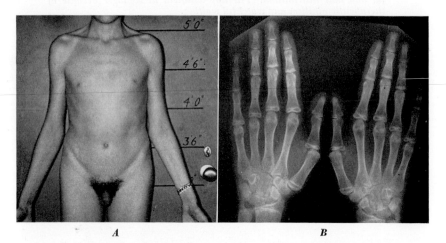

A   B

FIG. 318. Patient CB, age 27 years, height 70 inches. 17-Ketosteroids 8.2 mg. per 24 hours; FSH 6.6 mouse units per 24 hours; 17-hydroxysteroids 3.6 mg. per 24 hours; protein-bound iodine 3.1 gamma per cent. Patient with long-standing history of hypogonadism had received previous therapy with androgens. While there had been a regression of body hair after therapy was discontinued, the phallus has maintained its size. Further therapy with androgens produced excellent results, as was anticipated since the patient had open epiphyses. Note Figure 318B.

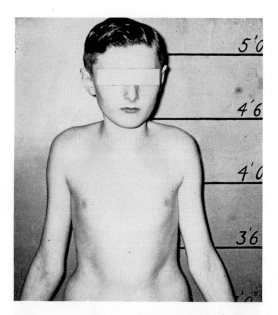

FIG. 319. Patient DH, age 14¼ years, height 62¼ inches. 17-Ketosteroids 3.1 mg. per 24 hours; FSH 26.4 mouse units per 24 hours; bone age normal. Marked hypogonadism with bilateral cryptorchism. The cryptorchid testes were completely atrophic and failed to respond to chorionic gonadotropin. Note the smooth skin, absence of acne, and general immature appearance.

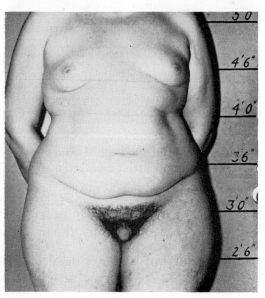

FIG. 320. Patient BS, age 30 years, height 71½ inches, span 76¾ inches. 17-Ketosteroids 16.5 mg. per 24 hours; FSH greater than 105 mouse units per 24 hours; chromatin negative. Note the marked feminine distribution of fat tissue. Both true and false gynecomastia were present. Despite weight reduction and androgen therapy, there was little change in general body configuration.

Skin. The skin of the adolescent patient with hypogonadism fails to show evidence of significant acne (Fig. 319); it is usually smooth and somewhat feminine in texture, appearing thinner than the skin of the normal male. Easy bruisability of the skin is usually noted. The ruddy

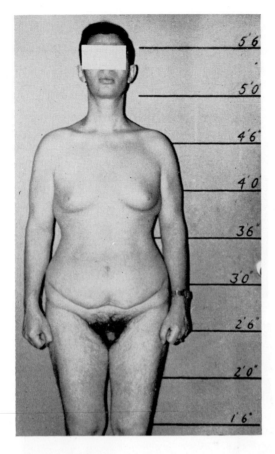

FIG. 321. Patient AG, age 35 years, height 67½ inches. 17-Ketosteroids 7.7 mg. per 24 hours; protein-bound iodine 4.8 gamma per cent; FSH increased; chromatin negative. Note the unusual feminine fat distribution, well-formed breasts containing an enormous amount of glandular tissue. With testosterone pellet implantation there has been some loss of fat in the hip and trochanteric area but not in the region of the breasts.

complexion of youth will persist for a prolonged period of time. In the adult with diminished testicular activity, there will usually be some difficulty in tanning.

Fat Distribution. Clinically, it may be noted that the hypogonadal patient has a characteristic feminine fat distribution, with an increase in fat deposition in the trochanteric areas of the body as well as in the region of the breasts (Figs. 320, 321). As a result, instead of the youth presenting a normal picture with wide shoulders and narrow hips, diagrammatically presented as ▽ , with the base representing the shoulders, the hypogonadal boy has narrow shoulders and wide hips resulting in a △ build with the base of the triangle representing the hip region. ▽ is the picture seen in the well-developed male.

Breasts. Increased fat deposition will usually be noted in the area of the breasts, bringing about some degree of false gynecomastia (Figs. 320, 321). In addition, increased amounts of glandular tissue also may be present so that the patient may show evidence of not only false but also true gynecomastia. There may be areolar accentuation in both true and false gynecomastia, but this is more prone to occur when glandular tissue is present in excessive amounts.

HORMONE EXCRETION STUDIES.   The biochemical changes are interesting and usually diagnostic.

17-KETOSTEROID FINDINGS.   *17-Ketosteroids—Adult.*   The normal 17-ketosteroid urinary excretion level in the male ranges from 10.0 to 24.0 mg. per 24 hours. The lower figure is usually noted in patients at around the time of puberty and again in the elderly age group. The 17-ketosteroid levels offer the physician the most valuable guide in determining relative androgenic function in the male. 17-Ketosteroid excretion is decreased in hypogonadism, whether primary or secondary in nature. The decrease in 17-ketosteroids may be only minimal in patients with primary gonadal failure inasmuch as two thirds of the ketosteroid levels are normally derived from the adrenal. The 17-ketosteroid level of adrenal origin may vary considerably, as evidenced by the fact that the normal range of 17-ketosteroid excretion in the female is 8.0 to 14.0 mg. per 24 hours and is derived only from adrenal precursors. This point is of utmost importance since in the male the 17-ketosteroids may still be within the lower limits of normal for the age of the patient, despite the clinical picture of gonadal failure. Thus, sufficient excretion of 17-ketosteroids of adrenal origin may occur in these patients to place them in the normal range for the male. However, if the patient has secondary hypogonadism associated with panhypopituitarism, the 17-ketosteroid excretion will be depressed to unusually low levels. On the other hand, secondary hypogonadism associated with only selective pituitary gonadotropic failure (hypogonadotropism) will be associated with a 17-ketosteroid level similar to that of a patient with primary testicular insufficiency.

17-Ketosteroids in Children.   In children, the level of 17-ketosteroid excretion depends on the age of the child. A convenient rule of thumb to follow in children is that they excrete approximately 0.50 to 0.75 mg. of 17-ketosteroid per 24 hours per year of life. Obviously, values at the lower limits of normal should be interpreted with some measure of suspicion. However, if these values are considerably below the lower limits of normal, the possibility of hypogonadism must be thought of, particularly if there is no evidence of decreased pituitary and/or adrenal cortical activity.

17-Ketosteroids in the Oriental and the Indian.   Low 17-ketosteroids may be noted in certain racial groups. This is particularly true in the Oriental and the Indian. Diet does not appear to play any specific role since the 17-ketosteroids do not appear to be increased appreciably when these individuals are maintained on a high protein diet. A low 17-ketosteroid excretion level in these persons is of no diagnostic importance.

17-Ketosteroids in Gout. Low 17-ketosteroid values are found in patients with gout and are no measure of their androgenic potential.[64] While the reason for the low 17-ketosteroid is not clear, one must consider this in assaying gonadal function when steroid excretion is obtained in a patient with a history of gout.

17-Ketosteroid Levels in the Addisonian Patient. The male with hypoadrenocorticoidism may show a significant depression of ketosteroids in the urine without having any disturbance in genital function. This may not be entirely true if the patient is an untreated Addisonian, since these patients may be so asthenic and fatigued as a result of their primary disease that all sexual function is secondarily affected and depressed due to lack of energy. In contrast, when they are maintained on appropriate corticoid therapy, normal genital function and activity is usually restored despite the persistent low 17-ketosteroid level.

GONADOTROPINS. If the patient has primary hypogonadism, he will show a definite increase in urinary gonadotropin excretion. An elevated gonadotropin points to testicular failure and helps to delineate the patients with primary from those with secondary hypogonadism. A decreased level of gonadotropic hormone secretion will be noted in the patient with secondary hypogonadism. Gonadotropic hormone study is a most important biologic test in determining whether the diminished gonadal function is primary or secondary to pituitary failure.

ESTROGEN LEVELS. Besides alterations in 17-ketosteroid and gonadotropin excretion, as a rule the hypogonadal patient will show no other specific chemical changes to aid in the diagnosis. While estrogen levels are usually normal, on rare occasion they may be elevated in patients with hypogonadism. Failure to find an elevated estrogen excretion in patients with hypogonadism is understandable when one considers the fact that it is the Leydig cells of the testes which are capable of excreting both androgens and estrogens. Hence, elevated estrogen levels would be unusual in hypogonadism where hypoleydigism is also predominant. In addition, the finding of increased estrogen levels does not necessarily imply that the patient has gonadal function.

X-RAY FINDINGS. *Epiphyses.* Examination of the epiphyses of the long bones may give a clue as to the endocrine status of the individual, particularly when there is some evidence of hypogonadism or hypothyroidism. A delay in epiphyseal development or closure will be noted in patients with decreased gonadal activity. Not only may there be a delay in epiphyseal fusion, but also the hypogonadal child examined prior to puberty may show a delay in appearance of some of the centers of ossification of the carpal bones. The hypogonadal male who is examined at an age significantly beyond the time that puberty would normally be anticipated may show considerable delay in epiphyseal closure. Such a delay in epiphyseal closure in a euthyroid individual points toward

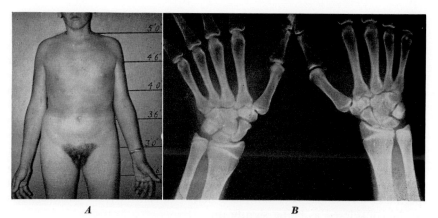

A   B

FIG. 322.   Patient SK (same patient as shown in Figure 316).   Note the tendency
for some enunuchoidal characteristics.   Muscle build and general characteristics
are entirely masculine at the present time due to androgen therapy.   However,
in Figure 322B note open epiphyses.   Patient had excellent response to steroidal
hormonal therapy.   Testes are larger, the phallus has reached considerable size
over and above the pre-treatment level, permitting satisfactory intercourse.   Good
response to androgens was anticipated inasmuch as epiphyses were still open.

hypogonadism.   Epiphyseal closure may be delayed to such a degree
that failure of fusion may be noted at times even in a 30 to 40 year
old hypogonadal male (Fig. 322).   However, the presence of open
epiphyses in a hypogonadal male of this age is a good prognostic sign
for an increase in size of the hypoplastic penis when appropriate therapy
is employed.   If the epiphyses are open, one can expect some increase in
size of the phallus in response to therapy, regardless of the age of the
patient.

Bone Texture.   The hypogonadal male also shows other x-ray
stigmata of his disease; namely, a tendency for minimal to significant
osteoporosis.   In addition, the heaviness in structure, anticipated in the
skeleton of the male, will usually be absent in the hypogonadal male so
that the x-ray appearance will be similar to that seen in the female.

Differentiation of Retardation of Bone Age.   It should be remembered that retardation of bone age may not be peculiar only to the male
with hypogonadism but may also be seen in other endocrinopathies,
particularly in patients with hypothyroidism and panhypopituitarism.
However, the specific x-ray findings noted in hypothyroidism are most
helpful in distinguishing this type of delay in bony maturation from
that noted in patients with hypogonadism. While most of the skeletal
changes noted in patients with decreased thyroid function are reviewed
in the chapter on hypothyroidism, the principal x-ray findings in these
patients are the irregular sites of ossification in the epiphyses, giving
the appearance of stippling or a moth-eaten effect.   Epiphyseal dysgenesis

is a characteristic finding of hypothyroidism and is not noted in other endocrinopathies associated with retardation of bone age. The failure of maturation of the epiphyses and the development of the carpal bones of the hands and wrists of the hypogonadal child may differ from other types of retardation of bone age. For example, the delay in bone age seen in hypogonadism is not so marked as that seen in patients with panhypopituitarism. The bony changes noted on x-ray in hypogonadism may be differentiated from the delay in bone age in children with decreased thyroid function by the specific abnormality of the epiphyses observed in hypothyroidism.

BONE AGE. Since knowledge of bone age is important in establishing evidence of delay, normality, or acceleration, it becomes apparent that specific criteria must be established before deviation from these criteria can be considered as being significant.

There are certain definite standards which one may use to determine the presence or absence of a delay in bone age. The older criteria which have depended on the standards described by Caffey[2] and others are perhaps somewhat below what the normal should be for a child of the present era. The apparent acceleration of development of the modern generation of children probably is due to the fact that the subjects on whom Caffey based his classical standards were studied four to five decades ago when children were still subjected to the ravages of serious childhood illness.[2] They experienced prolonged bouts of febrile illnesses and diarrheas, as well as diseases which now are considered medical curiosities, such as diphtheria, the debilitating pneumonias, etc. At the same time, the use of almost routine vitamin supplementation by the present-day pediatrician has no doubt been of importance in preventing retardation of bone age due to nutritional deficiencies. As a result, better nutrition and consequently better growth and development have come about so that the older classifications of bone age are now too conservative in determining the presence or absence of retardation of bone age. The normal bone age for a child in the early 1920's might well be considered as being somewhat retarded for a child in the early '60's. The standards suggested by Wilkins, in our experience, appear to be more appropriate for the classification of bone age of the modern child.[61] Attached to the back cover of this book is a sliding chart on the bone age of children. It may be used as a convenient way to determine with some degree of accuracy the approximate bone age of a patient.

PATIENT DIAGNOSIS. *Self-Comparison.* Another important diagnostic point in determining the presence of hypogonadism and the need for therapy in the adolescent boy is the impression that the developing boy has of himself in regard to his own genital development. Gross comparison of the size of their genitalia is frequently made by preadolescent and adolescent children. Those who do not come up to their expected standards may be subject to ridicule and contempt so that the child, poorly endowed from the point of view of size of his genitalia, may be exposed to criticism. It is for this reason that it is important to consider the child's concept of his own genital development when therapy is being contemplated. If the patient feels that his developmental processes are significantly retarded, this must then be considered as an important indication for therapy and a point of importance in favor of the diagnosis of hypogonadism.[30]

Psychological Requirements for Therapy. The psychological factors and aberrations in a child with hypogonadism are usually evident and need not be enlarged upon at the present time. However, since these factors may influence the patient's behavior and may be of intense concern to the child, it would be well to consider these psychological implications as a prime indication for treatment of the youth with hypogonadism. Many times, as a result of imagined or real insufficiency, a feeling of inferiority may develop which can lead to certain defense mechanisms on the part of the patient. Hence, we feel that it is necessary to stress the patient's mental anguish as much as the 17-KS and other laboratory or physical criteria in order to establish the need for a positive therapeutic approach. It is important to note that the ridicule to which such a hypogonadal youth is exposed may not only affect his psychic make-up, but may even influence his fertility later in life. A patient's apprehension over real or imagined genital inferiority may eventually lead to impotence. This may arise from a fear that he cannot be an effective male, since his small phallus might not be adequate for the satisfactory performance of coitus. In addition, there are youths who have prematurely discontinued their education because of their unwillingness to participate in compulsory physical education since exposure of their genitalia would be necessary in the shower, etc. The patient's feeling of genital inadequacy may thus start a cycle of events which may alter not only the future psycho-sexual life of the patient but also his socio-economic potentialities.

Therapy. WATCHFUL WAITING VERSUS HORMONAL THERAPY. The therapeutic management of a child with hypogonadism has been open to considerable question and criticism. Some physicians are nihilistic in their approach and condemn any form of treatment for hypogonadal patients. The nihilists claim that such therapy only achieves premature acceleration of genital development—an acceleration which, they state, is uncalled for inasmuch as normal development of the genitalia would eventually take place even without therapy.

The question posed to the therapist is: "Has any real benefit been accomplished by therapy?" The therapeutic nihilist would say *no* and advise a course of watchful waiting. His philosophy is, "Let us wait and see what will happen," with the assurance that most of the children will begin to develop later in life so that there is usually no need for therapy during adolescence.

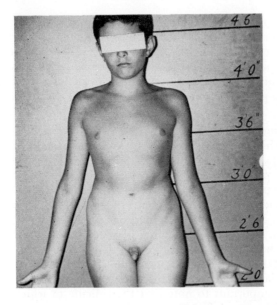

FIG. 323. Patient WG, age 10 years, height 56¾ inches. Protein-bound iodine 6.2 gamma per cent; 17-ketosteroids 3.9 mg. per 24 hours; FSH low; chromatin pattern negative. Despite the patient's young age, therapy was initiated because of the marked hypoplasia of the gonads and the general feminine fat distribution. His response to therapy has been excellent, associated with a general improvement in his psychosomatic make-up. He was accepted by his confreres and did well in school after treatment.

We feel that "watchful waiting" is uncalled for if the diagnosis of hypogonadism is made on the grounds of the clinical picture, the low 17-ketosteroids, and the psychological factors discussed above (Figs. 323-328). Delaying therapy may have adverse effects, particularly since one does not know what the future will disclose. Some patients have been damaged irreparably by the code of "watchful waiting," so that, when they attain their adult stature, their genital development is considerably below what one would normally anticipate in an adult male. Consequently, certain psychological aberrations may be projected upon the patient, resulting in an unhappy sexual, social and marital life. We feel that, if therapy is instituted at the time it is first needed, based on the criteria listed above, there will be no adverse effects as far as the patient's future genital development is concerned (Figs. 329-333).

EFFECT OF THERAPY ON BONE MATURATION AND GROWTH. In addition, it has been said at times that exogenous stimulation of the development of the gonads may bring about some acceleration of epiphyseal closure. As a result, the child will theoretically never reach the height he would have attained had he not received treatment; or, at best, while therapy may cause a spurt of growth, the over-all effect achieved will be no greater than that which would have occurred had therapy been withheld entirely. However, in our experience there is no evidence that gonadotropin therapy in the adolescent male will cause any abnormal acceleration of bone age. Our data indicates that, if anything, the growth achieved as a result of therapy is enhanced and not retarded.

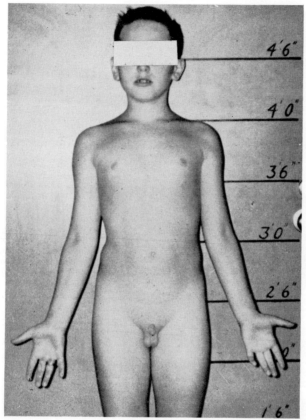

FIG. 324. *Patient RH, age 15 years, height 58 inches. 17-Keto-*
steroids 5.3 mg. per 24 hours; FSH less than 6.6 mouse units per 24
hours; chromatin negative. Patient shows same development as WG
(Figure 323) did at the age of 10. Therapy was withheld; the patient
is still immature and shows clinical signs of marked hypogonadism.
Epiphyses are open. Response to gonadotropic therapy has been
excellent. Earlier initiation of therapy would have prevented the
embarrassment to which this boy was exposed because of his preva-
lent hypogonadism.

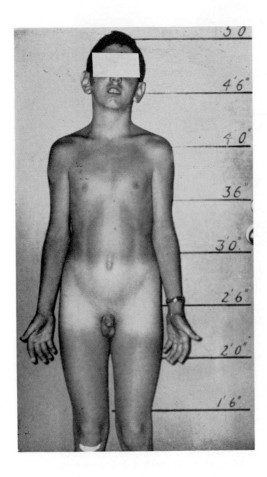

FIG. 325. Patient DL, age 15¼ years, height 60 inches, with retarded bone age and genital development as well as short stature. He was the product of "watchful waiting" and only recently has received chorionic gonadotropic therapy at the 1000 I.U. dose level with a good response. (See text for dose schedule.)

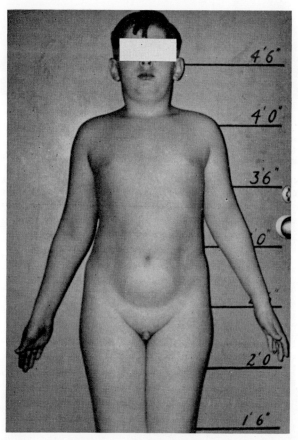

FIG. 326.   Patient MG, age 11 years, height 56½ inches; 17-keto-steroids 3.8 mg. per 24 hours. Note the marked gonadal hypoplasia and short stature. Therapy was instituted and child, who had been a retiring one seeking sedentary occupations, now partakes of the usual physical activities anticipated in a boy of this age.

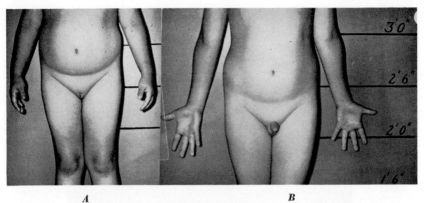

A   B

FIG. 327. Patient GB, age 9½ years, before (A) and after (B) chorionic
gonadotropin therapy. Despite his tender years the need for therapy was evident
by his clinical appearance and his own desire for more advanced maturation.
Note the unusually small phallus prior to therapy and normal response after the
prescribed course of "A.P.L." Prior to treatment the patient's height was 51½
inches and his weight 91 pounds. After treatment he was 54½ inches tall and
weighed 76¼ pounds; in addition he was a much more normal youth.

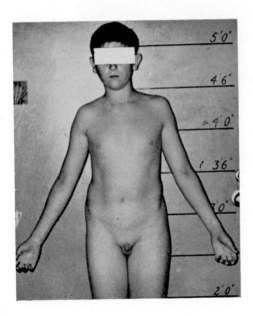

FIG. 328. Patient CS, age 13½
years, height 62¼ inches, 17-keto-
steroids 7.1 mg. per 24 hours. Note
the small genitalia. Child was
in a home for boys. He was
timid and did poorly in school. He
received the prescribed course of
therapy and matured well with
considerable improvement in school
grades and deportment. He became a much happier child.

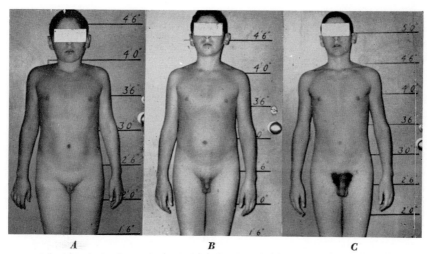

FIG. 329. Patient RS. Response of hypogonadal boy to therapy. A, Pre-treatment: age 11½ years, height 55½ inches; 17-ketosteroids 10.4 mg. per 24 hours; protein-bound iodine 5.5 gamma per cent; chromatin negative. Note hypogonadism and immature build. B, Age 12½ years, height 58¾ inches. Therapy given at age 11½ for 6 weeks as described in text. Note maturation of general build and normal genital development. C, Age 13¾ years, height 63¼ inches. Note continued maturation, well-developed phallus, and normal male physiognomy.

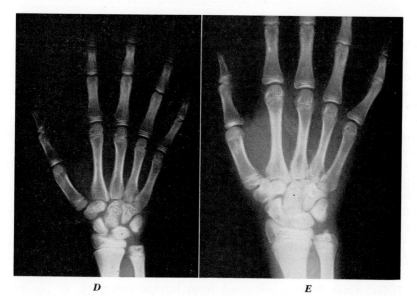

FIG. 330. Note epiphyses of patient in Figure 329 before treatment (A) and two years later (B), when excellent results had been achieved. Despite excellent growth of almost 8 inches, there was no evidence of acceleration of epiphyseal maturation.

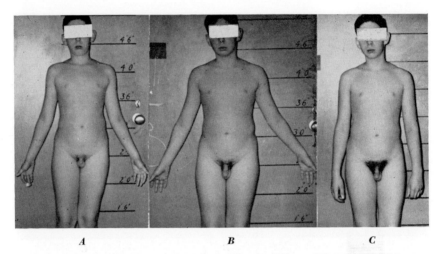

                    A   B   C

FIG. 331. Patient LB. A, Age 13, height 60 inches; 17-ketosteroids 7.2 mg.
per 24 hours; protein-bound iodine 6.7 gamma per cent; chromatin pattern negative. Note the general immature build and youthful-looking face. B, Seven months
later after patient received an initial course of gonadotropic hormone therapy
as described in text. Height 61¼ inches. Note the increase in size of the genitalia
and the more masculine build. C, Age 14, height 63¼ inches. No further treatment
given between B and C. Note continued maturation and normal body build and
configuration.

In order to refute such claims, a series of x-ray pictures have been
obtained before and after chorionic gonadotropin therapy in hypogonadal
children, some of whom have also received concomitant therapy with
norethandrolone or other anabolic steroids. Review of these x-ray pictures, some of which are presented here and others in Chapter 3, failed
to show any evidence of acceleration of epiphyseal closure or significant
advancement of bone age over and above that which would have accrued
due to the passage of time itself (Figs. 334-337). As far as can be seen,
there are no objective experimental data in the literature to the contrary,
to show that the doses recommended would have adverse effects on the
epiphyses. Thus, the warnings of the therapeutic nihilist appear to be
groundless when he denies the hypogonadal male the advantages of
appropriate therapy, since so-called disadvantages appear to be theoretical
rather than scientific.

CHORIONIC GONADOTROPIN THERAPY. The therapeutic management
of hypogonadism in the preadolescent or the adolescent male should at
first be dependent on the use of human chorionic gonadotropic hormone
(HCG). Since HCG is obtained from human sources—i. e., the urine
of pregnant women—it may be used with impunity as far as allergic
reactions are concerned. No immunologic phenomena or anti-hormone
formation will develop if its use is continued for several months. This

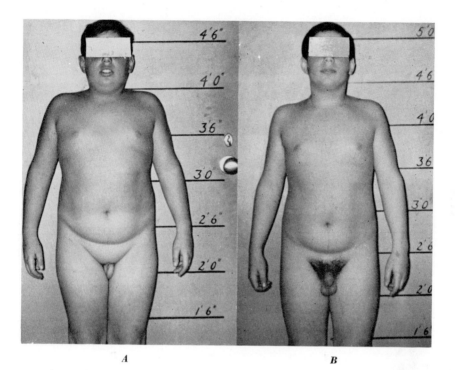

A   B

FIG. 332. Patient RC. A, Age 12½ years, height 56 inches; 17-ketosteroids
6.4 mg. per 24 hours; protein-bound iodine 4.8 gamma per cent; 17-hydroxy-
steroids 4.4 mg. per 24 hours. B, Age 14 years. The patient received a course of
human chorionic gonadotropin (HCG) at the 1000 I.U. dose level at the age of
12½ years. In 6 weeks his response was phenomenal. His growth of 3¾ inches
was far superior to his previous development. He is now well within normal
limits as far as genital development is concerned.

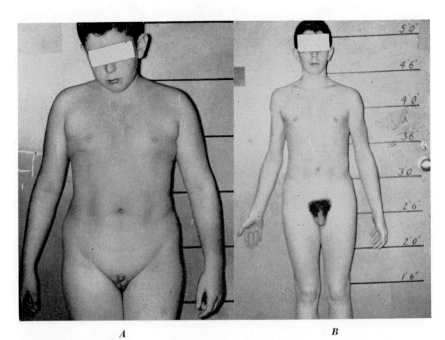

FIG. 333. Patient JG. A, Age 14 years, height 56½ inches; protein-bound iodine 5.0 gamma per cent; 17-ketosteroids 7.1 mg. per 24 hours; FSH = 6.6 mouse units per 24 hours; chromatin negative. B, Age 15¾ years, height 61¾ inches. Patient received initial course of HCG therapy at the 1000 I.U. level as described in the text. His growth response has been excellent, as has his genital growth.

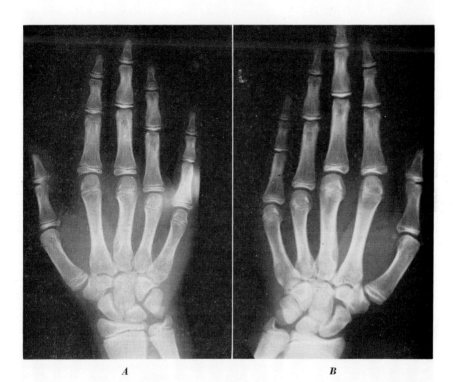

A   B

FIG. 334.   X-ray pictures of the hands and wrists of patient in Figure 333, pre-
treatment (A) and post-treatment (B).   There has been no evidence of acceleration of closure of the epiphyses over and above that seen with the change of
age alone.

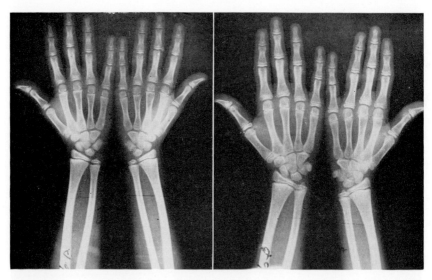

A   B

FIG. 335.   Patient NK, who received the course of HCG and norethandrolone
therapy as described in the text.   A, Age 12 years, height 55 inches, just prior to
therapy.   B, Age 13 years, one year later, height 60¼ inches.   Excellent genital
development and growth took place without encroachment upon the bone age
other than that associated with the passage of time alone.

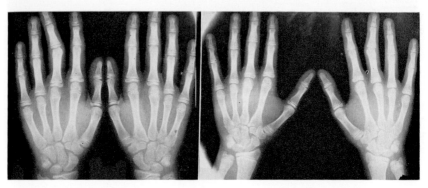

A   B

FIG. 336.   Patient DH.   A, Age 13 5/6 years, height 59¼ inches.   B, Age 14¾
years, height 62¾ inches.   Note the failure of any definite change to occur on
bone age maturation despite the excellent growth that followed the gonadotropic
hormone therapy given immediately after the control x-rays were obtained.

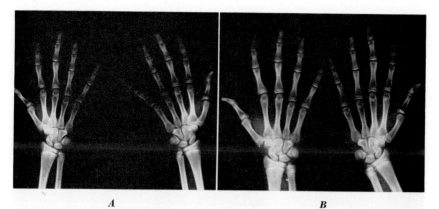

A   *B*

FIG. 337. *Patient DB. A, Age 13 years, height 55 inches; weight 99¼ pounds; 17-ketosteroids 6.4 mg. per 24 hours. B, Age 14¼ years; height 60 inches; weight 111 pounds. Patient received HCG and norethandrolone therapy at age 13 for 6 weeks. Note splendid growth (5 inches) without evidence of acceleration of bone age.*

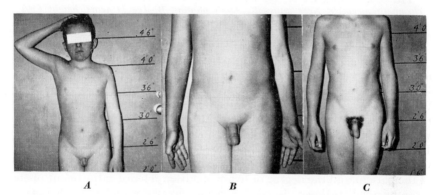

A   *B*   *C*

FIG. 338. *Patient EM. A, Age 12 years, height 57¾ inches; 17-ketosteroids 4.9 mg. per 24 hours; protein-bound iodine 4.5 gamma per cent. Note the hypogonadism and short stature. B, Age 12 5/6 years. The patient received the 6-week course of therapy described in the text at age 12. Note the splendid genital development. Height is now 60¾ inches. C, Age 13, height 61¼ inches. Continued improvement in genital development without further therapy.*

mode of therapy is physiologic in that the extract will be responsible for stimulating the patient's Leydig cells to secrete androgen. The androgen, in turn, should produce the desired physiologic increase in development and size of the secondary sex organs (Figs. 329-340). Since the androgens are of endogenous origin, they should not be present in unphysiologic levels or proportions when the recommended doses of chorionic gonadotropin are employed.

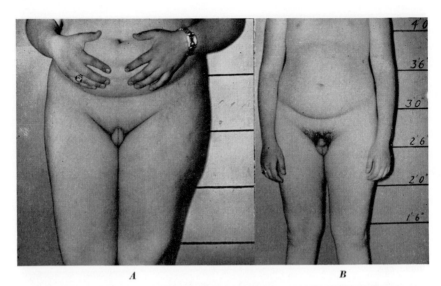

A   *B*

FIG. 339. Patient LA. A, Age 13 years, height 62½ inches; 17-ketosteroids low;
chromatin negative. Note unusually small phallus. B, Age 14 years, height 65¼
inches. Note excellent genital response and more normal muscle distribution
after treatment with HCG at the 1000 I.U. dose level.

Recommended Dose. An effective rule of thumb that has been
useful in determining the dosage of chorionic gonadotropin to be administered is as follows: children 10 years old or below receive a course of
therapy consisting of 500 international units of chorionic gonadotropin
three times a week for three weeks, followed by the same dose twice a
week for three weeks. If a child is above the age of 10, he will receive
1000 international units instead of the 500, in the same dosage schedule.[30]
Obviously, the dose should be regulated according to the size and weight
of the patient and the degree of hypogonadism. Hence, adjustment of the
recommended regimen is to be made according to the physician's
judgment.

Preparation. The preparation of choice is one available in powder
form so that solubilizing is accomplished just prior to the initiation of
treatment. The advantage of using the lyophilized material lies in the
fact that there will be little or no deterioration of the gonadotropin,
regardless of how long it stays on the shelf prior to use. However, regardless of the extract used, the physician should use the one with which he
is most familiar and which, in his experience, will offer him the best
predictability of response. The one we have found to be most reliable
is the "A.P.L." brand (Ayerst), which has yielded consistently satisfactory
results in most of the patients to whom this product has been administered.

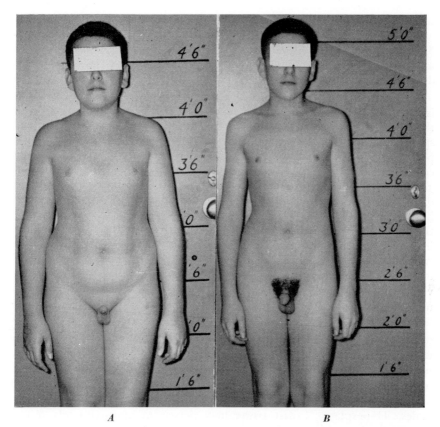

A   B

FIG. 340. Patient WE. A, Age 13½ years, height 57½ inches; protein-bound iodine normal; 17-ketosteroids 4.9 mg. per 24 hours; chromatin negative. B, Age 14¾ years, height 61½ inches. Splendid response with respect to both growth and development of genitalia. The patient received a course of HCG therapy for 6 weeks as described in the text at age 13½ years.

Among the preparations which have been recommended for the treatment of hypogonadism is "fortified" chorionic gonadotropin. This is a preparation of human chorionic gonadotropin to which thiamin hydrochloride and L (+) glutamic acid have been added.[13-15] The bizarre claims that have been made for this preparation have had no substantiation on qualified evaluation. This combination adds little, if anything, to the therapeutic efficacy of HCG and should not be included in one's armamentarium. The concept that such a combination is associated with a therapeutic response in castrated animals or humans is absurd.[13-15]

Associated Physiologic Effects. There have been no toxic manifestations attributed to chorionic gonadotropic hormone therapy. However, there are certain undesirable effects due to the HCG administration which the patients may exhibit during an appropriate course of therapy. Nevertheless, since these changes represent a physiologic expression of testicular stimulation to HCG, they cannot be considered as toxic effects despite their undesirability.

Gynecomastia. The principal objectionable side effect due to HCG is the development of true gynecomastia associated with accentuation of the areolae and breast tenderness. Gynecomastia also has been noted spontaneously in approximately 60 per cent of all boys going through puberty and has been attributed to endogenous production by the Leydig cells at the time of puberty. Breast enlargement after exogenous gonadotropic administration is no doubt due to the increased production of estrogen as a result of the stimulating effect the chorionic gonadotropin has on the Leydig cells. There may be an alternative explanation whereby the gynecomastia may be due to enhanced conversion to estrogens of the increased androgen secretion following the Leydig cell stimulation. Another possible source of the estrogens has been ascribed to the stimulatory effect of the chorionic gonadotropin on the Sertoli cells. However, in view of recent studies, it would appear that this latter possibility is unlikely.

Management of Iatrogenic Gynecomastia. Regardless of the source of estrogens, the gynecomastia occurring after chorionic gonadotropins is invariably temporary in nature and, in our experience, has always subsided spontaneously. Nevertheless, one might anticipate finding a few patients in whom the gynecomastia remains permanent in much the same manner as it does in the spontaneous gynecomastia of adolescent males. Hyperplastic breast tissue may persist in approximately 3 per cent of the boys developing gynecomastia (i.e., 3 per cent of the 75 per cent of all pubertal boys who develop gynecomastia). Since the gynecomastia presumably is related to the estrogen secretion stimulated by the effect of either the endogenous or the exogenous gonadotropins on the testes, one could anticipate the iatrogenic hypertrophy occasionally to persist and be of sufficient extent to cause some mental anxiety in the patient affected. However, the parents should be reassured that this is not an unusual response and that, in all probability, it would have occurred even with spontaneous testicular maturation. They should also be told that, in general, there is no specific medical treatment for this problem. If the gynecomastia persists, successful management may require an appropriate surgical approach, as will be discussed in more detail in Chapter 18, Gynecomastia.

Priapism. Another effect attributable to HCG therapy is a tendency for priapism to occur, with increased incidence of spontaneous erections taking place. The younger patient may show an increased tendency to fondle or manipulate his genitalia and initiate masturbation, or increase the frequency of masturbation if the practice had already been started. While a discussion of the mores of, and theoretical harm due to, masturbation is beyond the scope of this text, it may be stated categorically that there is no danger to the child either physically or mentally as a result of such practices. Untoward priapism will subside as soon as the therapy has been discontinued.

Hirsutism. The patient may also show an increased growth of pubic or scrotal hair. The new hair growth may be of a fine lanugo type or may actually represent acceleration of normal pubic hair growth. The pubarche (the presence of pubic hair) may normally appear in a child at the age of nine or ten. Significant development of pubic hair prior to this age is not a particularly adverse effect and can be anticipated in children with some degree of genital stimulation as a result of HCG therapy.

Personality Changes. There are other effects noted in children or young adults who have responded to chorionic gonadotropin, which are associated primarily with changes in the personality of the child and alteration of body build. The quiet, demure, recessive, docile, hypogonadal child may turn into the typical unpredictable, positive, aggressive adolescent exerting his prerogative by a belligerent attitude or actual physical combat. One such hypogonadal patient had been quiet and withdrawn and his greatest pleasure had been the opportunity to bake his mother a cake. After the prescribed course of HCG he refused to participate in any culinary duties, spoke back to his mother, and fought with his brothers—something he had never done in the past. The body build of the patient during and after therapy will be altered so that he will tend to lose his "baby" fat and will assume the more angular appearance of the normal male (Figs. 341-344). He may appear slimmer, not because the gonadotropin induces weight loss, but because his linear growth becomes accentuated with a redistribution of fat. It should be emphasized that chorionic gonadotropin has *no* role or place in the physician's armamentarium specifically for weight reduction alone.

CONCOMITANT ANABOLIC STEROID THERAPY. We have also administered anabolic steroids such as norethandrolone (Nilevar) together with the HCG. The rationale for the use of this steroid is to enhance the effect the HCG would have on growth and development of the patient.[30] The usual dose of norethandrolone with the larger dose of the HCG is 10.0 mg. twice a day for 10 days, followed by once a day thereafter until the course of HCG has been completed. When the smaller dose of gonadotropin is used, the dose of norethandrolone is reduced accordingly. Upon the completion of the course of gonadotropin, the need for further anabolic therapy will depend on the desire for additional growth in these patients. The growth effect of norethandrolone and other anabolic steroids will be discussed in a later chapter.

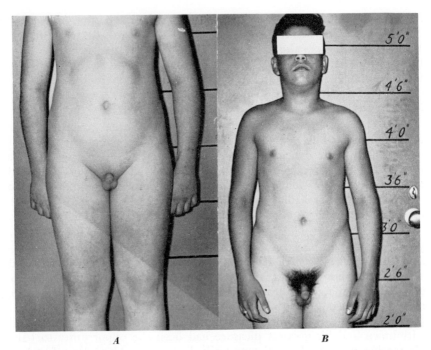

FIG. 341. *Patient ME. A, Age 14 years, height 57¼ inches. 17-Ketosteroids 6.7 mg. per 24 hours; chromatin negative. Patient required two courses of therapy. B, Age 15 1/3 years, height 62¼ inches. Note the maturation and normal genital development in a boy who is adequately matured for his age after the second course of treatment. Growth response is fair.*

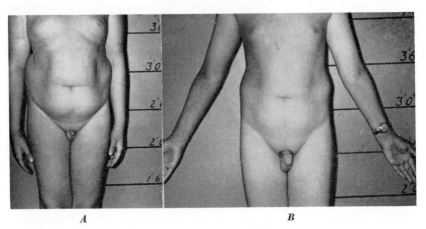

FIG. 342. *Patient EB. A, Age 13½ years, height 59¾ inches. B, Age 14 years, height 62¼ inches. Note the excellent genital response and reduction in adiposity. Therapy was given at age 13½ years and consisted of HCG administration.*

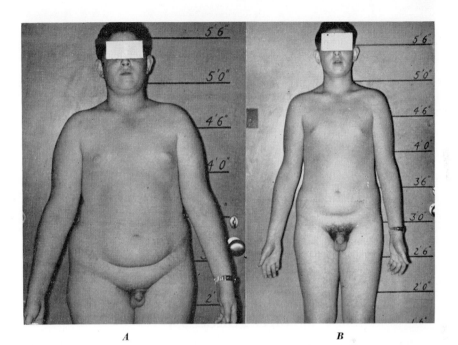

FIG. 343. Patient WP. A, Age 15 years, height 65½ inches, weight 175 pounds. 17-Ketosteroids 6.9 mg. per 24 hours; protein-bound iodine 9.3 gamma per cent. B, Age 15¾ years, height 68 inches, weight 156 pounds. Note the tremendous loss in weight, the general change in body build as well as increase in size of genitalia after the patient received the 1000 I.U. schedule of HCG at the age of 15. The weight loss is not ascribed to the gonadotropin but merely to better dietary control associated with a greater feeling of adequacy as far as the genitals are concerned.

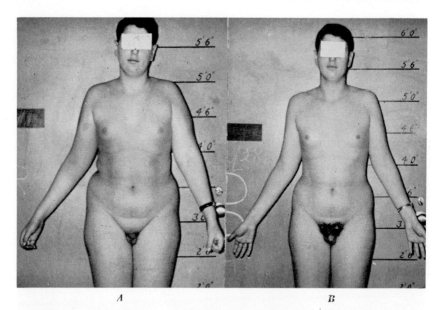

FIG. 344. Patient DP. A, Age 14½ years, height 70¼ inches, weight 191¾ pounds. 17-Ketosteroids 6.2 mg. per 24 hours; FSH greater than 6 but less than 13 mouse units per 24 hours; protein-bound iodine 6.4 gamma per cent; chromatin negative. B, Age 15-2/3 years, height 72¾ inches, weight 186¼ pounds. Note the general change in body build and genital maturation. Weight loss was based on dietary restriction. Hormonal response was not effective in causing weight loss per se but was merely responsible for producing a redistribution of fat. Patient received the standard (1000 I.U.) HCG regimen started at age 14½ years for one course only.

CRYPTORCHISM

The problem of the management of the undescended testicle has revolved around these questions: (1) When should the undescended testis be brought down to the scrotum? (2) If the testis should be brought down, should it be done by chorionic gonadotropic hormone therapy or by orchiopexy?

The answers to these questions reveal that there is no unanimity of opinion as to the most appropriate course to follow. Our concept requires the early administration of HCG. However, one must keep in mind that, while we feel that early therapy is wise and should be instituted as the age of four to six years, there are those who are equally positive that it is desirable to withhold both medical and/or surgical treatment until the post-pubertal phase of life.

Factors Involved in Testicular Descent. Many times failure of the testes to descend does not appear to be related to any specific hormone deficiency. Nevertheless, as described in the embryologic development of the testes, descent of the male gonad from its original abdominal position to its dependent resting place in the scrotum does appear to be a reflection of androgenic activity of the fetal testes. The gubernaculum apparently is not involved since cutting the gubernaculum has failed to prevent descent of the testes. While the prime factor causing descent is androgenic activity there must also be a tissue organizer or conductor peculiar to the testis itself, since androgens do not cause either the ovarian anlage or the ovary itself to descend. Mechanical factors such as a barrier in the path of descent of the testes might also play a role in the etiology of cryptorchism.

When Should Descent Be Attempted? The question arises as to the appropriate age when the undescended testis should be brought down into the scrotum. The answer depends, in part, on the answer to the following question: At what age does the abdominal position of the testis result in irreparable damage to the germinal epithelium, causing irreversible changes in the testis? In addition, the possibility of neoplastic alterations in the abdominal testis must also be considered in determining when and why the abdominal testis should be fixed in the scrotum. The need for early transposition of the abdominal testis to the scrotum appears to us to be paramount and is based on the following concepts:

1. The abdominal testis is incapable of sperm production. The longer the testis stays in the abdomen, the greater the damage to the germinal epithelium. Detectable damage to the germinal epithelium may be noted in the cryptorchid testis as early as four to five years of age.

2. The abdominal testis has a considerably greater neoplastic propensity than the scrotal testis.

3. The abdominal testis, while capable of secreting testosterone, may undergo premature failure so that complete absence of testicular activity may be noted as early as 35 to 40 years of age.

Diagnosis. The diagnosis of cryptorchism may or may not be difficult. The cremasteric reflex in children may be so active that, when examination is attempted, it may be almost impossible to palpate the testis due to the cremasteric muscle pulling it high in the scrotum in the region of the external canal. The small size of the testes in the preadolescent child also creates difficulties in examination. Before one can state positively that failure of either or both testes to descend has occurred, it is important to subject the child to one or both of the following procedures:

SPECIAL POSITION OR PROCEDURE TO DETERMINE POSITION OF TESTES. (1) Have the child squat on the floor or on a table. This position will usually make a previously undetectable testis more readily palpable in the scrotum, particularly if the gonad is high in the inguinal canal. (2) The second procedure is less practical but may be helpful in determining the presence or absence of a scrotal testis. The child is placed in a tub of warm water at a temperature of 100° to 101° F. Here, too, a scrotal testis previously not detectable may be readily palpable.

Another technique has involved having the child lie in a supine position and gradually but firmly attempting to "milk" the testis into the scrotum. This may be accomplished by stroking the pelvic area gently but firmly, going from the medial part of the iliac crest medially and inferiorly toward the scrotum. The examiner's fingers may be lubricated with soap to reduce the friction on the skin. Not infrequently the testis may be detected when it could not be felt before, particularly if it is high in the canal.

Therapy. Time for Its Initiation. The age at which to initiate therapy for cryptorchism has been open to some dispute. However, since damage to the germinal epithelium occurs early in life, it would appear to be essential to start treatment soon after the age of four to five, and preferably before the age of seven. Therapy may consist of either a hormonal (gonadotropin) or surgical (orchiopexy) approach, or a combination of the two. We feel that, initially, the hormonal mode of therapy is desirable and, if unsuccessful, then surgery should be done.

Medical or Gonadotropin Management. *Gonadotropins versus Androgens.* At no time should androgens be employed. Sex steroid therapy should be administered only when no testes are present, or if the gonads are so fibrotic and atrophied that they are incapable of responding to gonadotropin.

Rapid versus Chronic Gonadotropin Therapy. The gonadotropic hormonal approach may be achieved by one of two procedures, both of which utilize the administration of chorionic gonadotropin. The use of either one would depend on the clinician and the age of the patient. The rapid method has the advantage of producing less development of the secondary sexual characteristics. This form of treatment utilizes high doses of the gonadotropin over a shorter period of time whereby the patient receives 5000 I. U. every second day for four injections.

The chronic schedule of treatment not only has a greater degree of predictability in its effect but is also associated with a greater degree of development of the phallus and pubic hair. However, while there may be some degree of sexual maturation, there are no deleterious effects as far as premature epiphyseal closure is concerned. It is true that some youngsters may complain of priapism and pubic hair development; nevertheless, when therapy is discontinued, the priapism will subside. The pubic hair may diminish or may remain at the same state of development until spontaneous maturation of the testes occurs at the time that puberty would normally take place. The chronic method utilizes the same dosage schedule of chorionic gonadotropin recommended in the preadolescent male children with hypogonadism. The dose of HCG which is selected is administered by 15 injections spread over a period of six weeks.

If the testis or testes fail to descend following either course of treatment within the time of hormone administration or within seven to 10 days after the last injection, orchiopexy is necessary and should be done by one familiar with the technique. At the present time, it appears that the surgical procedure of Thorek is not the one of choice, being now held in disfavor by most urologic surgeons.

Advantages of Initial Medical Approach. The principal advantage of hormonal therapy in the younger child, even if surgical intervention becomes necessary, is that some degree of maturation of the genital tissue will occur. This may make the technical procedure easier for the surgeon and perhaps aid in the healing process by causing less tension upon the sutures.

Presence or Absence of Testes. The administration of chorionic gonadotropin also serves another distinct purpose. In the patient with bilateral cryptorchism, one may not know whether or not there are testes capable of functioning, or even whether the gonads are present at all. If the patient with bilateral cryptorchism fails to show any androgenic response to the chronic dose regimen advocated above, one may then conclude that there is no testicular tissue present at all, or that, if testicle-like organs are present, then they are so atrophic that they are incapable of function. A failure of response would be manifested by no change in penile size, absence of priapism and penile rubor, plus the fact that there will be no evident effect on pubic hair growth. If pubic hair is present, it will not increase in amount during the course of therapy; if pubic hair is absent, growth will not be initiated. In addition, there will be no evidence of scrotal stimulation or of any increase in redundancy. If no response is observed after the initial course of therapy, before one can state that the testes are absent or non-functional it would be wise to institute a second course of treatment, using two to three times the dose level initially employed. Here, again, a failure of any of the above criteria to be noted would be tantamount to a diagnosis of testicular failure or agenesis (Fig. 345). Since gonadal agenesis may be present in a chromatin negative patient with a male phenotype and high FSH, such a patient would not require an abdominal operation.

Management of Atrophic Testes. Failure to demonstrate functioning testicles points to the need for initiation of substitution therapy with androgen preparations. Institution of androgen therapy would depend, to a certain extent, on the age of the patient. Therapy is *not* indicated prior to the age that puberty would normally be anticipated. Indeed, excessive therapy given before the normal pubertal age would result in the possibility of premature closure of the epiphyses plus premature sexual precocity. The post-pubertal patient (past the age of 12 to 13) requires immediate treatment to develop his secondary sexual character-

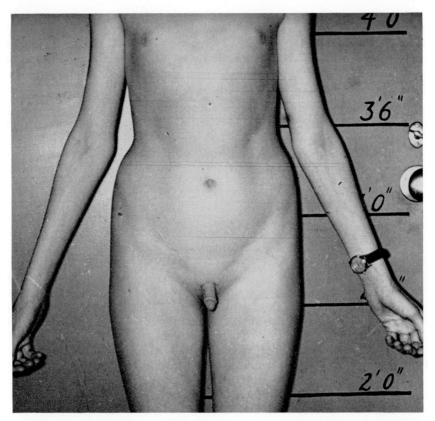

FIG. 345. *Same patient as shown in Fig. 319. Note the absence of testes and the small phallus. The penis did not increase in size when the patient received the gonadotropic hormone, indicating a lack of testicular action. The phallus responded excellently to androgen therapy.*

istics adequately, as well as to prevent eunuchoidal changes from taking place. The following parenteral or oral preparations may be used:

PARENTERAL PREPARATIONS.

1. Testosterone cyclopentylpropionate (Depo-Testosterone), 100.0 to 150.0 mg.

Testosterone enanthate (Delatestryl), 200.0 to 300.0 mg.

Testosterone phenylacetate (Perandren phenylacetate), 100.0 to 150.0 mg.

Any of these preparations may be administered every three to four weeks.

2. Pellet implantation of testosterone—nine pellets of 75.0 mg. each, implanted every six months.

ORAL PREPARATIONS.

1. Fluoxymesterone (Halotestin, Ultandren), 5.0 mg. b.i.d. to t.i.d.

2. Methyltestosterone, 10.0 to 15.0 mg. t.i.d. to q.i.d.

GUIDE TO TREATMENT.   An important guide to therapy would be the effect of such treatment on penile size, erection, and potentia. In other words, excessive stimulation or frequency of erections would be an indication to reduce the dose by giving the medication less frequently or by lowering the dose of material ingested or injected.

CHROMATIN STUDIES OF THE PATIENT WITH ABSENCE OF TESTICULAR FUNCTION.   The chromatin pattern of the patient with unilateral or bilateral cryptorchism should be studied. If the chromatin pattern is negative, in all probability one can expect the testes to be present in the vast majority of patients. Occasionally, agenesis of the testes may occur so that exploration may fail to disclose the presence of the male gonad. If the chromatin pattern is positive and scrotal testes are absent, theoretically the patient may have Klinefelter's syndrome with bilateral cryptorchism.   However, the probable diagnosis would be that of female pseudohermaphroditism of the congenital adrenogenital syndrome type. This diagnosis is to be favored, particularly if there is a well-developed phallus and scrotum, or a penis with some degree of hypospadias. An elevated urinary 17-ketosteroid and pregnanetriol excretion would be germane in establishing such a diagnosis. However, a positive chromatin pattern in a patient with unilateral cryptorchism may possibly indicate true hermaphroditism. In other words, what appears to be an undescended testicle may well be an ovary or ovarian anlage.

The abdominal gonad in such individuals could not be expected to respond to chorionic gonadotropin therapy as would the scrotal gonad. If the abdominal organ is an undescended Klinefelter's testis, because of normal Leydig cell function it would be as responsive to gonadotropic hormone therapy as any cryptorchid testis in a chromatin negative patient. Since one must determine the presence or absence of a possible ovarian anlage, plus the fact that degeneration of the interstitial elements as well as tubular structures will develop with the ever-present malignant potential of the intra-abdominal testis, it would be wise to have a laparotomy performed and to remove the gonad, regardless of whether it can or cannot be brought down successfully. The reason for this is that gametogenic function is unlikely and androgenic function of the organ could be readily substituted by the administration of the androgens cited above. The indication for surgery (orchiopexy), which is normally advised to aid normal spermatogenesis, would appear to be nil in this case. The same logic and therapeutic approach would also apply to the bilateral cryptorchid Klinefelter's syndrome.

The foregoing discussion has been concerned with a description of the interrelationships existing between the pituitary gland and the testes.

A definite and positive approach is recommended for treatment of the hypogonadal prepubertal or pubertal male. The advantages of such therapy have been extolled and x-ray evidence for the lack of any specific acceleration effect on bone maturation or epiphyseal closure has been offered. The need for a positive approach to the treatment of the cryptorchid male has been discussed. Other problems concerned specifically with the adult hypogonadal male will be described in Chapter 17 on the diagnosis and management of the male climacteric, Klinefelter's syndrome, and gynecomastia.

References

1. ASHBEL, R., COHEN, R. B., AND SELIGMAN, A. M.: Histochemical demonstration of ketosteroids in normal and neoplastic testes. Endocrinology 49:265-281, 1951.

2. CAFFEY, J.: Pediatric X-ray Diagnosis, 3rd ed. Year Book Publishers, Inc., Chicago, 1956.

3. CHARNY, C. W., AND WOLGIN, W.: Cryptorchism. Paul B. Hoeber, Inc., New York, 1957.

4. COHN, G. L., BONDY, P. K., AND CASTIGLIONE, C.: Studies on pyrogenic steroids. I. Separation, identification, and measurement of unconjugated dehydroepiandrosterone, etiocholanolone, and androsterone in human plasma. J. Clin. Invest. 40:400-407, 1961.

5. DORFMAN, R. I., AND SHIPLEY, R. A.: Androgens: Biochemistry, Physiology and Clinical Significance. J. Wiley & Sons, Inc., New York, 1956.

6. DVOSKIN, S.: Local maintenance of spermatogenesis in hypophysectomized rats with low dosages of testosterone from intratesticular pellets. Proc. Soc. Exp. Biol. Med. 54:111-113, 1943.

7. DVOSKIN, S.: Local maintenance of spermatogenesis by intratesticularly implanted pellets of testosterone in hypophysectomized rats. Amer. J. Anat. 75:289-327, 1944.

8. ENGLE, E. T.: Experimental induced descent of testis in Macacus monkey by hormones from anterior pituitary and pregnancy urine. Endocrinology 16:513-520, 1932.

9. ENGSTROM, W. W., AND MUNSON, P. L.: Continued studies on metabolism of testosterone in normal women in different phases of menstrual cycle. J. Clin. Endocr. 11:427-433, 1951.

10. FENNELL, R. H.: Endocrine pathology of the male reproductive system. In Velardo, J.: Essentials of Human Reproduction. Oxford University Press, Inc., New York, 1958, pp. 234-262.

11. FRAME, E. G., FLEISCHMANN, W., AND WILKINS, L.: Influence of a number of androgenic steroids on urinary excretion of neutral 17-ketosteroids. Bull. Johns Hopkins Hosp. 75:95-101, 1944.

12. GALLAGHER, T. F., BRADLOW, H. L., FUKUSHIMA, D. K., BEER, C. T., KRITCHEVSKY, T. H., STOKEM, M., EDINOFF, M. L., HELLMAN, L., AND DOBRINER, K.: Studies on the metabolites of isotopic steroid hormones in man. Recent Progr. Hormone Res. 9:411-434, 1954.

13. GOULD, W. L.: The male climacteric, report of a series of 120 cases using fortified gonadotropic hormone. Med. Times 79:154-161, 1951.

14. GOULD, W. L.: A new therapeutic approach to aging. Clin. Med. 4:865, 1957.

15. GOULD, W. L., AND STROSBERG, I.: Male senility, report of a series of 237 cases using the new fortified gonadotropin. Med. Times 79:622-628, 1951.

16. GREENBLATT, R. B., AND KUPPERMAN, H. S.: Further studies on the control of menorrhagia. J. Clin. Endocr. 6:675-687, 1946.

17. HAMILTON, J. B.: Male hormone substance: Prime factor in acne. J. Clin. Endocr. 1:570-592, 1941.

18. HELLER, C. G., AND NELSON, W. O.: The testis-pituitary relationship in man. Recent Progr. Hormone Res. 3:229-255, 1948.

19. HELLMAN, L., BRADLOW, H. L., ZUMOFF, B., FUKUSHIMA, D. K., AND GALLAGHER, T. F.: Thyroid-androgen interrelations and the hypocholesteremic effect of androsterone. J. Clin. Endocr. 19:936-948, 1959.

20. HERTZ, R., AND MEYER, R. K.: Effect of testosterone, testosterone propionate and dehydroandrosterone on secretion of gonadotropic complex as evidenced in parabiotic rats. Endocrinology 21:756-761, 1937.

21. JOST, A.: Hormone factors in the development of the fetus. The mammalian fetus: Physiologic aspects of development. Cold Spring Harbor Symp. Quant. Biol. 19:167-181, 1954.

22. JOST, A.: The role of fetal hormones in prenatal development. Harvey Lect. 55: 201-226, 1959-60.

23. KAPPAS, A., HELLMAN, L., FUKUSHIMA, D. K., AND GALLAGHER, T. F.: Pyrogenic effect of etiocholanolone. J. Clin. Endocr. 17:451-452, 1957.

24. KAPPAS, A., HELLMAN, L., FUKUSHIMA, D. K., AND GALLAGHER, T. F.: The thermogenic effect and metabolic fate of etiocholanolone in man. J. Clin. Endocr. 18: 1043-1055, 1958.

25. KLINEFELTER, H. F., JR., REIFENSTEIN, E. C., JR., AND ALBRIGHT, F.: Syndrome characterized by gynecomastia, aspermatogenesis, without A-Leydigism, and increased excretion of follicle-stimulating hormone. J. Clin. Endocr. 2:615-627, 1942.

26. KOCHAKIAN, C. D.: The role of hydrolytic enzymes in some of the metabolic activities of steroid hormones. Recent Progr. Hormone Res. 1:177-214, 1946.

27. KOETS, P.: The excretion of 17-ketosteroids in idiopathic hirsutism. J. Clin. Endocr. 9:795-800, 1949.

28. KUPPERMAN, H. S.: Hormones, Sex. In Ellis, Albert (ed.): Encyclopedia of Sexual Behavior. Hawthorn Books, New York, 1961.

29. KUPPERMAN, H. S., ARONSON, S. G., GAGLIANI, J., PARSONNET, M., ROBERTS, M., SILVER, B., AND POSTIGLIONE, R.: The value of various laboratory procedures in the comparative study of the duration of action of androgen. Acta Endocr. (Kbh.) 16:101-117, 1954.

30. KUPPERMAN, H. S., AND EPSTEIN, J. A.: Hormonal therapy versus watchful waiting in hypogonadism: The male. J. Amer. Geriat. Soc. 6:87-98, 1958.

31. KUPPERMAN, H. S., AND STUDDIFORD, W. E.: Endocrine therapy in gynecologic disorders. Postgrad. Med. 14:410-425, 1953.

32. LANMAN, J. T.: The adrenal fetal zone: Its occurrence in primates and a possible relationship to chorionic gonadotropin. Endocrinology 61:684-691, 1957.

33. LANMAN, J. T., AND DINERSTEIN, J.: The adrenotropic action of human pregnancy plasma. Endocrinology 64:494-502, 1959.

34. LEVIN, L.: The occurrence of α-estradiol in the urine of stallions: Its identification and isolation. J. Biol. Chem. 178:229-240, 1949.

35. LLOYD, C. W., AND WILLIAMS, R. H.: Endocrine changes associated with Laennec's cirrhosis of the liver. Amer. J. Med. 4:315-330, 1948.

36. LUDWIG, D. J.: Effect of androgens on spermatogenesis. Endocrinology 46:453-481, 1950.

37. MADDOCK, W. O., EPSTEIN, M., AND NELSON, W. O.: The assay of urinary estrogen as a test of human Leydig cell function. Ann. N. Y. Acad. Sci. 55:657-673, 1952.

38. MADDOCK, W. O., AND NELSON, W. O.: The effects of chorionic gonadotropin in adult men: Increased estrogen and 17-ketosteroid excretion, gynecomastia, Leydig cell stimulation and seminiferous tubule damage. J. Clin. Endocr. 12:985-1014, 1952.

39. McCULLAGH, D. R.: Dual endocrine activity of the testes. Science 76:19-20, 1932.

40. McCULLAGH, D. R., AND WALSH, E. L.: Experimental hypertrophy and atrophy of the prostate gland. Endocrinology 19:466-470, 1935.

41. McCULLAGH, E. P., AND HRUBY, F. J.: Testis-pituitary interrelationship. The relative inability of testosterone to reduce urinary gonadotropin in eunuchoid men. J. Clin. Endocr. 9:113-125, 1949.

42. MEYER, R. K., AND HERTZ, R.: Effect of oestrone on secretion of gonadotropic complex as evidenced in parabiotic rats. Amer. J. Physiol. 120:232-237, 1937.

43. NATHANSON, I. T., ENGEL, L. L., KELLEY, R. M., EKMAN, G., SPAULDING, K. H., AND ELLIOTT, J.: Effect of androgens on urinary excretion of ketosteroids, non-ketonic alcohols and estrogens. J. Clin. Endocr. 12:1172-1186, 1952.

44. NELSON, W. O.: Re-initiation of spermatogenesis in hypophysectomized rats. Amer. J. Physiol. 129:430-431, 1940.

45. PASCHKIS, K. E., CANTAROW, A., RAKOFF, A. E., HANSEN, L., AND WALKING, A. A.: Excretion in dogs of androgens, and estrogens in bile following injections of androgens. Proc. Soc. Exp. Biol. Med. 55:127-130, 1944.

46. PASCHKIS, K. E., RAKOFF, A. E., AND CANTAROW, A.: Clinical Endocrinology, 2nd ed. Paul B. Hoeber, Inc., New York, 1958, pp. 607-609.

47. REIFENSTEIN, E. C., JR., FORBES, A. P., ALBRIGHT, F., DONALDSON, E., AND CARROLL, E.: Effect of methyltestosterone on urinary 17-ketosteroids of adrenal origin. J. Clin. Invest. 24:416-434, 1945.

48. RUBIN, B. L., DORFMAN, R. I., AND MILLER, M.: Androgen excretion in human bile. Endocrinology 51:463-468, 1952.

49. RUBIN, D.: The question of an aqueous hormone from the testicle. Endocrinology 29:281-287, 1941.

50. SELYE, H.: On the protective action of testosterone against the kidney damaging effect of sublimate. J. Pharmacol. Exp. Ther. 68:454-457, 1940.

51. SELYE, H., AND FRIEDMAN, S. M.: Animal experiments concerning the hormonal therapy of testicular atrophy. Amer. J. Med. Sci. 201:886-894, 1941.

52. SMITH, P. E.: Maintenance and restoration of spermatogenesis in hypophysectomized rhesus monkeys by androgen administration. Yale J. Biol. Med. 17:281-287, 1944.

53. SOHVAL, A. R.: The anatomy and endocrine physiology of the male reproductive system. In Velardo, J.: The Endocrinology of Reproduction. Oxford University Press, Inc., New York, 1958, pp. 243-312.

54. TEILUM, G.: Estrogen-producing Sertoli cell tumors (androblastoma tubulare

lipoides) of human testis and ovary; homologous ovarian and testicular tumors. J. Clin. Endocr. 9:301-318, 1949.

55. TEILUM, G.: Oestrogen production by Sertoli cell in the etiology of benign senile hypertrophy of the human prostate. Testicular "lipoid cell ratio" and oestrogen-androgen quotient in human male. Acta Endocr. (Kbh.) 4:43-62, 1950.

56. TURNER, C. D.: General Endocrinology, 3rd ed. W. B. Saunders Company, Philadelphia, 1960.

57. VANVERTS, J.: L'ectopie inguinale du testicule n'est pas due à l'absence du gubernaculum testis. Nord. méd., Lille 12:217, 1906.

58. VIDGOFF, B., HILL, R., VEHRS, H., AND KUBIN, R.: Studies on the inhibitory hormone of the testes. II. Preparation and weight changes in the sex organs of the adult, male, white rat. Endocrinology 25:391-396, 1939.

59. WALSH, E. L., CUYLER, W. K., AND McCULLAGH, D. R.: Physiologic maintenance of male sex glands; effect of androtin on hypophysectomized rats. Amer. J. Physiol. 107:508-512, 1934.

60. WELLS, L. J., AND STATE, D.: Misconception of gubernaculum testis. Surgery 22: 502-508, 1947.

61. WILKINS, L.: The Diagnosis and Treatment of Endocrine Disorders in Childhood and Adolescence, 2nd ed. Charles C Thomas, Springfield, Ill., 1957.

62. WILKINS, L., AND FLEISCHMANN, W.: Effects of thyroid on creatine metabolism with a discussion of the mechanism of storage and excretion of creatine bodies. J. Clin. Invest. 25:360-377, 1946.

63. WILKINS, L., AND FLEISCHMANN, W.: The influence of various androgenic steroids on nitrogen balance and growth. J. Clin. Endocr. 6:383-401, 1946.

64. WOLFSON, W. Q., GUTERMAN, H. S., LEVINE, R., COHN, C., HUNT, H. D., ROSENBERG, E. F., KADOTA, L., AND TURNER, L.: An endocrine finding apparently characteristic of gout: Very low urinary 17-ketosteroid excretion with clinically normal androgenic function. J. Clin. Endocr. 9:497-513, 1949.

65. ZONDEK, B.: Oestrogenic hormone in urine of stallion. Nature 133:494, 1934.

66. ZWARENSTEIN, H.: Some aspects of the metabolism and excretion of androgens, 17-ketosteroids and oestrogens. Clin. Proc. 5:83-93, 1946.

chapter 17

The problem of decreased genital function in the adult male is similar to that in the preadolescent and adolescent youth and may cause the same psychological damage. However, in the adult there may be the additional problem of infertility which may accentuate the seriousness of the disease. Hypogonadism in the adult may be due to (1) a spontaneous onset of decreased testicular activity due either to primary testicular failure or to intrinsic testicular disease, or secondarily to selective pituitary hypogonadotropism, or (2) a carryover of the endocrinopathy responsible for hypogonadism observed during adolescence. In the adult male, hypogonadism may be classified under the several different types of gonadal insufficiency which will be discussed herein.

THE CLIMACTERIC

Male versus Female Climacteric. The question of the male climacteric and its actual designation as a clinical entity has not been agreed on nor has it been accepted by all as a specific clinical endocrinopathy. However, on the basis of various laboratory procedures and the presence of clinical stigmata, it now appears that definitive criteria may be formulated to define the syndrome designated as the male climacteric.[1-6, 9, 17, 28, 33, 34, 36] It should be emphasized that the number of patients experiencing the symptomatology attributed to the

Hypogonadism in the Adult Male

climacteric is considerably smaller in the male than in the female. In addition, it should be pointed out that, while vasomotor symptoms play such an important part in the diagnosis of the climacteric in the female, they are not so specific in the male and appear somewhat later in life than they do in the female. The sudden appearance of vasomotor symptoms associated with menstrual abnormalities emphasizes the climacteric syndrome in the female. There is nothing comparable in the male which gives the clinician such a dramatic clue pointing toward the onset of the climacteric.

Diagnosis. SYMPTOMATOLOGY. The principal symptoms of the male climacteric are nervousness, irritability, irascibility, and inability to concentrate, plus the characteristic vasomotor symptoms. These latter symptoms may be severe at night, and of such a degree as to disturb the patient's sleep. The patient lacks security and assurance, which prior to his climacteric may never have been a problem. He will also complain of angina pectoris[28] and various vague muscle aches and pains, as well as arthralgia without evident joint pathology. A most serious source of concern is the patient's diminished libido and potentia. Frequently, he is unable to achieve an erection readily, and when it does occur, usually it cannot be maintained. The patient tends to be less positive and forceful in his usual daily duties. He appears to lack the drive and initiative that may have characterized his behavior in the past and had been responsible for his achieving his position in his chosen profession or work.

LABORATORY FINDINGS.   Two important laboratory tests of value in establishing the diagnosis are:

1. *17-Ketosteroid excretion.*   This is usually below or at the lower limits of normal.

2. *Urinary gonadotropin (FSH) excretion.*   An increased level of excretion is invariably noted.

A third laboratory finding of diagnostic importance is a seminal fluid analysis. The male climacteric patient will usually exhibit oligospermia or azoospermia.

PHYSICAL FINDINGS.   There are no specific physical findings early in the onset of the syndrome. However, as it progresses, the testes tend to become somewhat smaller and flabby (Fig. 346) and may show varying degrees of atrophy (Figs. 346A, 347). There is usually an associated diminution in penile size (Fig. 346A). The skin may lose some of its turgidity, and a sallow complexion may prevail. Prostatic examination is not enlightening except that benign hypertrophy may be present and the residual urine volume increased. This may be due not only to the obstructive process of the prostatic enlargement itself, but also to

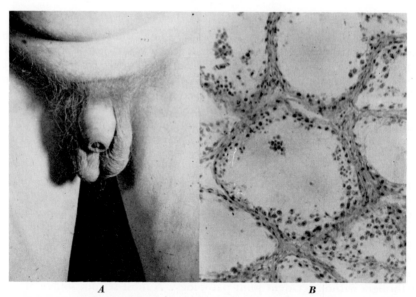

A   *B*

FIG. 346.   *A, Eunuchoidal male, age 50 years, with primary testicular atrophy associated with an elevated FSH. 17-Ketosteroids are low; gynecomastia is present. The prostate was not palpable. Note the relatively small penis and female escutcheon.*

B, Histologic section of testes of patient shown in A. Note the complete absence of spermatogenic elements. There is slight thickening of the tunica propria. Leydig cells are markedly diminished.

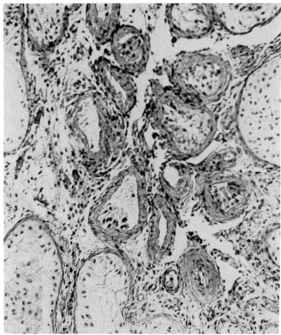

FIG. 347. Testis of a 55 year old male with low 17-ketosteroids and elevated FSH. Note the marked thickening of the tunica propria. Spermatogenic elements are absent. Sertoli cells are present. Leydig cells are decreased in number.

a decrease in the activity of the bladder muscle of Bell which is helpful in promoting efficient bladder contraction and expulsion of urine.

Therapy. When the diagnosis of the male climacteric has been made on the basis of both clinical and laboratory findings, the patient is placed upon appropriate androgenic therapy. The presence of a low 17-ketosteroid and elevated FSH would offer greater promise to the patient of a satisfactory response to therapy in contrast to poor or mediocre effects in patients with normal steroid or gonadotropin excretion.

ADVERSE EFFECTS. In considering therapy, one must keep in mind that the use of androgens is associated with the ever-present possibility of enhancing the growth of an anaplastic lesion of the prostate. While prostatic examination should precede the use of androgen therapy, there is no assurance that neoplastic lesions are not present, or could not develop, in a patient with negative prostate findings on rectal examination. Adequate precautions must be instituted and consist primarily of repeated prostatic examinations during the course of androgen therapy. The possible anaplastic-enhancing effect of androgens becomes more obvious when we realize that, in routine autopsy material, foci of anaplasia are noted in the prostate in a significant percentage of patients in whom prostatic disease was not suspected. While these lesions are silent and may remain silent, the potential effect of androgens in causing acceleration of their growth and spread must always be considered an ever-present threat.

METHOD OF THERAPY AND POSOLOGY. The therapeutic management of the male climacteric may be accomplished very readily by the use of either parenteral or oral therapy.

Parenteral Preparations:

1. Testosterone cyclopentylpropionate (Depo-Testosterone) in oil, 150.0 to 200.0 mg. every two to three weeks, will provide an excellent therapeutic effect.

2. Testosterone enanthate (Delatestryl), also an oil solution, is administered in a dose of 300.0 to 400.0 mg. every two to three weeks and will achieve the same effect.

3. Testosterone phenylacetate (Perandren phenylacetate) differs from the preceding two drugs in that it is an aqueous suspension; 150.0 to 200.0 mg. injected intramuscularly every two to three weeks will usually provide complete relief or symptomatology. It may be used in patients sensitive to oil solutions.

There is no question that these parenteral preparations are the ones of choice and are associated with minimal or no significant side effects. On the other hand neither testosterone propionate in oil nor an aqueous suspension of free testosterone, although well tolerated is now of little clinical value because the short-lived action of both drugs requires repeated and frequent administration. An aqueous suspension of testosterone propionate, while having a prolonged effect equal to that noted with the recommended preparations above, induces so much irritation at the site of injection (as well as sterile abscesses, induration, inflammatory changes, and febrile responses), that its use is specifically contraindicated.

Pellet Implantation. Pellet implantation may also be used as an effective means of maintaining patients with hypogonadism in an adequate physiologic state over prolonged periods of time. The usual procedure involves implantation of nine 75.0 mg. pellets of testosterone into the subcutaneous tissue of the subscapular area or the inguinal region. Hormonal effects due to implantation of pellets will usually persist for a period of six to nine months. However, there has been less need for such a regimen in recent years since the duration of action of the long-acting intramuscular preparations has been prolonged to such a degree that infrequent administration is required.

Oral Preparations. Oral therapy may also be employed, using methyltestosterone or fluoxymesterone. Both of these preparations are alpha-methylated, synthetic androgenic compounds which, unlike free testosterone or its esters, are effective when administered orally. A positive effect is noted fairly promptly when the following dose schedule is employed:

Fluoxymesterone (Halotestin, Ultandren), 5.0 mg. t.i.d. to q.i.d.
Methyltestosterone (Oreton M), 10.0 to 20.0 mg. t.i.d. to q.i.d.

JAUNDICE. Because methyltestosterone may induce jaundice[7-9, 20, 31, 35] through interference with biliary pigment transport and metabolism by the liver, fluoxymesterone, the 9-alpha fluorinated derivative, may be the preparation of choice. To date, there have been no reported cases of jaundice associated with its use. For equal effects, much more of the methylated but nonfluorinated testosterone must be administered than of the fluorinated compound, and the size of dose of the methyltestosterone may be the reason for its occasional association with jaundice. The increase in bilirubin levels usually is accompanied by a decreased BSP excretion, but with normal cephalin flocculation, thymol turbidity, total protein, and A/G ratio. These findings point toward a defect in biliary pigment transportation rather than to hepatic cellular disease. When hyperbilirubinemia occurs, it is usually only transitory and invariably reverts to normal when the medication is discontinued.

Oral versus Parenteral Administration. While it is difficult to quantitate the therapeutic response, we have found that the parenteral preparations appear to be more effective than the oral ones. This, perhaps, may be attributed in part to the psychosomatic effects of administering a drug by injection, or to the use of an inadequate dose of the oral preparation.

Another advantage of the parenteral preparations is that they appear to have a better anabolic effect. Indeed, methyltestosterone actually induces an increased creatine output which may be associated with increased muscle catabolism.

Linguet Administration. Our own experience with linguet medication has indicated that it is a relatively unpredictable form of treatment. While the theoretical advantages are plausible—i.e., the steroid being absorbed via the oral mucosa and bypassing liver inactivation—the practical aspects are somewhat different. Enough of the material is swallowed through the process of salivation so that inactivation occurs in much the same manner that it would if the preparation were swallowed *in toto.* Secondly, the taste of the sublingual preparation has generally been found to be objectionable so that there has been sufficient patient resistance to this mode of therapy.

THERAPEUTIC TEST WITH PLACEBOS. Since many of the symptoms for which the hypogonadal male is treated are subjective in nature and difficult to evaluate, and since therapy must be administered over a prolonged period of time, the clinician should eliminate the possible psychosomatic effects of oral or parenteral medication by noting the patient's response to a placebo. It is pointless to continue the active androgen if a placebo will accomplish the same effect. Indeed, a therapeutic test with a placebo is an additional diagnostic procedure that can be employed to substantiate the presence of a true endocrine deficiency or to uncover the psycho-

somatic aspects of a "placebo responder." An equivalent response to
both the androgen and the placebo would raise some question as to
the need for androgen therapy and the existence of a deficiency syndrome.

EUNUCHOIDISM

Primary or Secondary Gonadal Failure.   The eunuchoidal individual
may have primary or secondary gonadal failure; that is, the diminished or
absent testicular function is due to either (1) primary testicular failure
(Figs. 348, 349) or (2) selective pituitary gonadotropic insufficiency
(Figs. 350-353). These may be differentiated one from the other not only
by the clinical appearance of the patient in certain select examples, but
also by appropriate laboratory and functional tests.

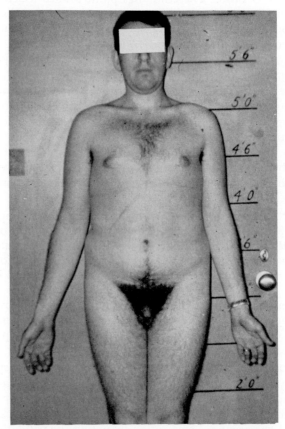

FIG. 348.   Patient HK, male, age 27½ years, with primary testicular failure. Weight 195, height 71½ inches, span 76½ inches, azoospermia, FSH = 105 mouse units per 24 hours, 17-ketosteroids = 10.2
mg. per 24 hours, chromatin negative. Note the small phallus and
the tendency for eunuchoidal build.

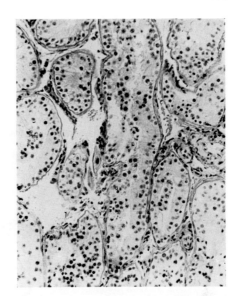

FIG. 349. Patient G, age 23 years, with primary testicular failure associated with a high FSH and low 17-ketosteroid excretion. Seminiferous tubules contain Sertoli cells. Patient is chromatin negative.

FIG. 350. Patient JN, age 32 years, weight 152½ pounds, height 71 inches, span 74 inches, with hypogonadotropic hypogonadism. FSH less than 6.6 mouse units per 24 hours, 17-ketosteroids 15.2 mg. per 24 hours; chromatin pattern is negative. Note the tall eunuchoidal build, female escutcheon, and diminution of bodily hair.

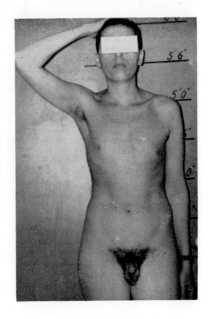

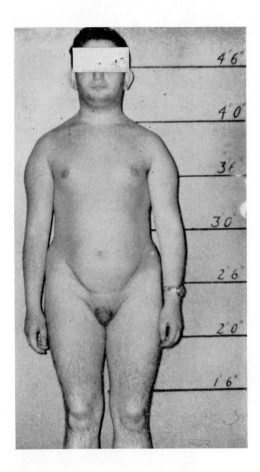

FIG. 351. Patient GE, age 25 years, weight 111½ pounds, height 56¾ inches, span 56 inches, with hypogonadotropic hypogonadism. Patient had received intensive therapy with androgens followed by premature epiphyseal closure. Note the hypoplastic genitalia.

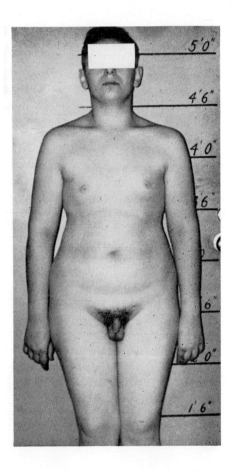

FIG. 352A. Patient AM, age 18 years, with hypogonadotropic hypogonadism. Height 61¾ inches, span 65 inches, weight 140½ pounds. FSH less than 6.6 mouse units per 24 hours. 17-Ketosteroids 17.8 mg. per 24 hours. Note the eunuchoidal build and the hypoplasia of the external genitalia.

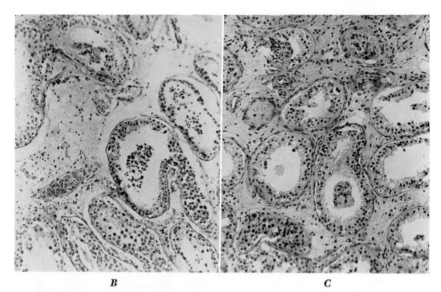

B   C

FIG. 352. B, Testicular biopsy of patient AM shown in Figure 352A. Note the atrophy of the spermatogenic elements of the tubules. The tunica propria is not thickened. Leydig cells are significantly diminished in number.

C, Biopsy of opposite testis. Note essentially the same morphology as that described for Figure 352B.

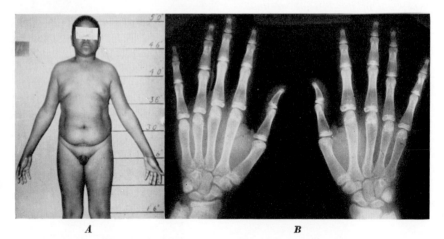

A   B

FIG. 353. A, Patient AC, age 27 years, weight 115 pounds, height 59½ inches, span 62 inches. 17-Ketosteroids 4.9 mg. per 24 hours, FSH less than 6.6 mouse units per 24 hours, chromatin negative. Note the marked hypoplasia of the gonads, short stature, and immature appearance. Clinical picture is one of decreased pituitary activity.

B, X-rays of patient AC, shown in Figure 353A. Note the open epiphyses, which is most unusual for a patient of this age. Prognosis for growth is good.

DIFFERENTIAL RESPONSE TO GONADOTROPIC HORMONE THERAPY. One such functional test is the positive response of the patients with pituitary failure to the exogenous administration of gonadotropic hormone. Administration of pregnant mare's serum, 500 I.U. three times per week (t.i.w.) for six weeks, to the adult male with hypogonadism would theoretically increase the sperm count without materially affecting 17-ketosteroid excretion. On the other hand, human chorionic gonadotropin (HCG), 2000 I.U. t.i.w. for six weeks, enhances 17-ketosteroid output associated with clinical evidence of increased androgenic function. In addition, elevation of estrogenic excretion may be noted as a result of stimulation of the Leydig cells which appear to be bipotential in their response to gonadotropin; i.e., they may be stimulated to secrete both androgenic and estrogenic precursors. Patients with primary testicular failure or agenesis will show no evidence of a clinical or ketosteroid response to chorionic gonadotropin. The use of human pituitary gonadotropin would also provide the physician with an effective preparation for differentiating between primary and secondary testicular failure. Unfortunately, the use of this material is still limited so that it is relatively unavailable for either therapeutic or diagnostic purposes. Its advantage over the pregnant mare's gonadotropin is that the likelihood for antihormone formation with continued or prolonged use of the human material is highly improbable.

CLINICAL DIFFERENCES. Clinically, there may be another differentiating point—the patient with testicular failure will always appear eunuchoidal (Fig. 354) (as described below) in contrast to the variable

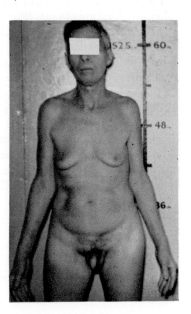

FIG. 354. Patient SR, age 62 years, with primary testicular failure. Note the gynecomastia and the hypoplasia of the gonads together with the typical eunuchoidal picture.

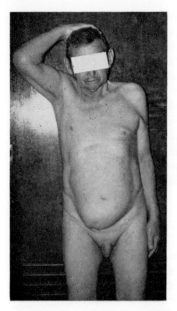

FIG. 355. Patient JK, age 53 years, with pan-hypopituitarism. Note the hypoplasia of the gonads with the complete absence of body hair. The eunuchoidal picture has been altered by the pan-hypopituitarism.

picture that may be presented in the patient with gonadotropic insufficiency. If there is selective gonadotropic insufficiency, one would anticipate the same clinical picture as noted in primary gonadal failure. However, if there were also other tropic insufficiencies, then the stigmata of these deficiencies would be prevalent with the eunuchoidal habitus being minimal or absent (Fig. 355).

Iatrogenic testicular failure may be induced in a male by the administration of large doses of estrogen. The histologic appearance of the testes would be akin to that noted in hypopituitary gonadotropism due to suppression of pituitary gonadotropin by the exogenous estrogen. Such a picture was seen in a transvestite who took large doses of stilbestrol in an attempt to feminize his figure (Fig. 356).

Clinical and Laboratory Features. The clinical stigmata of a eunuchoidal male are (1) absence of beard and bodily hair growth, (2) feminine-type habitus with narrow shoulders and wide hips, (3) span greatly exceeding his height, (4) small penis, (5) little or no prostatic development, and (6) atrophic testes. In addition, laboratory findings are (1) low 17-ketosteroids, (2) high urinary gonadotropin if he has primary testicular failure, or (3) a low urinary gonadotropin if he has selective pituitary gonadotropin failure.

Gynecomastia may be present in the male with primary testicular failure (Fig. 354) but is rarely seen in patients with selective gonadotropic insufficiency.

Therapy.   Regardless of the primary or secondary nature of the patient's disease, he will require the same therapy as outlined for the climacteric male.

Therapy will usually correct the loss of potentia and cause some growth of facial and body hair. It will tend to increase muscle mass and, to a certain extent, reverse the feminine type of habitus. The relationship of span to height will not be altered unless the epiphyses are open. In this case, there will be some reduction in eunuchoidal build, as well as an increase in penile size. As a rule, patients with closed epiphyses will show little, if any, penile growth in response to androgen therapy, regardless of the degree of hypoplasia of the penis (Fig. 357).

GONADOTROPIN VERSUS ANDROGEN THERAPY.   While the use of gonadotropic hormone in patients with pituitary insufficiency is, theoretically, the correct approach, it would be impractical because of the need for repeated parenteral administration. In addition, parenteral administration of gonadotropins prepared from sources foreign to the human body may lead to antihormone formation. This would tend to nullify any benefit the gonad-stimulating treatment might have and, indeed, eventually it would inhibit endogenous pituitary gonadotropin. The use of human pituitary gonadotropin, when available in adequate amounts, would be helpful in restoring testicular function in those males with selective gonadotropic insufficiency.

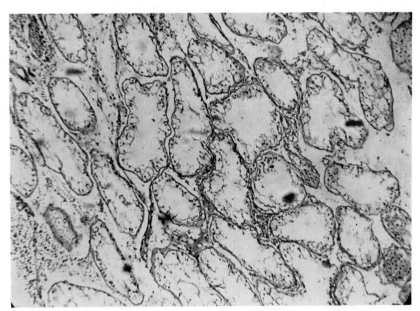

FIG. 356. Testicular biopsy of patient receiving high doses of stilbestrol. Note the complete distortion of the cyto-architecture of the testes.

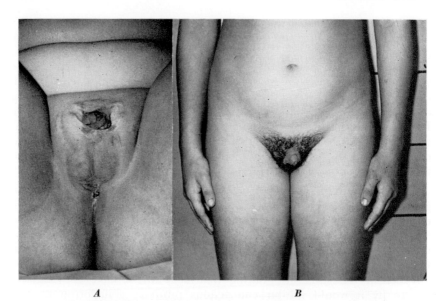

A   B

**FIG. 357. Patient MC. A, Age 10 years, height 55 inches, span 56 inches.
Note the indifferent external genitalia with an unusually small penis and scars
due to numerous operations for hypospadias. The patient failed to respond to
comparatively large doses of HCG. B, Same patient at the age of 12 years. Height
is 63 inches, span 63½ inches. Patient has had appropriate therapy with androgens. Note the increase of pubic hair and the marked enlargement of the phallus,
albeit still hypoplastic.**

NEED FOR ANDROGEN THERAPY.   The futility of gonadotropic therapy
is illustrated in patient MC (Figs. 357A and B), in whom administration of human chorionic gonadotropin (HCG) failed to achieve any
satisfactory response. This patient, who had indifferent genitalia as an
infant and was chromatin negative, was reared as a boy despite the
fact that he had a third-degree hypospadias and bilateral cryptorchid and
hypoplastic testes. Figure 357A reveals the negligible response noted
after repeated use of large doses of HCG. Orchiopexy had been unsuccessful and resulted in the testes being almost entirely destroyed by the
operative procedures and resulting scar formation. An excellent response
to testosterone cyclopentylpropionate (Depo-Testosterone) was noted
when large doses of 150.0 mg. every seven days were administered for four
to five months (Fig. 357B). This is the only type of therapy that can be
used in this patient in order to achieve some measure of success as far
as penile length and development of the secondary sexual characteristics
are concerned.

NEED FOR THERAPY IN THE YOUNG PRE-ADULT.   On the other hand, hypogonadism may be noted in a male who had previously been treated as a youth with good response. One such patient is depicted in Figures 358A, B, C. Figure 358A depicts the state of gonadal development prior to treatment.

HCG THERAPY.   The excellent response to the initial and standard dose of HCG is well demonstrated in Fig. 358B. However, five years later, without additional therapy in the interim, there was no further advancement of genital development (Fig. 358C). Consequently, he was found to be in need of another course of HCG. This patient exemplifies very well the concept that watchful waiting would have been ill advised since his initial response to exogenous gonadotropins was not implemented by his own endogenous gonadotropins in the following four to five years. The spontaneous development anticipated by the therapeutic nihilist has not taken place. In contrast, patient EW, shown in Figure 359, responded well after an initial course of HCG and continued to show good additional development and progress without further treatment.

It is interesting to note the clinical state of patient DG, shown in Figure 360, which is precisely the same as that of patient LA prior to treatment (Fig. 358A). In view of our experience with patient LA, we will definitely insist upon immediate HCG treatment for patient DG in order to prevent hypogonadism as an adult. There will be no therapeutic procrastination or "watchful waiting."

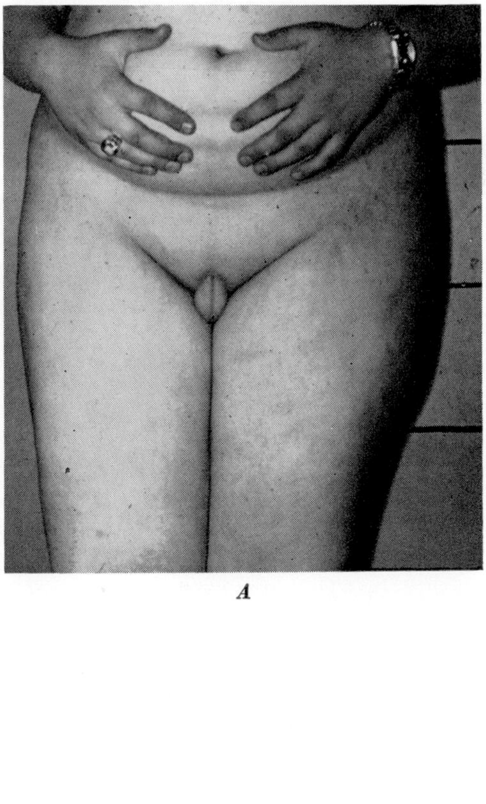

FIG. 358A. Patient LA, age 13 years, height 62¼ inches, weight 167¾ pounds. Note marked hypoplasia of the gonads with female fat distribution.

A

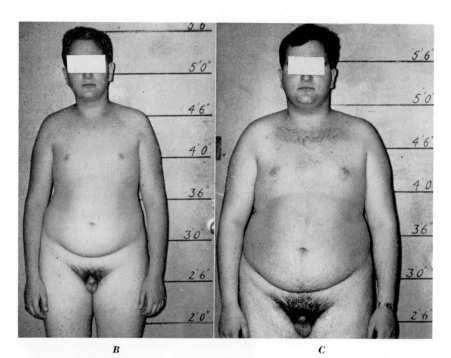

B   C

FIG. 358. *B, Same patient as shown in Figure 358A, 1 year later, after a single course of chorionic gonadotropin as recommended in the text. Note the excellent response as far as testicular size is concerned, with the testes and the penis still being hypoplastic.*

C, Five years after Figure 358B was photographed. Note no further progress in size of either penis or testes; thus, the increase in size achieved after 1 year was not followed by further progression. There has been no resumption of gonadal stimulation; thus, the patient would have had unusually hypoplastic genitalia if therapy had not been instituted earlier. Waiting for spontaneous maturation would have been disastrous.

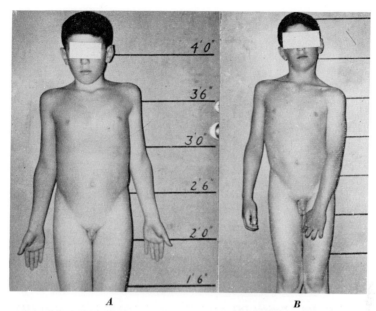

FIG. 359. Patient EW. A, Age 11 years, prior to gonadotropic therapy. Height 53¼ inches. Note hypoplasia of the gonads.

B, Age 11½ years, height 54¼ inches. Note excellent response to HCG.

FIG. 359C. Patient EW, shown in Figures 359A and B, age 13-2/3 years, height 60 inches. Note continued growth of phallus and development without further HCG therapy. Not infrequently, an initial course of therapy will be followed by such continued improvement in genital development.

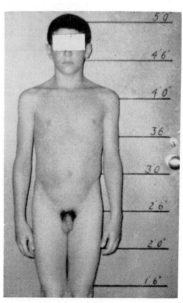

C

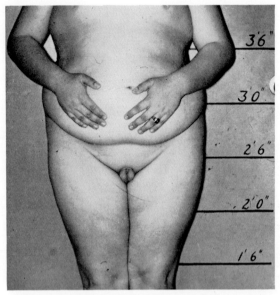

FIG. 360. Patient DG, age 14¾ years, height 61 inches, span 62¼ inches, weight 189½ pounds. FSH less than 6.6 mouse units per 24 hours, 17-ketosteroids 9.6 mg. per 24 hours. Note the marked hypoplasia of the gonads, very similar to the patient shown in Figure 358. This patient is an ideal candidate for therapy with HCG to thwart hypogonadism as an adult. Watchful waiting and withholding gonadotropic therapy in such a patient, in light of our experience, would be most unwise.

KLINEFELTER'S SYNDROME

Diagnostic Criteria. Klinefelter's syndrome, or gonadal dysgenesis, in the male is an unusual and interesting clinical entity first described by Klinefelter, Reifenstein, and Albright in 1941[23] and later elaborated upon by others.[11-13] The syndrome, as originally discussed, was characterized by:

1. High FSH excretion.

2. Azoospermia with hyalinization of the seminiferous tubules without absence or diminution of Leydig cells (Fig. 361). The testicular picture is said to be characteristic of the syndrome.[30] However, this may not be so since the testicular cyto-architecture may vary from one with only absence of the spermatogenic cells to hyalinization of all tubular elements and, indeed, to complete distortion of the testicular morphology, so that the tissue can not be recognized as of testicular origin (Figs. 362-364).

3. Usually, a normal 17-ketosteroid and 17-hydroxysteroid excretion.

4. The presence of gynecomastia in the majority of the patients (Figs. 365-368) (or, if absent, not infrequently one sees areolar accentuation [Fig. 369]).

5. Normal estrogen excretion (despite the gynecomastia that may be present).

6. A tendency for eunuchoidal build with increased fat distribution in the trochanteric areas (Figs. 365-367).

7. Some degree of impotence in most of the patients (Fig. 370).

CHROMATIN PATTERN. More recently, it has been shown that this syndrome may be easily identified by determining the chromatin pattern of the patient.[15-24] Indeed, early recognition of the syndrome can be obtained in the infant or the very young male by a study of the chromatin pattern before any of the classic clinical stigmata are noted.[4, 5, 24] In general: (1) Most patients are chromatin positive (gonadal dysgenesis); (2) however, some are still chromatin negative, but show the typical physical stigmata seen in the chromatin positive patient with Klinefelter's syndrome.

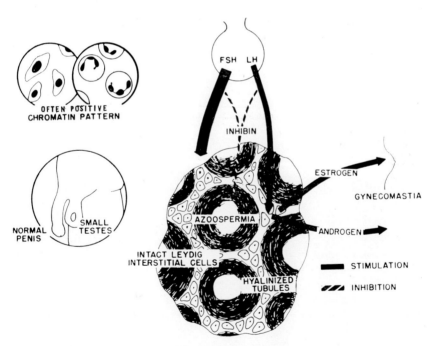

FIG. 361. Diagrammatic presentation of the physiopathology seen in patients with Klinefelter's syndrome.

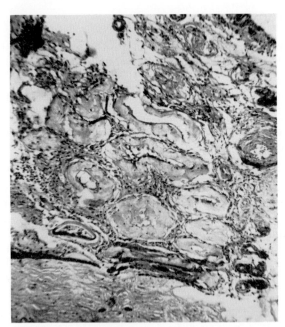

FIG. 362. Testes of a chromatin positive patient with Klinefelter's syndrome. Note the complete destruction of tubular elements and their replacement by hyalinization. Leydig cells appear
normal.

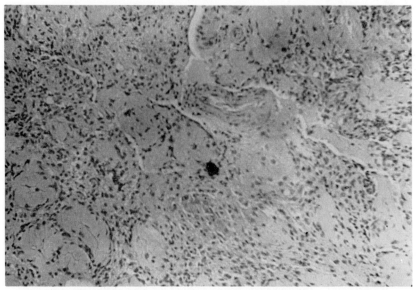

FIG. 363. Testes of patient KM, who was chromatin positive. Note almost
complete distortion of testicular cyto-architecture with the testicular structure
still being recognizable. The tubular hyalinization is marked. The Leydig
cells appear to be increased in number.

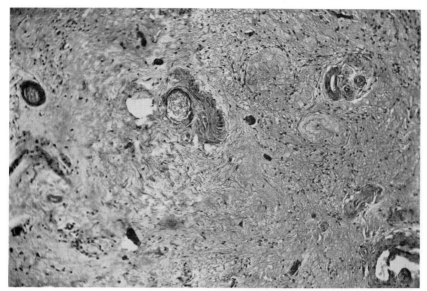

FIG. 364. Testes of patient N, having positive chromatin pattern. Note the complete distortion of testicular cyto-architecture so that it is difficult to recognize the tissue as being of testicular origin. Hyalinization of some tubules may be seen.

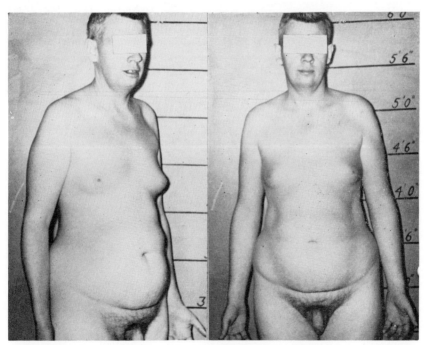

FIG. 365. Patient US, age 36 years, positive chromatin pattern. Note the eunuchoidal build, gynecomastia, and female fat distribution. A female escutcheon is present.

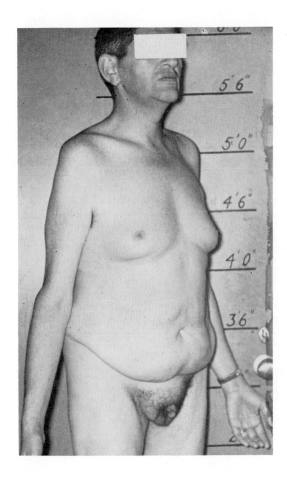

FIG. 366. Patient WG, age
53 years, chromatin positive.
Normal FSH, low 17-keto-
steroids. Note the gynecomastia, female fat distribution, and genital hypoplasia.

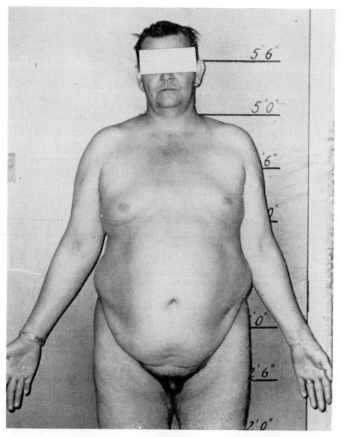

FIG. 367. Patient JL, age 48 years, chromatin positive. Note obesity, female escutcheon and hypoplasia of the gonads. Libido said to be adequate.

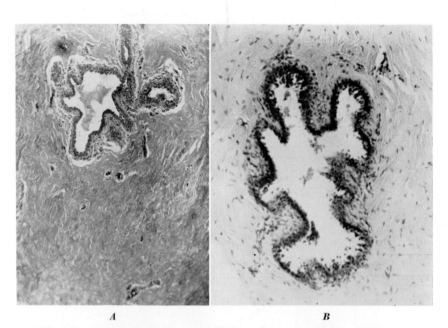

A   B

FIG. 368. *A and B, Biopsy of breast of chromatin positive patients with Klinefelter's syndrome. Note the marked stimulation of glandular elements with little effect on the stroma.*

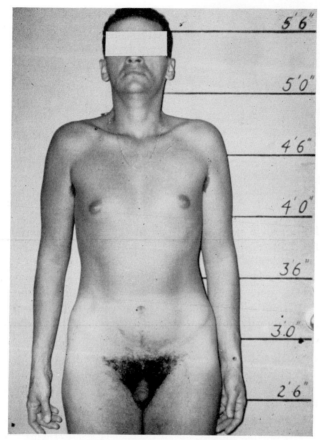

FIG. 369.   Patient AV, age 34 years, chromatin positive. Increased
FSH excretion. Note the general muscular build with normal phallus.
Note areolar accentuation without true gynecomastia.

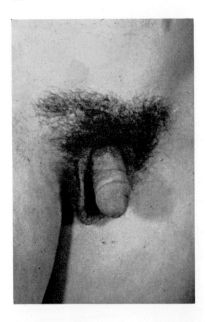

FIG. 370. Patient ML, age 25 years, chromatin positive, elevated FSH. Note the normal phallus but the complete absence of detectable scrotal testes. On palpation the testes were represented by two small fibrotic, pea-like structures.

The finding of a positive chromatin pattern in a phenotypic male establishes the diagnosis of Klinefelter's syndrome. However, a negative chromatin individual with azoospermia, tubular hyalinization, and normal Leydig cells in a male with high FSH and normal 17-ketosteroid excretion, with or without gynecomastia, would also be classified in the same syndrome. The patient with the positive chromatin pattern may be described as one of gonadal dysplasia with seminiferous tubular dysgenesis or testicular dysplasia.

CLASSIC CLINICAL STIGMATA. Clinically, the diagnosis may also be suspected in a phenotypic male whose testes are unusually small and firm. The penis in these individuals is invariably normal (Fig. 370) or on the smaller side of normal (Fig. 371A). When such a paradoxical combination exists in a normal or eunuchoidal male with or without gynecomastia, Klinefelter's syndrome should be suspected (Figs. 371-379). Not infrequently, general physical inspection, not including the genitalia, would fail to disclose any evidence of the syndrome since some patients with testicular dysplasia are perfectly masculine in their outward appearance and show a male escutcheon accompanied by adequate potentia and libido (Figs. 380, 381). Indeed, in some the penis may be inordinately enlarged (Fig. 381) despite considerable hypoplasia of the testes. The chromatin pattern should be obtained in a male with azoospermia, adequate penile development and small, firm testes. A positive chromatin pattern confirms the diagnosis and points to the hopelessness

for fertility if the patient's major complaint has been failure or inability
to procreate. It should be noted, however, that Bradbury has described
the presence of sperm in serial sections of a testis obtained from a male
with Klinefelter's syndrome with a positive chromatin finding. In addition, spermatogenesis and spermatozoa have been reported in other
chromatin positive males and, indeed, sperm has been found in the
seminal fluid of several patients.[3, 12, 21] Nevertheless, the statement
still holds that a male phenotype with a positive chromatin pattern
is probably incapable of procreating. While sperm has been found in
the seminal fluid of such patients, albeit rarely, there has been no
reported case of pregnancy following insemination with such semen.

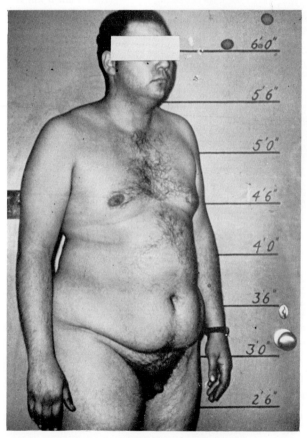

FIG. 371A. Patient ME, age 28 years, weight 300 pounds, height 73¾
inches, chromatin positive, normal FSH. Note the obesity, but in general
a masculine-like habitus. Body hair is normal.

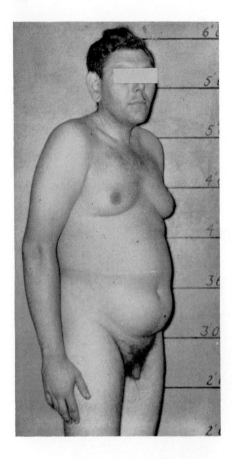

FIG. 371B. Patient WB, age 32 years, weight 203 pounds, chromatin negative. Patient has Klinefelter's syndrome with azoospermia and gynecomastia. FSH = 52 mouse uits per 24 hours, 17-ketosteroids = 8.4 mg. per 24 hours.

The most constant findings in Klinefelter's syndrome are the azoospermia and the high FSH. In the rare patients with this syndrome in whom sperm may be found, however, the FSH may be low or normal. The variable characteristics or findings are:

1. A chromatin pattern that is either positive or negative, without any distinctive clinical features in either type.

2. Gynecomastia that may or may not be present and that appears to be related to the elevated FSH. (Gynecomastia is rarely, if ever, seen in eunuchoidal males with pituitary insufficiency.)

3. Diminished androgenic function that may or may not be associated with low 17-ketosteroids.

4. Eunuchoidal build that may or may not be present but is invariably noted in patients with low 17-ketosteroid excretion.

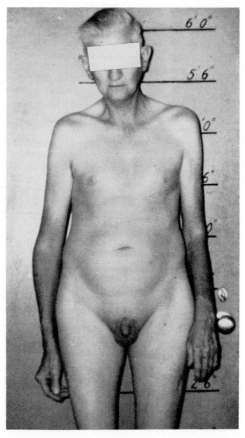

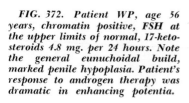

FIG. 372. Patient WP, age 56 years, chromatin positive, FSH at the upper limits of normal, 17-keto-steroids 4.8 mg. per 24 hours. Note the general eunuchoidal build, marked penile hypoplasia. Patient's response to androgen therapy was dramatic in enhancing potentia.

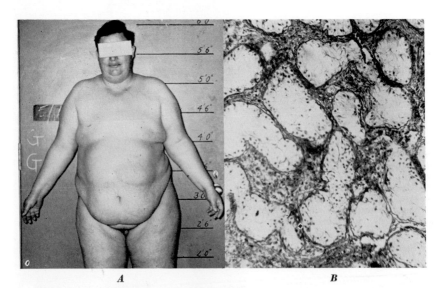

FIG. 373.   A, Patient GG, age 39 years, weight 333½ pounds, height 69¾ inches.
Chromatin positive, 17-ketosteroids 18.2 mg. per 24 hours. Note the marked obesity.
Patient has marked genital hypoplasia. His potentia is poor. B, Histologic picture
of testicular biopsy showing no evidence of tubular hyalinization. Leydig cells
appear normal.

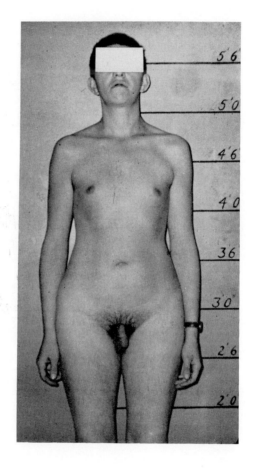

FIG. 374. Patient SC, age 28 years, chromatin positive, high FSH, low 17-ketosteroids. Note the eunuchoidal build, absence of gynecomastia, and hypoplasia of the gonads. This is the only Klinefelter patient seen who had homosexual tendencies.

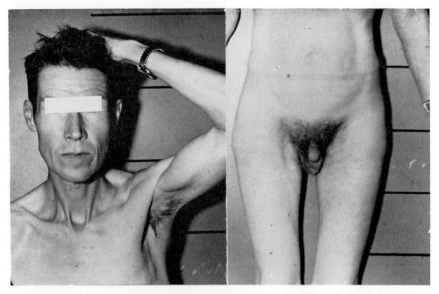

FIG. 375. Patient BS, age 48 years. Chromatin positive, elevated FSH, 17-ketosteroids 15.3 mg. per 24 hours. Note absence of facial hair, female escutcheon, the phallus at the lower limits of normal with respect to size. The testes are markedly hypoplastic.

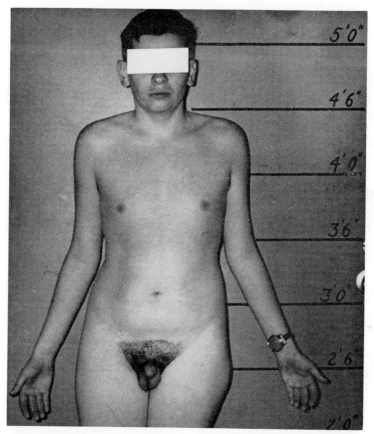

FIG. 376. Patient EM, age 20½ years, weight 114 pounds, height 61½ inches, chromatin positive. FSH = 52 mouse units per 24 hours. Note immature appearance, absence of gynecomastia, cubitus valgus and genital hypoplasia, female escutcheon with absence of facial hair.

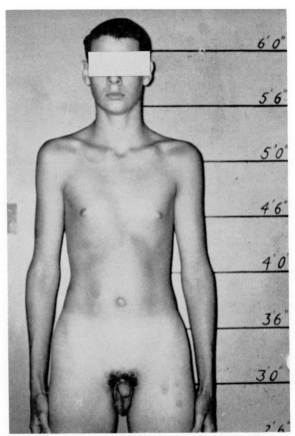

FIG. 377. Patient CO, age 17 years, chromatin positive, FSH greater than 105 mouse units per 24 hours, 17-ketosteroids 7.1 mg. per 24 hours. Note the absence of gynecomastia, the marked hypoplasia of the testes and the small phallus. The failure of secondary sex characteristics to develop has been partially corrected by administration of androgens.

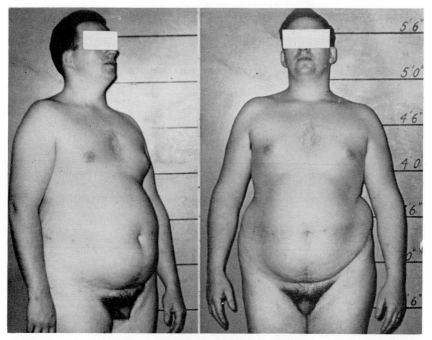

FIG. 378. *Patient DH, age 28 years, chromatin positive, FSH = 13.2 mouse units per 24 hours, 17-ketosteroids 19.3 mg. per 24 hours. Note the obesity, hypoplasia of the genitalia, but normal body hair distribution.*

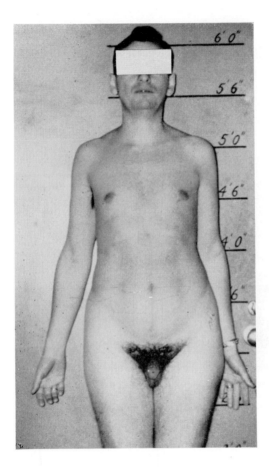

FIG. 379. Patient SW, age
34 years, weight 175 pounds,
height 71 inches, chromatin positive. Infertility problem, azoospermia. Note the tendency for
normal genitalia with a female
escutcheon.

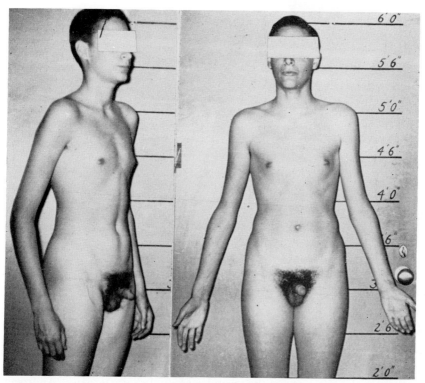

FIG. 380. Patient JC, age 20 years, chromatin positive, FSH = 105 mouse units per 24 hours, 17-ketosteroids 8.3 mg. per 24 hours. Phallus is normal. The testes are hypoplastic. Gynecomastia is absent. Patient's physical status made more masculine by administration of androgens.

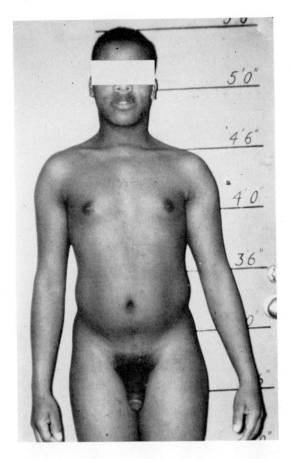

FIG. 381. Patient WN, age 20 years, weight 142 pounds, height 64¾ inches, chromatin positive. Note the well-developed phallus and the normal masculine build. The patient shows minimal gynecomastia.

Therapy. ANDROGEN.   Therapy in Klinefelter's syndrome always depends on the relative size and function of the testes and the phallus, as well as the development of the secondary sexual characteristics. Androgen therapy is indicated if there are diminished potentia and clinical manifestations of hypogonadism or testosterone insufficiency, regardless of the chromatin pattern of the patient. Such therapy when needed would be the same as that suggested for the climacteric male. However, it should be emphasized that, except for the small testes, not all males with Klinefelter's syndrome show clinical stigmata of the disease. Many of these patients have normal 17-ketosteroids and androgen therapy usually is not needed. As far as is known to date, there is no specific therapy to ameliorate the azoospermia in these patients.

Early recognition of the patient with Klinefelter's syndrome may be facilitated by a high suspicion index, carefully checking for a discrepancy between the size of the testes (small) and that of the phallus (normal), plus the finding of a positive chromatin pattern (Fig. 381). The presence of gynecomastia in a young male with poorly developed genitalia also should lead one to examine the chromatin pattern to establish if possible the presence of seminiferous tubular dysgenesis (Figs. 382-384). The urinary gonadotropin level (FSH) may not be elevated in prepubertal boys and occasionally may be normal in the adult (see Fig. 378).

Early diagnosis, then, permits initiation of appropriate therapy as a prophylaxis against the development of some of the bizarre characteristics of the syndrome.

PLASTIC REPAIR OF GYNECOMASTIA. The gynecomastia will not respond to any type of hormonal therapy and can be treated, if it is of sufficient magnitude, only by plastic surgery. Certain types of androgen therapy may actually induce or accentuate the gynecomastia. This is particularly true of orally administered methyltestosterone, although it

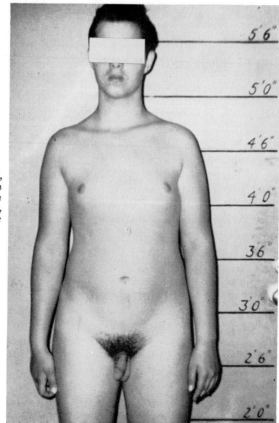

FIG. 382A. Patient GK, age 14½ years, chromatin positive. The patient has a normally developed phallus, small testes and no evidence of gynecomastia.

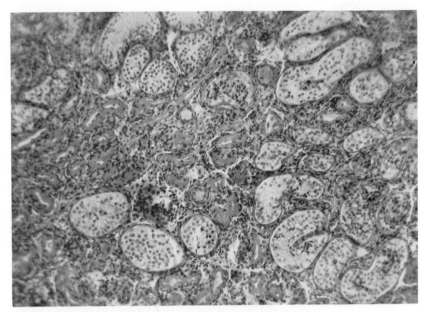

FIG. 382B. Testicular biopsy in patient GK does not show hyalinization of tubules. The only tubular elements present are Sertoli cells.

may rarely be noted after administration of parenteral testosterone or its esters.

In some patients with minimal gynecomastia, a trial course of norethandrolone may be of some value in diminishing breast size. The use of 20.0 to 30.0 mg. per day has decreased the size of the breast in some patients after three to four weeks of treatment. If there is no response within this period of time, it is useless to continue the medication. When there is marked resistance to surgery, the same medical approach may be attempted, but one should not offer the patient much hope for improvement.

The plastic procedure of choice (see Chapter 18, Gynecomastia) is one involving a subareolar semicircular incision. The glandular tissue should be removed without disturbing the anatomic relationship of areolae and nipples. A good cosmetic effect removes many of the psychological aberrations previously associated with the breast enlargement. This is particularly important in the younger male where the presence of significantly enlarged breasts serves as a serious stigma and may lead to ridicule by his peers. Fear of such derision has led to behavior problems and the discontinuance of all physical activity where disrobing is necessary. A corrective surgical procedure readily restores the patient to normal activity for one of his age. It is usually wise for the surgeon to remove enough breast tissue so that there is a concavity at the site of removal of the breast tissue. The reason for this is that, in the process of healing, fibrous tissue will fill in the depression left by removal of the glandular tissue and restore normal anatomic relationships.

Cause of Gynecomastia. The etiology of the gynecomastia does not appear to be related to the presence of increased estrogen levels. A possible mechanism for the gynecomastia has been suggested on the basis of the destruction of the tubular elements, where it is assumed that inhibin, an aqueous-soluble, nonsteroidal substance with pituitary inhibiting properties, is produced. Hyalinization of the tubules results in destruction of the elements necessary for inhibin secretion (Fig. 362)

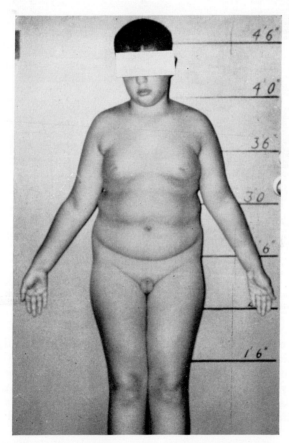

FIG. 383. *Patient DP, age 10 years, FSH greater than 105 mouse units per 24 hours. Diagnosis of Klinefelter's syndrome was suspected on the basis of hypoplasia of testes and gynecomastia, and confirmed by finding a positive chromatin pattern. Therapy with androgens will be used later to prevent eunuchoidal changes.*

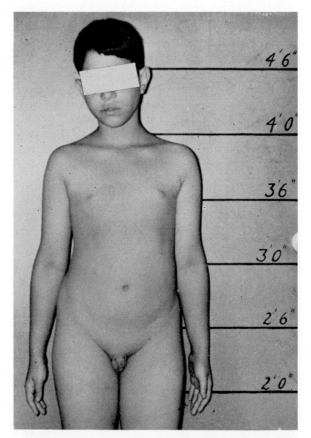

FIG. 384. Patient NC, age 9 years, chromatin positive. Note essentially normal build. While the phallus was normal in size for the
patient's age, his testes were unusually small. This was sufficient to
warrant further investigation so that a chromatin pattern was
obtained. His bone age is normal.

(possibly the Sertoli cells) so that pituitary secretion is uninhibited. This
is reflected in the high FSH excretion level these patients show. It has
been assumed that, whatever mammotropin factors may be present in
the pituitary gland, their secretion is likewise uninhibited and excessive.
The postulated excess secretion of these mammotropins may then
adversely affect the breast to produce the gynecomastia and mazoplasia.

ABNORMALITIES OF POTENTIA AND LIBIDO

Diagnosis. The endocrine management of patients with deficiency
of libido and potentia has frequently been associated with failure

or inadequate responses. Paradoxically, the female with absence or diminution of libido will usually show a more predictable response in enhancement of libido than the male after the use of androgens. Androgen therapy in the male complaining of loss of sexual drive is frequently initiated empirically without attempting to establish the presence or absence of an androgen deficiency syndrome. Consequently, the great majority of men so treated will fail to show a therapeutic response. In most, if a response *does* occur, it may be attributed to the psychosomatic effects of the administered pills or injections rather than to the physiologic effects of the preparation itself. In order to place the management of libido deficiencies in the male on a more physiologic footing, it is necessary to perform two diagnostic laboratory tests to demonstrate the presence of hypogonadism. The laboratory procedures and their interpretation are the same as those described for the male climacteric. In addition, placebo therapy alternated with the administration of active androgenic preparations, with clear demonstration of a good response to the active steroid and none or a poor response to the placebo, would also confirm the presence of an endocrine deficiency.

LABORATORY DIAGNOSIS. The laboratory procedures which establish the diagnosis of testicular insufficiency as the cause responsible for the decreased potentia include determination of 17-ketosteroid and/or urinary gonadotropin excretion levels. In addition, a seminal fluid analysis will be helpful in establishing the presence or absence of some measure of testicular failure. If the patient has a demonstrable deficiency of androgenic production by the testes the 17-ketosteroid excretion should be low while the FSH output would be increased. Similarly, beginning testicular failure will be associated with a diminished production of sperm so that the seminal fluid count would show either oligospermia or azoospermia. The failure to demonstrate any hormonal deficiency of androgens as evidenced by normal 17-ketosteroid excretion, or the failure to demonstrate diminished testicular activity as evidenced by a normal seminal fluid count and FSH assay, would make it highly improbable that the patient would show any more than a "placebo response" to replacement therapy with androgenic preparations.

PLACEBO RESPONSE. If none of the above laboratory procedures can be employed, one may then check the accuracy of the therapeutic effect of androgens by noting the response of the patient to identically administered placebo therapy. The importance of such testing cannot be overemphasized since there is such a marked psychological overlay in the patient with potentia difficulties. Except in the aged, loss of potentia in the male on a psychic basis far exceeds in incidence the loss on an endocrine deficiency basis. A good or equal response to a placebo would raise some doubt as to the validity for continued androgen treatment. On the other hand, if the active androgenic material will produce an amelioration of the specific complaint followed by a resurgence of the patient's complaints when placebo therapy is used, the physician has important clinical evidence pointing to the testes as the cause of the patient's loss of libido. Such findings would support the need for continued use of androgen therapy.

Therapy. When the diagnosis has been supported by the laboratory procedures outlined above, the same therapy as prescribed for the male climacteric may be employed. It should be emphasized, as previously noted, that the use of methyltestosterone, if prolonged and continuous, may result in some of the treated patients showing evidence of biliary stasis. This may be more prone to occur in the older than the younger age group. The advantage of the parenteral medication over the oral is that, to date, there has been no reported case of biliary stasis due to parenteral androgens.

IMPOTENCY OF PSYCHOGENIC ORIGIN. If the patient does not show the laboratory stigmata listed above, not infrequently a transitory improvement in potentia may be noted after the initial administration of androgen therapy. However, the beneficial effects will be short-lived and the patient will revert to his original complaints, thus implying the absence of testicular insufficiency. In this type of patient, there is no question that the psychiatric approach is a wise one, although here, too, such therapy is prolonged and often fraught with failure. There is little reason to expect a beneficial synergistic effect with the combined use of both psychiatric and hormonal therapy.

The sex-hormone deficiency state in the adult male readily responds to therapy when androgens are appropriately administered. Invariably, the use of these steroids in psychogenic disease without endocrine stigmata is associated with poor results. Adequate diagnostic procedures not only enhance the clinical acumen of the physician but also, when corroborating androgen insufficiency, almost guarantee an excellent response to appropriate steroid therapy.

MANAGEMENT OF SPERMATIC DEFECTS

Seminal Fluid Analysis. COLLECTION OF SPECIMEN. *Interval Between Ejaculation.* In the analysis of seminal fluid for evaluation of potential fertility, fact and fiction have prevailed concerning the appropriate method of collection of seminal fluid and the precise values that are commensurate with fertility. Abstinence from intercourse for a certain period of time prior to obtaining the specimen has not proved to be as important a factor as once thought. Abstaining from sexual intercourse will result in an increase in the number of sperm that are present per cc. However, there will also be a corresponding increase in the number of immotile and dead sperm (Fig. 385). Collection of seminal fluid specimens within 24 hours of previous intercourse may result in less numbers than

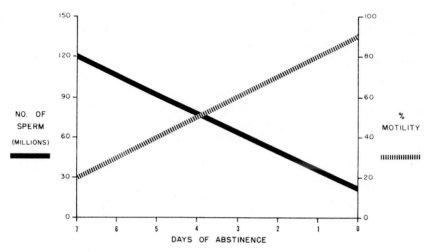

FIG. 385. *The relationship between frequency of ejaculation and the number and motility of sperm.*

would be seen if abstinence had been practiced for seven days, but the number of variable sperm would be increased significantly.

Appropriate Method. The appropriate method of collection of the sperm is by masturbation. The withdrawal procedure may be inadequate because of possible loss of some of the initial portion of the ejaculate, which is by far the most important with respect to both numbers and motility of the sperm. It is for this reason that accidental loss of a portion of the specimen in delayed withdrawal may give an inaccurate picture as to the fertility potential of the semen. Ejaculation should always be made into a clean glass jar, and transport of the specimen to the laboratory should be accomplished as rapidly as possible when motility is to be checked. There is no need to take special precautions as to temperature regulation during transportation of the specimen to the laboratory. It should not be exposed to extreme cold or heat and may be kept in the pants pocket or purse until delivered. Seminal fluid collection in a rubber container is entirely unsatisfactory if motility is to be studied, for the ingredients in the rubber material (probably the sulfur) result in death of the sperm. Thus, an inaccurate picture of the fertility potential of the seminal fluid would be gotten, although an accurate count of the number of sperm per cubic centimeter could be obtained by this method.

Normal Values. The concept of the number of sperm which is commensurate with fertility has diminished from a minimum of 60 million per cubic centimeter in the past to the present minimum of only 20 million per cubic centimeter. The lower count has been based on the fact that a significant number of men who have fathered children were found to have sperm at this level. Obviously, in addition to the numbers, one must also be cognizant of the fact that motility plays an important part in the fertility index. Hence, a count at the lower limits of normal should have a high degree of motility to be associated with a good fertility index. Normal motility should be in the range of 80 per cent or better. Normal volume may range from two to five cubic centimeters.

Staining Methods. No attempt will be made to outline the procedures for counting the sperm or for the usual staining methods, inasmuch as these techniques are readily available in any of the many excellent clinical laboratory texts. However, it would be well worth while to describe a relatively simple staining procedure which gives the physician an adequate morphologic demonstration of the sperm, permitting one to delineate morphologic abnormalities of the head, neck, and tail, as well as to estimate vitality.[2] This technique involves the use of the following reagents: aqueous eosin Y 5 per cent, and nigrosine 10 per cent. One drop of semen is well mixed with two drops of eosin, following which three drops of nigrosine are added and the combined mixture is spread across a slide in the form of a thin film. It has been said that the sperm which are viable will not take a stain and will stand out as relatively light forms outlined against the semi-dark nigrosine background. Dead sperm which have lost their ability to resist membrane penetration by the eosin will be stained pink and are also well visualized against the darkness of the nigrosine stain. Regardless of whether or not this is a vital staining technique, implying that only the dead sperm take the stain, the presenting morphologic picture of the stained and unstained sperm is usually adequate for most studies of abnormalities of the sperm head, neck, or tail.

Management of Abnormal Seminal Fluid Findings. Sperm Agglutination. Occasionally, upon examination of the seminal fluid, one may note a significant degree of agglutination of the heads of the various sperm forming a rosette with the tails radiating toward the periphery.[36, 37] This phenomenon is thought to be due to agglutination of the sperm as a result of the presence of agglutinins in the supernatant material. It has been claimed that the seminal fluid contains both anti-agglutinins and agglutinins.[27] In order for the agglutinins to be inactivated, active anti-agglutinins must be present. Hence, the presence of agglutination would imply that anti-agglutinins are absent or do not exist in an active form. The anti-agglutinins are activated by the process of reduction as well as by exposure to an increased amount of light.[22] When reduction fails to take place, relatively poor to no anti-agglutinin activity is noted. The therapeutic management of these patients is based on the oral administration of ascorbic acid, a very potent reducing agent,[25, 27] in doses of 100 mg. t.i.d. This will result in activation of the anti-agglutinins, with diminution of agglutination and reappearance of a normal seminal fluid picture and motility.

DECREASED MOTILITY. Diminution of motility of the sperm may be helped considerably by the addition of androgens, according to the method of McLeod.[29] He has recommended the use of 25 mg. of methyltestosterone twice per day in patients with a significant decrease in sperm motility. The use of this steroid enhances motility and will diminish the degree of necrospermia. The doses used will not inhibit pituitary gonadotropin so that the numbers of sperm will not be diminished. Therapy may be continued for a period of several months.

OLIGOSPERMIA. The presence of oligospermia may be the result of inadequate maturation of the germinal epithelium or diminished activity of the seminiferous tubules. Inasmuch as human follicle stimulating hormone (FSH) is still not available for clinical use, the patient who shows a significant degree of oligospermia may be placed on a course of pregnant mare's serum (Equinex). This gonadotropin is rich in FSH activity. The gonadotropin may be instrumental in stimulating the germinal epithelium to significantly increase the numbers of sperm in the ejaculate. In conjunction with this, the patient also is given an androgen to help potentiate the action of the gonadotropin.[25] The doses used are as follows:

1. 500 I.U. of pregnant mare's serum three times a week for three weeks, followed by twice a week for three to six weeks. At least 20 to 40 days are required for a complete spermatogenic cycle to take place; hence, changes in spermatogenesis are not anticipated before three weeks of therapy with gonadotropins.

2. Androgens:
      Testosterone cyclopentylpropionate, 100 mg.
      Testosterone enanthate, 200 mg.
      Testosterone phenylacetate, 100 mg.

Any one of the androgen preparations noted above may be administered every two or three weeks.

This regimen has been helpful in enhancing the numbers of sperm so that an infertile specimen may be changed into a fertile one. One cannot continue the pregnant mare's serum indefinitely because of its theoretical potentiality of antihormone formation. Pregnant mare's serum is derived from sources foreign to the human body and thereby can result in antibody formation. Consequently, if improvement in sperm count occurs with the use of this gonadotropin, it may be continued until a peak response is reached, or until signs appear of a decrease in number of sperm. At this time, antihormone formation may have taken place so that further administration of pregnant mare's serum gonadotropin would be ill advised.

We have never seen an allergic reaction to pregnant mare's serum in the past six or seven years due to its highly purified nature. A second course of pregnant mare's serum may be given with impunity as far as sensitizing reactions are concerned. However, the possibility of antihormone formation, as discussed above, must always be kept in mind.

The purpose of the androgen is to enhance the response of the testes to the gonadotropin. This possibility has been described in the case of the ovary as far as estrogen and gonadotropin are concerned. In addition, it has been noted that androgens may maintain spermatogenesis in the testes of a hypophysectomized animal, pointing to the potential spermatogenic effect of androgens in certain instances.

THE REBOUND PHENOMENON.   Several years ago, Heller, et al.,[19] and later, Heckel[14, 15] and Charny,[7] suggested that the administration of androgens in high doses would effectively inhibit gonadotropic hormone secretion, thereby bringing about a diminution in sperm count. However, when the androgen was discontinued, this was then followed by a marked increase in the number of sperm per cubic centimeter to levels said to be higher than those recorded prior to institution of the androgen. The resurgence of the seminal fluid analysis under these conditions has been referred to as the rebound phenomenon. In our experience, the rebound phenomenon has been one of theory rather than of fact. However, the procedure may be tried in those patients where a marked oligospermia exists with or without necrospermia. One must always keep in mind that there is the ever-present potential that, after complete suppression of sperm has been accomplished, it may persist for a period of several months after the androgen has been discontinued. This would be unfortunate in the patient who originally had a subnormal sperm count where fertility could still have been possible.

Miscellaneous Factors.   One need not be totally pessimistic as far as improvement of a deficient seminal fluid is concerned. Specific therapeutic procedures as outlined above may be employed. The possibility of the role of factors other than those just described being involved in oligospermia must be considered. The physiologic alterations noted in the adrenogenital syndrome may reduce significantly the sperm count. The diagnosis and management of this syndrome is discussed in Chapter 20 and will not be repeated here.

VAGINAL FACTORS.   *Vaginal Flora.*   Another point to be emphasized is that, while the seminal fluid may be more than satisfactory as far as count and viability of the specimen are concerned, the vaginal environment may be hostile and completely inactivate the semen. This may be due, in part, to vaginal flora or pH which is incompatible with viable semen. Here the use of douches containing physiologic nutrients may change a hopeless picture to a fertile one. At times the use of an appropriate antibiotic may rid the vagina of those pathogens that are responsible for having an adverse effect on the sperm. The sensitivity of these bacteria to specific antibiotics may be ascertained by the plate technique.

ABO (blood group) incompatibilities may also be a serious factor in the inactivation of sperm deposited intravaginally.[1] This may be checked by the usual *in vitro* techniques employed for such tests. Therapy includes the use of corticoids in the female in doses equivalent to 25 mg. of cortisone four times a day for four days, starting about two days before the anticipated day of ovulation. This procedure may create a sufficiently high tissue level of corticoid in the vagina to diminish the degree of ABO incompatibility.

Recently, Heller, *et al.*,[16] has reported on the inhibiting effect that bis (dichloroacetyl) diamines have on spermatogenesis with prolonged use. While these preparations may have some use as an oral contraceptive in the human, the use of related compounds for other therapeutic modalities might conceivably have an adverse effect on spermatogenesis. Thus, the use of new chemical compounds, particularly those with amebicidal effects, should be considered as potential inhibitors of spermatogenesis and appropriate precautions taken.

References

1. BEHRMAN, S. J., BUETTNER-JANUSCH, J., HEGLAR, R., GERSHOWITS, H., AND TEW, W. L.: ABO (H) blood incompatibility as a cause of infertility: A new concept. Amer. J. Obstet. Gynec. 79:847-855, 1960.

2. BLOM, E.: A one minute live-dead sperm stain by means of eosin-nigrosin. Fertil. Steril. 1:176-177, 1950.

3. BRADBURY, J. T., BUNGE, R., AND BOCCABELLA, R. A.: Chromatin test in Klinefelter's syndrome. J. Clin. Endocr. 16:689, 1956.

4. BRIGGS, D. K., EPSTEIN, J., AND KUPPERMAN, H. S.: The place of chromatin sex determinations in Klinefelter's syndrome. J. Urol. 80:57-61, 1958.

5. BRIGGS, D. K., AND KUPPERMAN, H. S.: New concepts in the evaluation of intersex and infertility. Amer. J. Med. 24:915-928, 1958.

6. BUNGE, R. G., AND BRADBURY, J. T.: Newer concepts of the Klinefelter syndrome. J. Urol. 76:758-765, 1956.

7. CHARNY, C. W.: The use of androgens for human spermatogenesis. Fertil. Steril. 10:557-570, 1959.

8. DEL CASTILLO, E. B., TRABUCCO, A., AND DE LA BALZE, F. A.: Syndrome produced by absence of the germinal epithelium without impairment of the Sertoli or Leydig cells. J. Clin. Endocr. 7:493-502, 1947.

9. DOUGLAS, R. J.: The male climacteric: Its diagnosis and treatment. J. Urol. 45:404-410, 1941.

10. EPSTEIN, J. A., BRIGGS, D. K., AND KUPPERMAN, H. S.: The use of chromatin sex determinations in the assessment of fertility and intersex infants. Fertil. Steril. 9:521-532, 1958.

11. FERGUSON-SMITH, M. A., LENNOX, B., MACK, W. S., AND STEWART, J. S. S.: Klinefelter's syndrome: Frequency and testicular morphology in relation to nuclear sex. Lancet 2:167-169, 1957.

12. FERGUSON-SMITH, M. A., AND MUNRO, I. B.: Spermatogenesis in the presence of female nuclear sex. Scot. Med. J. 3:39-42, 1958.

13. GRIBOFF, S., AND LAWRENCE, R.: The chromosomal etiology of congenital gonadal defects. Amer. J. Med. 30:544-563, 1961.

14. HECKEL, N. J., AND McDONALD, J. H.: The rebound phenomenon of the spermato-
    genic activity of the human testis following the administration of testosterone
    propionate. Fertil. Steril. 3:49-56, 1952.

15. HECKEL, N. J., ROSSO, W. A., AND KESTEL, L.: Spermatogenic rebound phenomenon
    after administration of testosterone propionate. J. Clin. Endocr. 11:235-245, 1951.

16. HELLER, C. G., MOORE, D. J., CLERMONT, Y., AND PAULSEN, C. A.: Dichotomous
    effect of Bis-(dichloroacetyl) Diamines upon spermatogenesis, Leydig-cell and
    gonadotropin function in man. Abs. 37, Endocrine Soc. 43rd Meeting, 1961.

17. HELLER, C. G., AND MYERS, G. B.: Male climacteric: Its symptomatology, diagnosis,
    and treatment. J.A.M.A. 126:472-477, 1944.

18. HELLER, C. G., AND NELSON, W. O.: Hyalinization of the seminiferous tubules
    associated with normal or failing Leydig cell function. Discussion of relationship
    to eunuchoidism, gynecomastia, elevated gonadotropins, depressed 17-ketosteroids
    and estrogens. J. Clin. Endocr. 5:1-12, 1945.

19. HELLER, C. G., NELSON, W. O., HILL, I. B., HENDERSON, E., MADDOCK, W. O., JUNGCK,
    E. C., PAULSEN, C. A., AND MORTIMORE, G. E.: Improvement in spermatogenesis
    following depression of the human testis with testosterone. Fertil. Steril. 1:415-
    420, 1950.

20. KAPLAN, A. A.: Jaundice due to methyltestosterone therapy. Gastroenterology 31:
    384-390, 1956.

21. KAPLAN, N. M., AND NORFLEET, R. G.: Hypogonadism in young men (with emphasis
    on Klinefelter's syndrome). Ann. Intern. Med. 54:461-481, 1961.

22. KIHLSTRÖM, J. E.: Effect of artificial light upon male sperm antiagglutinin produc-
    tion. Fertil. Steril. 9:114-119, 1958.

23. KLINEFELTER, H. F., JR., REIFENSTEIN, E. G., JR., AND ALBRIGHT, F.: Syndrome
    characterized by gynecomastia, aspermatogenesis without A-leydigism and in-
    creased excretion of follicle-stimulating hormone. J. Clin. Endocr. 2:615-627,
    1942.

24. KUPPERMAN, H. S.: Endocrinologic implications and clinical value of chromatin
    sex determination. Trans. N.Y. Acad. Sci. 20:505-515, 1958.

25. KUPPERMAN, H. S., AND EPSTEIN, J. A.: Endocrine therapy of sterility. Amer. Practit.
    9:547-563, 1958.

26. LANDAU, R. L.: Concept of male climacteric. Med. Clin. N. Amer. 35:279-288, 1951.

27. LINDAHL, P. E., AND KIHLSTRÖM, J. E.: An antiagglutinic factor in mammalian
    sperm plasm. Fertil. Steril. 5:241-255, 1954.

28. McGAVACK, T. H.: Angina-like pain: A manifestation of the male climacterium.
    J. Clin. Endocr. 3:71-80, 1943.

29. McLEOD, J.: The effect of methyltestosterone upon sperm motility. Presented at
    15th Annual Meeting Amer. Soc. for Study of Sterility, 1959.

30. NELSON, W. O., AND HELLER, C. G.: Hyalinization of the seminiferous tubules
    associated with normal or failing Leydig-cell function. Microscopic picture in the
    testis and associated changes in the breast. J. Clin. Endocr. 5:13-26, 1945.

31. PETERS, J. H., RANDALL, A. H., MENDELOFF, J., PEACE, R., COBERLY, J. C., AND
    HURLEY, M. B.: Jaundice during administration of methylestrenolone. J. Clin.
    Endocr. 18:114-115, 1958.

32. RABOCH, J.: Thirty-one men with female sex chromatin. J. Clin. Endocr. 17:1429-
    1439, 1957.

33. WERNER, A. A.: Male climacteric: Report of 54 cases. J.A.M.A. 127:705-710, 1945.

34. WERNER, A. A.: Male climacteric: Report of 273 cases. J.A.M.A. 132:188-194, 1946.

35. WERNER, S. C., HANGER, F. M., AND KRITZLER, R. A.: Jaundice during methyl testosterone therapy. Amer. J. Med. 8:325-331, 1958.

36. WILSON, L.: Sperm agglutinins in human semen and blood. Proc. Soc. Exp. Biol. Med. 85:652-655, 1954.

37. WILSON, L.: Sperm agglutination due to autoantibodies: A new cause of sterility. Fertil. Steril. 7:262-267, 1956.

chapter 18

Development of breast tissue in the male, although unphysiologic, may be seen in a considerable number of adolescent boys at the time sexual maturation is being initiated. Enlargement of the breasts in the male (gynecomastia) may also occur as a result of a pathologic process and as a consequence of therapy with certain cyclopentanophenanthrene steroids (Table 16, page 618).

Physiologic Gynecomastia. GYNECOMASTIA OF THE ADOLESCENT. In the normal development of the male at puberty, not infrequently, breast enlargement takes place and is associated with significant hypertrophy of true glandular elements (Figs. 386-392). As a rule, the gynecomastia is bilateral. Occasionally, it may be unilateral (Fig. 393) in much the same fashion that unilateral breast growth can take place in the normally developing female at the time of the menarche. The enlargement of the breasts in the adolescent male occurs to some degree in more than three fourths of the males going through puberty. Less than 5 per cent of the patients with adolescent gynecomastia will be left with permanent gynecomastia of significant proportions (Figs. 394, 395).

Physiopathology. Gynecomastia is believed to be due to the increased production of endogenous estrogen by the steroid secreting cells in the testes. The increased estrogen levels may be due to direct estrogen secretion by the Leydig cells (as previously suggested in the section on the physiology of the testes) or may be due to an increased breakdown of etiocholanolone precursors into estrogenic substances. In either case, the end result is the same—stimulation of the glandular development of the male's mammary tissue, resulting in slight to marked enlargement of the breasts. Histologic examination of the breast tissue

Gynecomastia

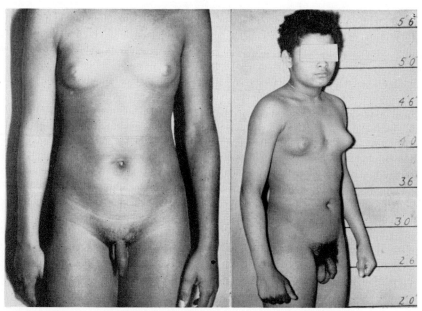

FIG. 386   FIG. 387

FIG. 386. Patient FS, age 13 years, with adolescent gynecomastia of some one to two years' duration. Endocrine work-up was normal. Note the well-developed phallus, beginning growth of pubic hair, and the well-formed breasts.

FIG. 387. Patient PR, age 15 years, weight 105½ pounds, height 67½ inches, normal 17-ketosteroids (8.2). Note the well-developed genitalia and equally well-developed breasts. Male secondary sex development outside of the breasts is normal for the patient's age.

617

TABLE 16

Conditions Associated with Abnormal Mammary Development in the Male*

Drug Therapy	Tumors	Testicular Alterations	Pituitary Syndromes	Other Endocrine Diseases	Neurologic Syndromes	Hepatic and Alimentary Alterations	Pulmonary Alterations	Miscellaneous
Estrogens Androgens Desoxycorticosterone Corticoids Chorionic gonadotropin Digitalis Isoniazid Amphetamine	Chorionepithelioma Hydatid mole Teratoma Testicular interstitial-cell tumor Adrenal tumor Renal tumor Mediastinal dysembryoma	Eunuchoidism Castration Klinefelter's syndrome Hermaphrodism Pseudohermaphrodism Chronic infection (tuberculosis, lues, leprosy)	Acromegaly Gigantism Cushing's syndrome Chromophobe tumors	Adrenal hyperplasia Hyper- and hypothyroidsm Diabetes mellitus	Parkinsonism Syringomyelia Meningoencephalitis Skull trauma Transverse myelitis Medullary trauma Paraplegia	Cirrhosis Infectious hepatitis Chronic hepatitis Starvation Dietary deficiency	Tumors Tuberculosis Bronchiectasis Hydatid cysts Abscesses Polycystic lungs Spontaneous pneumothorax Nonspecific lung infection Emphysema	Trauma to breast Pubescence in male Perinatal

* After Brambilla, Epstein, and Kupperman.[5]

618

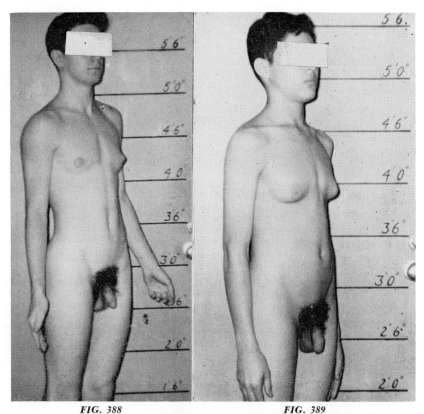

FIG. 388   FIG. 389

FIG. 388. Patient WM, age 13½ years, weight 149¾ pounds, height 70 inches, 17-ketosteroids 9.1 mg. per 24 hours. Note the well-developed phallus and testes, also the moderate gynecomastia. There is some degree of areolar accentuation.

FIG. 389. Patient MM, age 15¾ years, weight 121 pounds, height 64¾ inches, 17-ketosteroids 6.5 mg. per 24 hours, estrogen less than 8.1 rat units per 24 hours. Note the well-developed genitalia. Breast development is moderate to marked and is associated with areolar accentuation.

will show the typical changes seen in the prepubertal breast development in the female. This may range from only modest alveolar development (Fig. 396) to profound hypertrophy and hyperplasia of all glandular elements (Fig. 397).

The laboratory determination of estrogens in these patients will usually fail to show any significant elevation of estrogen excretion by biologic tests, but will disclose elevated levels when chemical methods are employed. It should be stressed that the increased estrogen output from the testes may occur only for a relatively short period of time; hence, most of these patients have evanescent gynecomastia which is followed by spontaneous regression when the endogenous estrogen levels fall to normal values (Fig. 398).

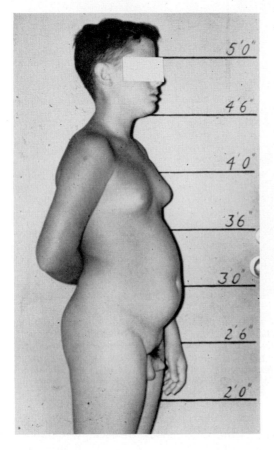

FIG. 390. Patient RR, age 16 years, weight 121¼ pounds, height 64 inches, 17-ketosteroids 15.7 mg. per 24 hours, estrogen less than 6.5 mouse units per 24 hours. Note the well-formed breasts seen in the adolescent youth and normal genital development for a boy of his age.

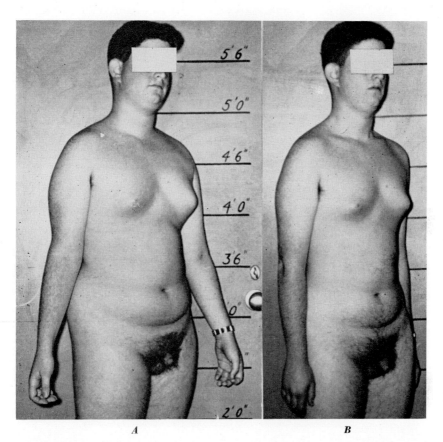

A   B

FIG. 391. A, Patient SB, age 14½ years, weight 199 pounds, height 68½ inches, 17-ketosteroids 12.4 mg. per 24 hours, estrogen less than 15 mouse units per 24 hours. True gynecomastia present.

B, Age 15, weight 167 pounds, height 69¼ inches. Note that the gynecomastia remained unchanged despite the loss of weight. The patient's genital development is normal for a patient of his age.

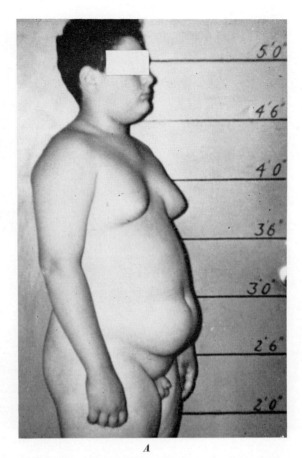

A

FIG. 392A. *Gynecomastia in young adolescent males. A, Patient JF, age 14 years, weight 187 pounds, height 63 inches, 17-ketosteroids 10.9 mg. per 24 hours. Note small genitalia in an obese boy with marked gynecomastia. The gynecomastia is partially adipose tissue, although true glandular tissue is present. This represents gynecomastia of the adolescent boy where genital development is comparatively poor.*

FIG. 392B. Patient JD, age 14 years, weight 142½ pounds, height 61½ inches. 17-Ketosteroids, 11 mg. per 24 hours; estrogen, less than 10 rat units per 24 hours. Chromatin negative. Note true gynecomastia in young obese male. Glandular tissue was markedly stimulated.

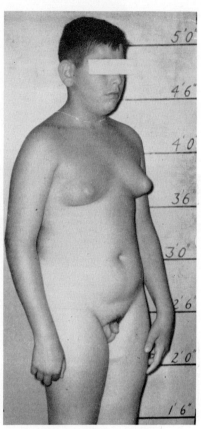

B

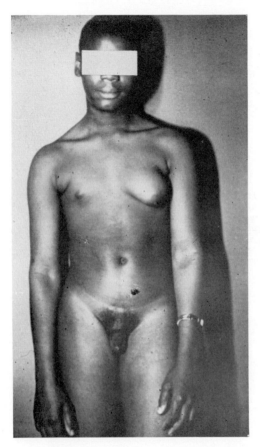

FIG. 393. Patient AG, age 14 years, weight 100½ pounds, height 61 inches. FSH = 13.2 mouse units per 24 hours. Note the unilateral gynecomastia in a boy with normal genitalia.

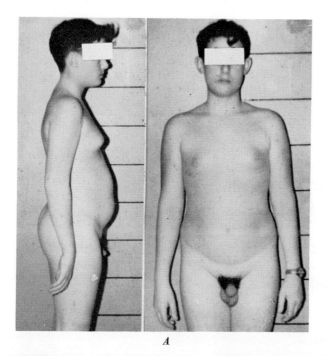

FIG. 394. *Patient WK at ages 14 (A) and 19 (B) years. Note that the gynecomastia present at age 14 did not resolve and was still present at age 19. If spontaneous disappearance of the gynecomastia does not occur in one year, a surgical plastic procedure would be wise if breast enlargement is of sufficient magnitude to be psychologically disturbing to the patient.*

625

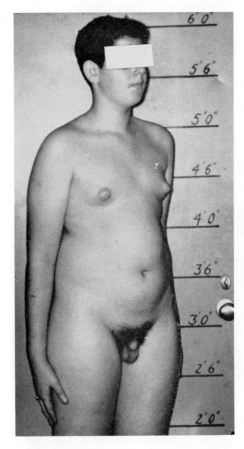

FIG. 395. Patient GK, age 17 years. Adolescent gynecomastia. 17-Ketosteroids, 13.1 mg. per 24 hours; FSH more than 13 but less than 26 mouse units per 24 hours. Testes are normal. Patient required a plastic resection since there were no signs of spontaneous resolution three to four years after the initial development of the gynecomastia.

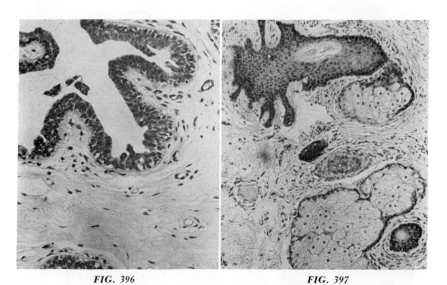

FIG. 396   FIG. 397

FIG. 396. Breast biopsy of patient AG (shown in Figure 393) with marked gynecomastia. Note the dilatation of the alveolar structures and the hypertrophy of the epithelium.

FIG. 397. Patient RM. Breast biopsy. Note the marked development of the duct and alveolar structure of the breast in a male with considerable gynecomastia associated with Klinefelter's syndrome.

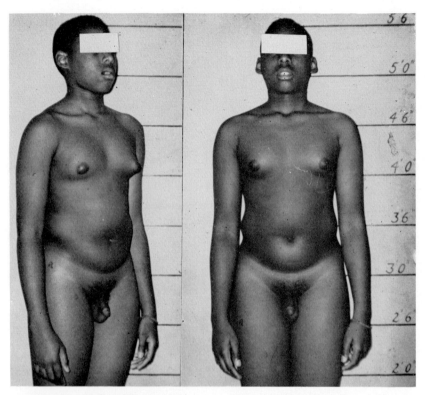

FIG. 398.   Patient RT, age 12½ years.   17-Ketosteroids, 6.5 mg. per 24 hours; estrogens, less than 5.8 mouse units per 24 hours.   Adolescent gynecomastia.   No therapy required.   There was spontaneous resolution.

KLINEFELTER'S SYNDROME. The second form of physiologic gynecomastia is seen in some patients with Klinefelter's syndrome (Fig. 399).[20]
The physiopathology in this syndrome has already been described and
will not be elaborated upon here. Suffice it to say that, as has been noted
in some patients with adolescent gynecomastia, there is no evidence of
increased estrogen excretion in these men despite the presence of excellent
breast growth. The physiologic mechanism responsible for the breast hypertrophy has been explained upon the basis of uninhibited secretion of a
pituitary breast stimulating factor; the uninhibited secretion takes place
as a result of the absence of inhibin from the hyalinized tubules of the
Klinefelter testes. Rarely is gynecomastia noted in the prepubertal Klinefelter. However, it may occur in these children prior to the time that
hyalinization of the tubules takes place (Fig. 400).

NEONATAL BREAST HYPERTROPHY. The third type of physiologic
gynecomastia is seen in the neonatal period when both male and female
infants may show some breast hypertrophy as a result of exposure to the
maternal hormones during pregnancy. This is invariably of a temporary
nature, and indeed may be associated with some galactorrhea ("witch's
milk"). The precociously stimulated breasts rapidly resolve without treat-

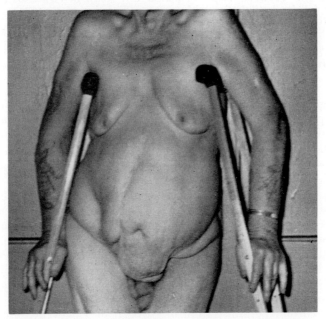

FIG. 399. A, Patient CN, age 67 years. Chromatin positive. Note
the marked degree of gynecomastia in a male with Klinefelter's syndrome. There has been a loss of glandular elements due to the
patient's age very similar to that seen in the female of this age group.

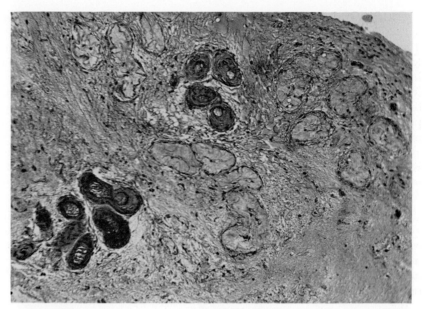

FIG. 399B. Testicular biopsy of patient CN, shown in Figure 399A, demonstrating tubular hyalinization with complete distortion of the cyto-architecture of the testes.

ment during the early postnatal period, as does the secretion of milk if present.

Pathologic Breast Enlargement. Pathologic causes for gynecomastia may be placed under two categories: (1) that associated with a primary pathologic process (as breast anaplasia) and (2) that due to trauma.

NEOPLASTIC DISEASE OF THE BREAST. While adenoma and carcinoma of the breast are beyond the scope of this book, it should be noted that such disease is comparatively rare in the normal male not receiving estrogen therapy. However, when present, anaplasia is of a highly malignant nature and is rapidly progressive. The mass is usually unilateral and characterized by a stony hardness quite different upon palpation from the firm gynecomastia that is physiologic in origin. The sudden appearance of a unilateral firm, hard, nodular hypertrophy in a postpubertal male without lung or hepatic disease, and with no history of steroid ingestion, should be looked on with suspicion and subjected to prompt surgical investigation to rule out the possibility of anaplastic disease.

The chronic administration of estrogen to a male because of metastatic prostatic carcinoma will induce breast enlargement. These males tend to show a higher incidence of mammary carcinoma than that seen in the male population as a whole.

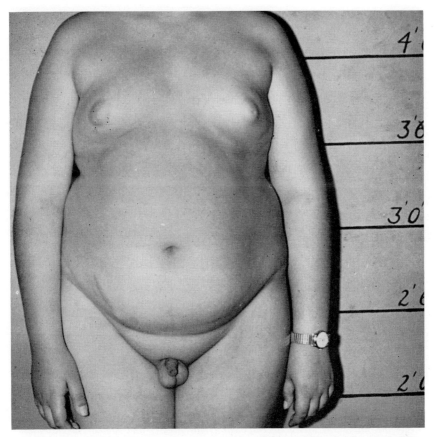

FIG. 400. Patient JB, age 13 years, weight 171½ pounds, height 62 inches. FSH less than 6.6 mouse units per 24 hours, 17-ketosteroids 6.5 mg. per 24 hours. Young male with Klinefelter's syndrome. Chromatin negative. Diagnosis of Klinefelter's syndrome made by testicular biopsy. Note the areolar accentuation and moderate development of the breasts.

GYNECOMASTIA SECONDARY TO TRAUMA. Gynecomastia due to trauma is comparatively rare (Figs. 401, 402), but, when present, may have serious import due to the possibility of subsequent anaplasia. Consequently, if significant hypertrophy occurs and spontaneous resolution does not take place, removal of the enlarged breast which had been injured is usually a wise prophylactic procedure against the development of possible mitotic changes. In traumatic gynecomastia the history is specific and is the most important diagnostic clue. These patients show no alteration of genital function. Their endocrine status is usually completely normal. Removal of the offending mass of mammary tissue should be accomplished in much the same manner that a mammoplasty is done

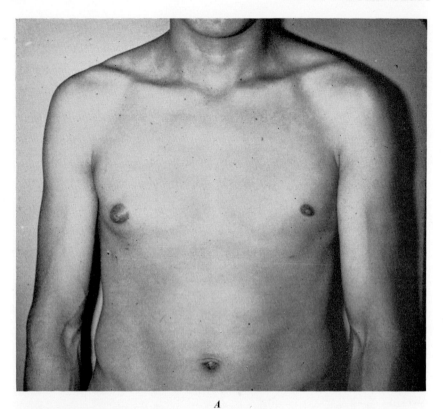

A

FIG. 401A. Unilateral gynecomastia due to trauma. A, Patient WU, age 19 years, weight 160¼ pounds, height 69 inches, 17-ketosteroids 18.8 mg. per 24 hours. Note the unilateral breast development (right breast) and areolar accentuation. The patient injured his right breast several weeks prior to the time this photograph was made. True gynecomastia was present.

for bilateral gynecomastia, with the end result of preservation of the areolae.

Gynecomastia Secondary to Systemic Disease. HEPATIC DISEASE. The most common systemic disease frequently leading to gynecomastia in the adult is liver disease, particularly that associated with chronic alcoholism. However, gynecomastia may also be noted in postnecrotic cirrhosis as well as in hepatic insufficiency where destruction of the liver parenchyma has occurred as a result of chemical intoxication or parasitic infection. The association of gynecomastia with hepatic disease is presumably due to the role of the liver in the inactivation of the endogenous estrogen normally circulating in the male. One of the functions of the liver, which is lost earliest in hepatic disease, is the ability of the liver to metabolize the steroid hormones. This deficit is manifested very

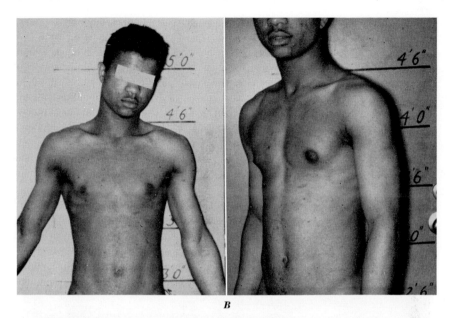

FIG. 401B. *Patient BG, age 19 years, weight 124 pounds, height 63¾ inches. Note unilateral enlargement of the left breast which followed a traumatic episode. True glandular tissue and gynecomastia were present in this breast only. Endocrine work-up revealed no abnormality.*

promptly as far as 17-ketosteroid excretion is concerned. There is a lowering of 17-ketosteroid levels in the urine in hepatic insufficiency, the reason being that the liver is unable to convert the endogenous androgens into their neutral 17-ketosteroid excretory products. Similarly, the normal estrogen level, which is usually low in the male, becomes elevated when the liver is incapable of inactivating this steroid. The increased estrogen level causes gynecomastia, as well as oligospermia or azoospermia, a diminution of bodily hair and beard growth, plus the fact that the skin in these patients tends to become somewhat smooth and feminine in character. The depressed spermatogenic response no doubt is due to the inhibiting effect the elevated estrogen level has on pituitary gonadotropic secretion. This, in turn, is followed by diminution in testicular function and eventually by atrophy.

PULMONARY PATHOLOGY. For some unknown reason, gynecomastia is frequently associated with a variety of types of lung disease. Gynecomastia has been observed in patients with bronchiogenic cancer, emphysema, bronchiectasis, and tuberculosis.[1, 4, 7-9, 13, 22, 25, 29, 31, 34] In the latter disease, it has also appeared following treatment with INH[13] and disappeared as rapidly when treatment was stopped. The relationship of these various pulmonary entities to the initiation of gynecomastia is vague. At times the gynecomastia may be unilateral, occurring on the

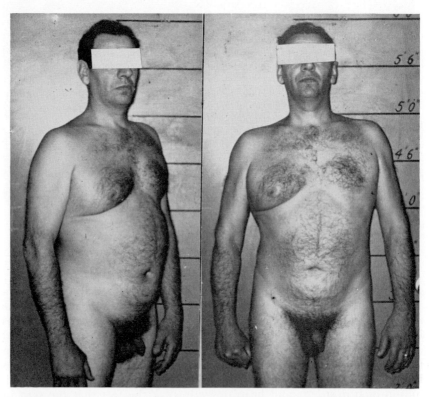

FIG. 402. Patient BG, age 45 years, height 70 inches, weight 201 pounds. Note the unilateral hypertrophy of tissue of right side of the chest, which was thought to be due to unilateral gynecomastia. This occurred as a result of repeated traumatic episodes due to occupational habits. The patient is a metal worker and is known as a spinner. His job compelled him to apply pressure to his instrument with his body. The pressure was exerted by pressing the right side of the chest forcibly against his instrument. Hypertrophy occurred after 10 years of such work. The mass was removed and revealed no evidence of glandular tissue but consisted primarily of fatty infiltration.

same side as the diseased lung. However, more frequently it is bilateral, unrelated to the site of pulmonary pathology. Similar breast hypertrophy has been known to occur in young females with comparatively benign types of lung pathology. For example, breast growth has been described in a pre-adolescent girl who had an associated upper respiratory infection.[5] The mechanism responsible for the breast hypertrophy in both males and females with lung disease is obscure. The endocrine status of these patients is usually normal. There is no evidence of any disturbance of estrogen levels in these patients, nor is there any manifestation of mechanical blockage and swelling due to venous or lymphatic obstruction.

GYNECOMASTIA DUE TO MALNUTRITION. Starvation or malnutrition per se may be associated with enlargement of the breast.[21, 33] The mechanism of action is not understood and may be due in part to impaired liver function. Peculiarly enough, when male volunteers, previously subjected to starvation, are permitted to recover, they too will show an increase in breast size.[30] Why recovery from starvation is associated with breast enlargement is not known. The liver may be implicated in these patients. Thus, the failure of estrogen inactivation reported to take place in vitamin-B deficient animals[2, 3] might well be attributed to the inanition associated with such a deficient diet[10, 18, 19] and not due to any specific vitamin deficiency. When adequate protein intake was maintained despite the B deficiency, adequate metabolism of estrogen occurred since liver function was maintained at a normal level.[18, 19]

Estrogen Secreting Tumor of Testis or Adrenal. Obviously, breast enlargement may occur as a result of the presence of an estrogen-secreting tumor of either the adrenals or the testes (Fig. 403).[6, 14, 15, 17, 32, 35] Unusual and rapid enlargement of the breast in a male, without apparent cause and regardless of age, should be considered as being induced by an estrogen-producing tumor. Removal of the tumor invariably results in diminution in size of the gynecomastia. An adrenal tumor with estrogenic properties is unusually rare and would be associated with hypoplasia of both testes. On the other hand, a testicular feminizing tumor is associated with one atrophic testis and one of normal or increased size.

Iatrogenic Gynecomastia. CYCLOPENTANOPHENANTHRENE DRUGS. The administration of many different types of substances may cause a significant degree of breast growth (Fig. 404). Inasmuch as these substances all have the structural form of the cyclopentanophenanthrene nucleus, it appears that there may be a general or common metabolic breakdown product from all which may be estrogenic-like in activity and is responsible for stimulating breast growth. Gynecomastia obviously may be induced by the administration of estrogen but also may occur after androgen therapy,[23, 27] particularly methyltestosterone,[27] as well as after

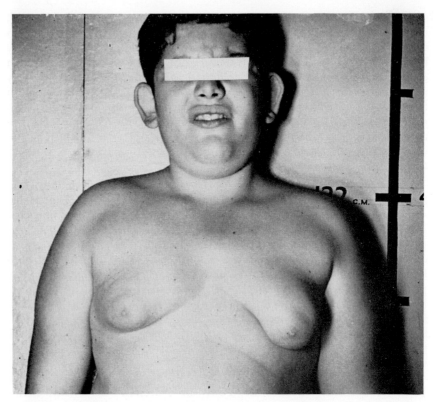

*FIG. 403A. Patient CS, age 11 years, weight 130 pounds, height 57¾ inches.
Note the markedly enlarged breasts and accentuation of the areolae usually associated with estrogenic secreting neoplasms.*

adrenocorticosteroids (Fig. 405)[11, 23, 26] or with increased endogenous
adrenal function.[28] Gynecomastia has also been reported after digitalis
medication.[23, 24] Although it might appear logical to employ androgens
for their theoretical anti-estrogenic effect and potential inhibiting action
on breast growth, the fact that androgens can induce gynecomastia would
obviate their use as a therapeutic agent in male patients with breast
hypertrophy.[21] This is particularly true of the active androgens.

GONADOTROPINS. Gynecomastia has also been observed after the
use of human chorionic gonadotropic (HCG) hormone (Fig. 406)[23] in
the human, and has also been noted in monkeys after gonadotropin
administration.[12] While this is not a steroid substance in itself, HCG is
responsible for stimulating hormone production by the Leydig cells of
the testes in patients having gonads capable of responding. The presence
of gynecomastia following this type of therapy is of no more importance
than that which is usually seen in the young male going through normal

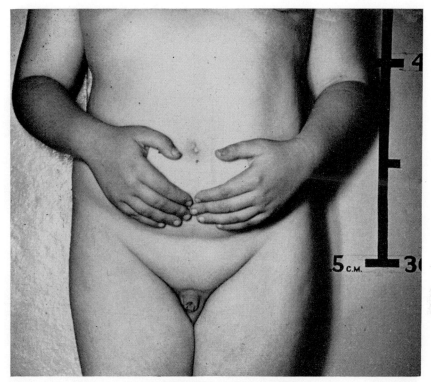

FIG. 403B.   Note small genitalia.

puberty. In these individuals, once the chorionic gonadotropin is discontinued, spontaneous resolution of the hypertrophied breast tissue will usually take place. However, as is seen in the spontaneously occurring condition, theoretically one can anticipate that 3 per cent of the patients showing breast stimulation after chorionic gonadotropin therapy might have permanent gynecomastia. Fortunately, we have never yet seen a case of permanent gynecomastia occur when it developed during the course of HCG treatment in any one of the many patients with undescended testes or hypogonadism who have received such therapy.

Occasionally, gynecomastia may be seen prior to the institution of HCG therapy. While one must alert the parents to the possibility of accentuation of the gynecomastia after HCG administration, this must be considered as a calculated risk where such treatment is indicated. On the other hand, the gynecomastia may not be accentuated after HCG and, indeed, the tendency for a more masculine build (loss of "baby fat") after HCG may result in a decrease in the degree of breast hypertrophy, or at best there may be no accentuation of growth of breast tissue (Fig. 407A and B).

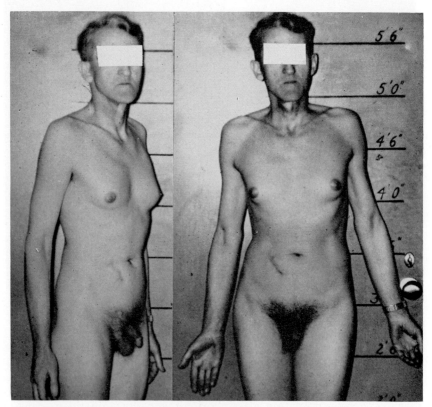

FIG. 404. Patient TG, age 53 years. 17-Ketosteroids, 18.7 mg. per 24 hours; FSH, less than 6.6 mouse units per 24 hours; estrogen, more than 50 rat units per 24 hours. Iatrogenic gynecomastia. Patient worked as a chemist with organic compounds that were not known to be estrogenic. His libido was decreased as was his hair growth on the body. When he changed his place of work his estrogen level fell to normal, his gynecomastia subsided and libido returned.

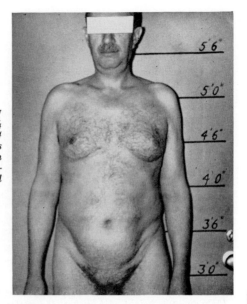

FIG. 405. Patient WTB, age 57 years, weight 188 pounds, height 72¾ inches, 17-ketosteroids 10.1 mg. per 24 hours. Patient had been on continuous doses of corticoid because of collagen disease. The breast development occurred after the initiation of corticoid therapy.

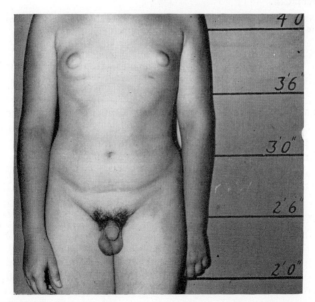

FIG. 406. Patient AW, age 12½ years, weight 122¼ pounds, height 61¼ inches. Note adequately developed genitalia and gynecomastia which developed following treatment with HCG. The gynecomastia subsided within a period of several months after HCG therapy was discontinued.

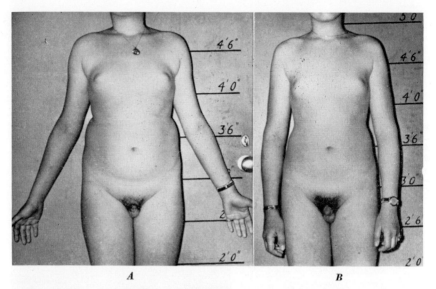

FIG. 407. A, Patient HS, before treatment with HCG: age 14 years, weight 151¾ pounds, height 66½ inches, 17-ketosteroids 8.4 mg. per 24 hours. Note the hypoplastic genitalia for a boy of patient's age. The gynecomastia was present prior to treatment.

B, Post-treatment picture. Note the well-developed genitalia. The gynecomastia in this case was not increased with HCG therapy.

Diagnosis.   The diagnosis of gynecomastia is relatively easy and is based on the demonstration of true glandular tissue by either inspection or palpation.

TRUE VERSUS FALSE GYNECOMASTIA.   One must, of course, differentiate between false and true gynecomastia.   False gynecomastia refers simply to the deposition of adipose tissue and hypertrophy of muscle tissue in the mammary area simulating breast growth. Adipose deposition is usually seen in the obese or aging male where there has been sufficient loss of pectoral muscle tissue with fatty infiltration to give the clinical impression of breast hypertrophy. In these patients, areolar accentuation is rarely seen.

True glandular tissue may be demonstrated readily by physical examination. The most appropriate method for this is to place the index finger squarely in the middle of the nipple with the thumb and the third finger grasping the adjacent tissue. If there is only adipose tissue, no firm mass of tissue will be felt. If glandular tissue is present, a significant density of underlying tissue is palpable and can easily be differentiated from adipose tissue. However, one must keep in mind that, not infrequently, there may be both false and true gynecomastia in the same breast. In such individuals, the enlargement of the breast is usually great and is similar to the adipose glandular breast of the prepubertal female (Figs. 408-410). Such breasts may assume unusual proportions (Fig. 410). The early growth of breast tissue of true gynecomastia may be associated with some tenderness and discomfort. Adipose tissue is rarely tender.

AREOLAE.   The second most important diagnostic point is that the areolae are invariably accentuated (Fig. 411) and may even be puffy in appearance (Fig. 412) in patients with true gynecomastia. This is an important diagnostic clue to differentiate adipose from true glandular growth, since areolar accentuation is not a prominent component of the enlarged fatty breast. In addition, there may be increased areolar pigmentation (Fig. 413) in patients with true gynecomastia as contrasted with the absence of such pigmentation when adiposity is responsible for the breast enlargement.

FIRMNESS AND SHAPE OF TISSUE.   In true gynecomastia, one will usually feel a small firm disk of tissue beneath the areolae, with the broad base pointing toward the rib cage and the conical end directed toward the

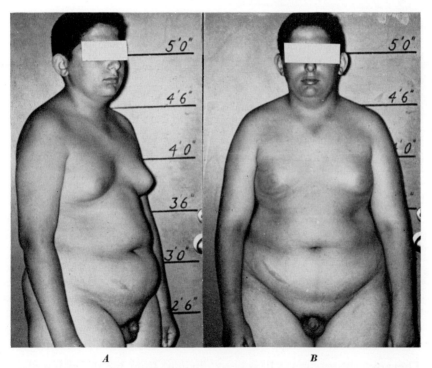

A   B

FIG. 408 A and B.   Patient BK, age 13 years, weight 183 pounds, height 63½ inches, 17-ketosteroids 12.9 mg. per 24 hours, FSH less than 6.6 mouse units per 24 hours. Note false gynecomastia associated with true glandular development. Much of the gynecomastia subsided when the patient's weight was decreased.

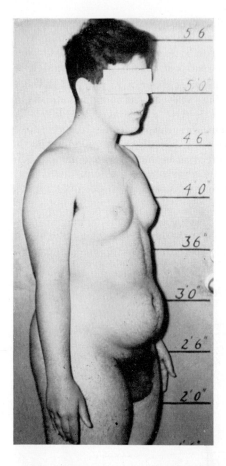

FIG. 409. Patient TP, age 15 years, weight 200 pounds, height 65 inches, 17-ketosteroids 21.8 mg. per 24 hours. Note the false and true gynecomastia. The adipose tissue was due in part to the patient's excessive weight. Note the well-developed genitalia and normal 17-ketosteroids.

nipple. Glandular tissue is always firm but never hard. The presence of any hard nodules or any hard lymphatic glands in the axillary region would point toward anaplasia of the breast and the need for biopsy for diagnosis.

NATURE OF BREAST ENLARGEMENT. One should keep in mind that, occasionally, supernumerary tissue may be present, representing an atavistic trait of ontogeny. These extra mammary areas may be confused with lymph nodes, particularly if there is no superficial nipple or areolae. However, they are usually multiple in number and bilateral, and may be associated with a tuft of hair growth in the center of the anlage.

Therapy. ANDROGENS. It appears obvious, from the discussion above, that since androgens may cause an increased amount of breast growth in some patients, their use in the management of gynecomastia is contra-indicated. Of all the androgens that have been used, methyltestosterone has been the one most frequently indicted as causing breast development.

Its use should never be advocated in patients with gynecomastia. However, if breast growth does occur during therapy with methyltestosterone, it will invariably subside completely after cessation of drug administration.

MAMMOPLASTY. The only specific corrective form of therapy for gynecomastia is the plastic surgical removal of the underlying breast tissue. Surgery is relatively simple and involves removal of the glandular elements no matter what their extent, through a semicircular incision around the inferior border of the areolae. This will be associated with minimal scar formation. Any scar tissue which does form would be in the line of cleavage between the areolae and the skin, and thereby be inconspicuous. It is usually advisable to excise enough underlying tissue so that a slight concavity in the breast area results postoperatively. This is of some importance since when complete healing takes place, there is usually an infiltration of fibrous tissue to completely fill any defect in this portion of the chest wall. Hence, if a perfectly flat surface was achieved with the mammoplastic procedure, the infiltrating connective tissue might eventually create significant prominence in the breast at the site of surgery, creating the impression of recurrence of the gynecomastia (Fig. 414 A and B).

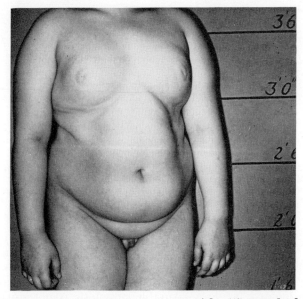

FIG. 410. Patient CG, age 8 years, weight 107 pounds, height 52¼ inches, 17-ketosteroids 7.3 mg. per 24 hours, estrogen less than 4.2 mouse units per 24 hours. Note enormous development of breasts consisting of both glandular and adipose tissue. Weight reduction was responsible for a diminution in size of the breasts. However, glandular elements persisted.

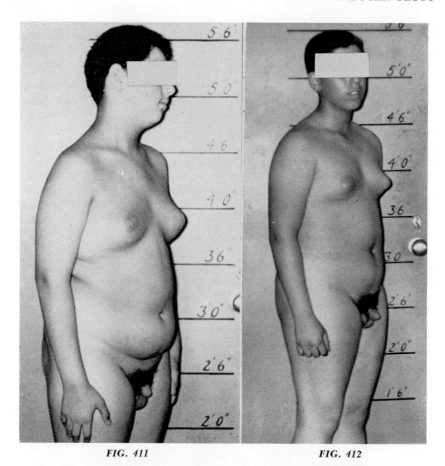

FIG. 411   FIG. 412

FIG. 411. *Patient MN, age 13 years, weight 170 pounds, height 65¼ inches, 17-ketosteroids 9.6 mg. per 24 hours. Note the marked areolar accentuation in a patient with marked gynecomastia of the adolescent.*

FIG. 412. *Patient HM, age 14½ years, weight 178½ pounds, height 64½ inches. Note marked gynecomastia and puffiness of the areolar area. The normal genital development and 17-ketosteroids indicate that the gynecomastia is associated with the process of adolescence.*

NORETHANDROLONE THERAPY. At times, it has been noted that there are some males with gynecomastia in whom diminution in breast size occurred after norethandrolone therapy (Fig. 415). This has been observed in several patients with a considerable degree of breast enlargement. Consequently, while a favorable prognosis is not usually anticipated, the use of norethandrolone may be worthy of a therapeutic trial prior to the institution of surgery. The usual dose of norethandrolone would be 10 mg. b.i.d. to t.i.d. The benefit which occurs is probably due to the action of norethandrolone in inhibiting any pituitary factors that may be responsible for producing breast hypertrophy. A trial with this steroid should not exceed a period of more than six to eight weeks. If there is no significant decrease in breast size, then plastic removal of the breast should be accomplished by surgery. Use of the steroid for longer periods of time would not be any more effective.

Conclusion. Gynecomastia is a single diagnostic entity with multiple factors as far as etiology is concerned. One must differentiate between false (adipose tissue) and true gynecomastia. The latter is characterized by the aberrant growth of true glandular tissue plus areolar accentuation. Not infrequently, pubescence is associated with temporary but true breast hypertrophy in the male. Where this remains permanent and is a cause of discomfort, from both the mental and the physical points of view, then a mammoplastic procedure is the one of choice. Pulmonary and hepatic

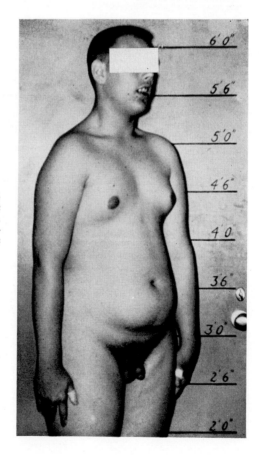

FIG. 413. Patient WK, age 14½ years, weight 240 pounds, height 71½ inches, 17-ketosteroids 14.1 mg. per 24 hours. Note the areolar accentuation and pigmentation in a patient with normal genitalia.

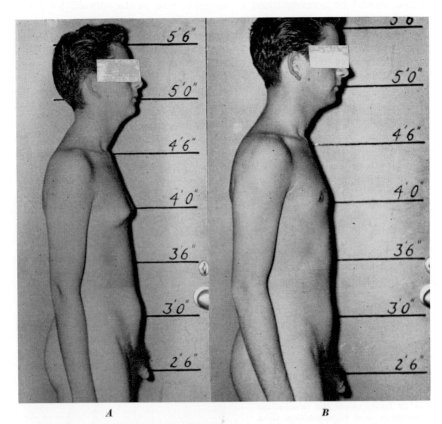

FIG. 414. *A, Patient SH with Klinefelter's syndrome. Age 21 years, weight 130¼ pounds, height 65¾ inches. Note the well-developed gynecomastia present prior to surgery.*

B, Postoperative picture showing the excellent cosmetic result achieved with the technique described in the text. Note preservation of the areolae plus some depression of the peri-areolar tissue. This will prevent the appearance of false gynecomastia when the surgical site is infiltrated with fibrous connective tissue.

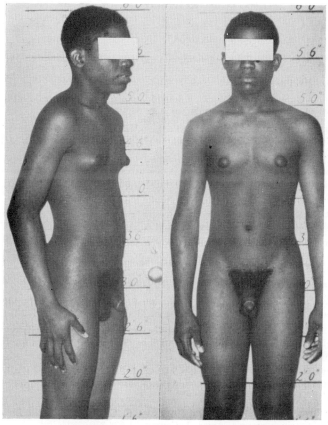

FIG. 415.   Patient GT, age 14½ years. 17-Ketosteroids 9.1 mg. per
24 hours. Estrogen less than 15 rat units per 24 hours. Adolescent
gynecomastia, tender and painful. Pain and size of breasts diminished
with norethandrolone (Norlutin) 10 mg. t.i.d. for 20 days.

disease may be associated with gynecomastia. There is no specific explanation why breast enlargement occurs in pulmonary disease. However,
hepatic insufficiency may be associated with incomplete steroid inactivation, resulting in increased endogenous estrogenic activity bringing about
testicular suppression and feminization. Anaplasia of the male breast,
while relatively infrequent, is of such a malignant nature that not infrequently metastases are present when the primary disease is recognized.
Therefore, it is absolutely necessary to differentiate between benign
gynecomastia (usually bilateral in position and firm to soft on palpation)
and anaplasia of the breast (unilateral in location and stony hard in
consistency).

References

1. ALTSCHUL, A.: Gynecomastia in lung tumor associated with pulmonary tuberculosis. New York J. Med. 38:637-640, 1938.

2. BISKIND, M. S.: Nutritional therapy of endocrine disturbances. *In* Harris, R. S., and Thimann, K. V.: Vitamins and Hormones, Vol. 4. Academic Press, New York, 1946, pp. 147-185.

3. BISKIND, M. S., AND BISKIND, G. R.: Effect of vitamin B complex deficiency on inactivation of estrone in liver. Endocrinology 31:109-114, 1942.

4. BOULARD, C., PORTIER, A., CHEVROT, L., AND MASSONNAT, J.: Gynécomastie, hippocratisme digital et maladie polykystique du poumon. Alergie Med. 55:1041-1046, 1951.

5. BRAMBILLA, F., EPSTEIN, J. A., AND KUPPERMAN, H. S.: Intermittent precocious breast development associated with mild bronchitis. J. Clin. Endocr. 21:80-90, 1961.

6. COHEN, J., AND DIAMOND, I.: Leontiasis ossea, slipped epiphyses and granulosa cell tumor of testis with renal disease. A.M.A. Arch. Path. (Chic.) 56:488-500, 1953.

7. CRESPO SANTILLANA: Sobre un caso de ginecomastia postgranúlica. Acta Pediat. Esp. 10:1037-1048, 1952.

8. DEL CASTILLO, E. B., DE LA BALZE, F. A., AND REFORZO MEMBRIVES, J.: Ginecomastia y cáncer del pulmón. Semana Med. 1:1419-1423, 1941.

9. DEL CASTILLO, E. B., DE LA BALZE, F, A., AND REFORZO MEMBRIVES, J.: Ginecomastia y carcinoma pulmonar. Ensayo Patogen. Med., Buenos Aires 4:176-184, 1944.

10. DRILL, V. A., AND PFEIFFER, C. A.: Effect of vitamin B complex deficiency, controlled inanition and methionine on inactivation of estrogen by the liver. Endocrinology 38:300-307, 1946.

11. EDWARDS, R. A., SHIMKIN, M. B., AND SHAVER, J. S.: Hypertrophy of the breasts due to injection of adrenal cortex extract in a man with Addison's disease. J.A.M.A. 111:412-414, 1938.

12. GESCHICKTER, C. F., LEWIS, D., AND HARTMAN, C. G.: Tumors of the breast related to the oestrin hormone. Amer. J. Cancer, 21:828-859, 1934.

13. GUINET, P., GARIN, J. P., AND MORNEIX, A.: Un cas de gynécomastie chez un tuberculeux pulmonaire grave en cours de traitment par l'hydrazide de l'acide isonicotinique. Lyon Med. 188:281-284, 1953.

14. HEIDEMAN, M. L., JR.: Transient recurrent gynecomastia after removal of an estrogen-secreting interstitial-cell tumor of the testis. J. Clin. Endocr. 19:1331-1343, 1959.

15. HUGGINS, C., AND MOULDER, P. V.: Estrogen production by Sertoli cell tumors of the testis. Cancer Res. 5:510-514, 1945.

16. HUGUENIN, R., FAUVET, J., PIERART, A., AND DE LEOBARDY, J.: Le syndrome "cancer broncho-pulmonaire périotite des os longs, gynécomastie." Bull. Soc. Med. Hop. Paris 70:986-991, 1954.

17. HUNT, V. C., AND BUDD, J. W.: Gynecomastia associated with interstitial-cell tumor of the testicle. J. Urol. 42:1242-1250, 1939.

18. JAILER, J. W.: Effect of inanition on inactivation of estrogen by liver. Endocrinology 43:78-82, 1948.

19. JAILER, J. W., AND SEAMAN, L.: Estrogen inactivation by liver as modified by dietary protein. Proc. Soc. Exp. Biol. Med. 73:70-72, 1950.

20. KLINEFELTER, H. F., JR., REIFENSTEIN, E. C., JR., AND ALBRIGHT, F.: Syndrome characterized by gynecomastia, aspermatogenesis, without A-leydigism and increased excretion of follicle-stimulating hormone. J. Clin. Endocr. 2:615-627, 1942.

21. KLATSKIN, G., SALTER, W. T., AND HUMM, F. D.: Gynecomastia due to malnutrition. 1. Clinical studies. Amer. J. Med. Sci. 213:19-30, 1947.

22. LACHAPELE, A. P., BIRABEN, J., AND LACOSTE, G.: Le syndrome cancer pulmonaire, périostite des os longs, gynécomastie. J. Med. Bordeaux 135:499-500, 1958.

23. LEWIN, M. L.: Gynecomastia: Hypertrophy of the male breast. J. Clin. Endocr. 1: 511-514, 1941.

24. LEWINN, E. B.: Gynecomastia during digitalis therapy, report of eight additional cases with liver function studies. New Engl. J. Med. 248:316-320, 1953.

25. MAGGI, A. L. C., REMOLAR, J. M., AND MEEROFF, M.: Sindrome de hipertensión bronco-alveolar, osteoartropatía y ginecomastia por neoplasia endobronquial. Prensa Med. Argent. 36:2383-2390, 1949.

26. MAMOU, H., GRIMBERG, J., AND SAMAMA, A.: Signification clinique des gynécomasties. (A propos d'un cas de gynécomastie par le traitement à la desoxycorticostérone.) Sem. Hop. Paris 26:2724-2732, 1950.

27. McCULLAGH, E. P., AND ROSSMILLER, H. R.: Methyl testosterone. I. Androgenic effects and production of gynecomastia and oligospermia. J. Clin. Endocr. 1:496-502, 1941.

28. MENVILLE, J. G.: Gynecomastia. Arch. Surg. (Chic.) 26:1054-1083, 1933.

29. MOLINA, C., ABERKANE, B., AND CONQUY-DOUARD, T.: Les gynécomasties chez les tuberculeux pulmonaires; a propos de cinq observations. Maroc Med. 36:635-643, 1957.

30. PLATT, S. S., SCHULZ, R. Z., AND KUNSTADTER, R. H.: Hypertrophy of male breast associated with recovery from starvation. Bull. U. S. Army Med. Dept. 7:403-405, 1947.

31. PODESTÁ, H., ALURRALDE, P., AND ARLA, J. E.: Asociación ginecomastia-osteoartropatia hipertrofiante néumica en las neoplasias broncopulmonares. Prensa Med. Argent. 45:152-156, 1958.

32. POMER, F. A., STILES, R. E., AND GRAHAM, J. H.: Interstitial-cell tumors of the testis in children. New Engl. J. Med. 250:233-237, 1954.

33. SALTER, W. T., KLATSKIN, G., AND HUMM, F. D.: Gynecomastia due to malnutrition. II. Endocrine studies. Amer. J. Med. Sci. 213:31-36, 1947.

34. SEQUERA TAMAYO, A.: Gynecomastia en el cancer del pumón. Rev. Policlin. Caracas 15:90, 1946.

35. WARD, J. A., KRANTZ, S., MENDELOFF, J., AND HALTIWANGER, E.: Interstitial-cell tumor of the testis: Report of 2 cases. J. Clin. Endocr. 20:1622-1632, 1960.

chapter 19

Hypofunction of the adrenal glands may range in severity from a mild to a marked degree. In the comparatively mild state, it may result in disability of such a minor degree to make the patient slightly less capable of doing his usual daily duties, but the severely deficient individual may be so affected that his very existence is endangered whenever he is depleted of salt or exposed to any stressful situation. The diagnosis of profound hypoadrenocorticoidism is usually an obvious one, in contrast to the difficulty in recognition of the patient with subclinical or minimal hypoadrenocorticoidism, particularly in the early stages of adrenal insufficiency when there is only minimally decreased activity of the adrenal glands. In the latter case, the associated symptoms and findings may simulate unrelated disease entities, and, because of the prevailing asthenia, the patient, at times, may even be classified as psychoneurotic. Since an error in diagnosis is an ever-present possibility, it is imperative that adequate diagnostic measures be used before patients and their complaints are cast into the wastebasket of modern-day diagnosis—a "psychoneurotic." Furthermore, it is necessary to delineate between bona fide adrenal disease and psychosomatic disturbances, since the patient with decreased adrenal activity, although minimal at first, may face a fatal outcome if his disease progresses unrecognized and untreated. Therefore, it is important that the physician be cognizant of the fact that hypoadrenocorticoidism may mimic psychosomatic disease such as inadequacies or asthenia.

Adrenal
Insufficiency

Adrenal insufficiency was first characterized as a specific clinical entity by Addison in 1855.[1] His classic clinical description of the disease cannot be improved upon more than a century later. The acuteness of Addison's description is made all the more apparent since Bright himself had described one of the cases discussed by Addison, but he apparently failed to comprehend or correlate the clinical significance of adrenal atrophy and the associated syndrome. Neoplastic invasion of the adrenals and anemia, which were considered by Addison to be the major etiologic factors of his disease, are regarded as relatively uncommon elements in the physiopathology of the adrenal glands in Addison's disease.

Anatomy, Physiology, and Morphology of the Adrenal Gland. ANATOMY. The adrenal glands cap the superior pole of each kidney and have a combined weight of 8 to 11 Gm. The right adrenal, shaped like a truncated pyramid, is situated somewhat lower (due to the overlying liver) than the left adrenal, which is more elongated and semilunar in appearance (Fig. 416). The lower pole of the left adrenal may extend down to the hilar portion of the left kidney. The blood supply to the adrenal is derived via three arteries arising from the inferior diaphragmatic (phrenic) artery, aorta, and renal artery, respectively. The nerve supply to the adrenal gland arises from the splanchnic plexus from a large number of roots, presumably from the sixth to the sixteenth segments of the spinal cord. These nerves join to form the suprarenal plexus and

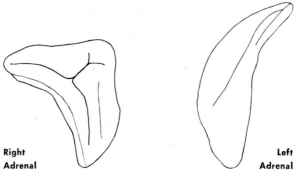

Right
Adrenal

Left
Adrenal

FIG. 416.   Gross appearance of the adrenal glands.

connect with the renal and celiac plexuses as well as with the celiac
ganglia. They are preganglionic medullated fibers and run without
synaptic interruption to the cells they innervate. The fibers pass through
the cortex and terminate in the medulla, where clawlike terminations
can be seen in the region of the medullary cells. The preganglionic nature
of these fibers and their intimate relationship with the medullary cells
lend credence to the thought that the cells of the medulla are modified
ganglion cells—a concept supported by the embryologic development of
this region of the adrenal. There do not appear to be any definite
nerve connections with the cells of the cortex.

MORPHOLOGY. Morphologically, the adrenal gland is made up of
the outer cortex and the inner medulla. The cortex is divided into three
zones—the zona glomerulosa lying beneath the capsule, the zona fasciculata
or middle zone layer, and the zona reticularis lying adjacent to the
medulla.[2] The zona glomerulosa is the thinnest of the three cortical zone
layers and contains cells arranged in whorls or in hooked or coiled
columns which connect with the linear columns of cells of the fasciculata
(Fig. 417). Occasionally, a cross section of the glomerulosa cells, because
of their particular configuration, produces an appearance similar to the
acinar grouping of cells such as in the thyroid. The middle zone layer,
the zona fasciculata, is the widest of the three layers of the cortex and
consists of linear columns of cells arranged parallel to one another and
perpendicular to the capsule (Fig. 417). The cells are rich in lipid-like
material and are polygonal in shape with vesicular nuclei. The parallel
columns are separated from one another by sinusoids lined partly with
reticulo-endothelial cells. The zona reticularis is the innermost zone
layer of the cortex whose cells are also polygonal in shape but are arranged
in criss-cross fashion, forming a reticulum of linear cellular elements in
the form of an anastomosing network (Fig. 417) .

Some investigators suggest that the cells of the adrenal cortex originate near the capsule adjacent to the zona glomerulosa and then migrate

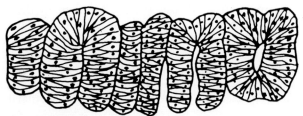

Zona Glomerulosa

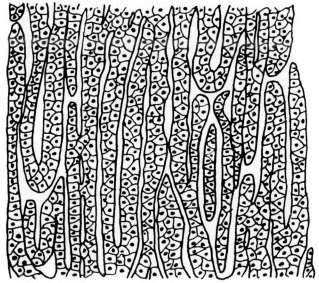

Zona Fasciculata

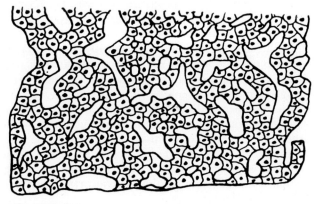

Zona Reticularis

*FIG. 417. Diagrammatic presentation of the cellular alignment
of the three zones of the adrenal cortex.*

down toward the reticularis. Mitosis is most frequent in the portion of the glomerulosa adjacent to the fasciculata. It diminishes as one proceeds down toward the reticularis. Regeneration and growth of the adrenal cortex may originate in the zona glomerulosa, while the lipoid material is most abundant in the fasciculata and least in the reticularis. This latter zone layer contains the largest number of degenerative cells. Pigment is abundantly present in the zona reticularis, particularly after the age of 20.

The X-Zone or Fetal Layer.   It is interesting to note that, in rodents, the reticularis zone layer is especially prominent and has been referred to as the X-zone.[24] It has been suggested that this zone layer may be the source of adrenal androgen in rodents. The X-zone layer, which is more prominent in male mice, normally disappears as the animal approaches sexual maturation; however, it will persist if the mice are castrated early, but can be made to disappear by the administration of exogenous androgens.[40]

Fetal Zone in the Human.   The human fetus has a similar fetal or X-zone layer which makes up by far the largest portion of the fetal adrenal cortex. It is this structure which is responsible for the enormous size of the fetal adrenal, comparatively speaking. The X-zone in the human fetus appears to be distinct from the three classic zone layers described above. This layer, whether or not it is related to the zona reticularis, is responsible for the adrenal gland being larger than the kidney in a four week old human embryo. At birth the adrenal becomes one third the size of the kidney, while in the adult it is only 3 to 4 per cent of the kidney's size. The fetal zone layer seen in the embryo of the human and of other primates appears to be dependent on chorionic gonadotropin (HCG) for its existence.[30] The precise role of this zone layer in the normal development of the fetus or its importance in the development of androgenic syndromes is not known. However, one may state categorically at the present time that this zone layer (fetal zone) in the human plays no part in the initiation of the adrenogenital syndrome (AGS), although through its possible relationship to the zona reticularis its potential androgenic role may be indirectly stimulated in the AGS.

PHYSIOLOGY.   Our concepts of the physiology of the adrenal cortex have gone through tremendous change in the past decade. Knowledge of the basic mechanisms concerned with the production and the secretion of the adrenocortical hormones permits us to comprehend the physiopathology of the adrenal cortex. While this may not appear to be particularly important in order to understand the pathogenesis of hypofunction of the adrenal cortex, it is certainly necessary to have some knowledge of the factors responsible for regulation of the adrenocortical secretion to be able to prescribe appropriate therapy.

STEROID NUCLEUS.   Some points concerning nomenclature and numbering of the carbon atoms in the structure of the nucleus common to all

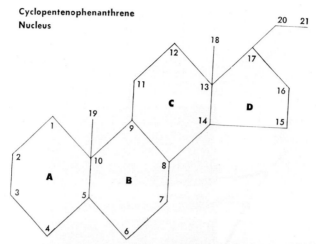

FIG. 418. *Basic structural configuration of all steroid nuclei. Each number refers to the presence of a carbon atom and is identified by that number.*

steroid hormones should be considered. All the steroids are composed of the cyclopentenophenanthrene nucleus (Fig. 418). There are four rings in this structure, designated as A, B, C and D, which have their carbon atoms numbered as indicated in Figure 418. Hence, when one mentions 17-ketosteroids, he does not refer to 17 different steroids but just to those steroids with a ketone group at the 17 carbon atom. Oxygenation at carbon 21 would mean that the two hydrogen atoms at this carbon have been replaced by a $= 0$ (double-bond oxygen). The symbol $\triangle 1$ (delta-one), or $\triangle 3$ refers to the fact that carbon 1 and 2 (for $\triangle 1$) or 3 and 4 (for $\triangle 3$) are unsaturated and are connected with a double bond such as $C = C$.

Aldosterone Secretion. Adrenocorticotropic hormone (ACTH) is responsible for maintaining the function and the integrity of the two innermost zone layers of the adrenal cortex. The zona glomerulosa and its secretory product, aldosterone, do not appear to be under direct ACTH control (Fig. 419).[7, 18] Aldosterone controls salt and water metabolism of the body. This hormone may be present in one of two forms (Fig. 420). The factors controlling aldosterone secretion are in the blood levels of sodium and potassium and the degree of hydration (Fig. 419).[8, 33] Aldosterone secretion is increased when blood sodium is low, blood potassium is high, or the patient is dehydrated.[13] On the other hand, aldosterone secretion is diminished when blood sodium is high, potassium is low or the patient is well hydrated or edematous.

GLOMERULOTROPIN. It is thought that this substance controls aldosterone output through a chemoreceptor area in the diencephalon

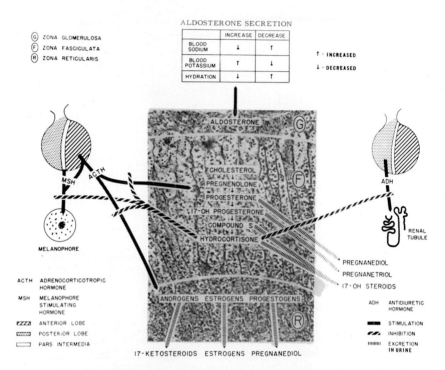

FIG. 419. *Interrelationship existing between the pituitary and adrenal cortex.*
Inhibition of ACTH, MSH, and ADH secretion by hydrocortisone is appropri-
ately indicated. The secretion of aldosterone is determined by serum electro-
lyte activity.

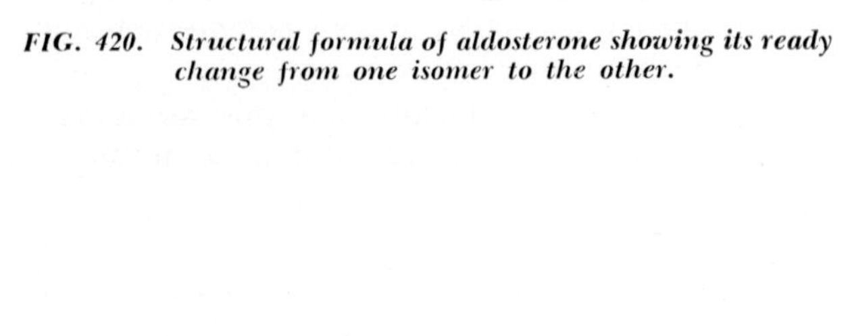

Aldosterone

FIG. 420. *Structural formula of aldosterone showing its ready*
change from one isomer to the other.

or, more specifically, in the pineal gland.[12] The chemoreceptors supposedly are responsible for releasing or inhibiting the release of a substance termed glomerulotropin, which in turn controls the secretory activity of the zona glomerulosa.

However, the entire story is not this simple and is discussed more fully in Chapter 22. A few remarks on aldosterone secretion are included here for reference purposes. The statement that aldosterone secretion or the zona glomerulosa is not under ACTH control[34] may not be precisely true, inasmuch as there has been evidence to show that increased aldosterone secretion can be induced with ACTH.[5] A more comprehensive view may be that, under normal circumstances, glomerulotropin controls the secretion of aldosterone. However, in cases of increased need or stress, further aldosterone secretion may be stimulated by ACTH.[26] Unlike desoxycorticosterone acetate (DCA), aldosterone requires the presence of glucocorticoids to achieve its physiologic effect.[9] Aldosterone may be ineffective in the adrenalectomized dog or in the human without adrenal function unless hydrocortisone or other glucocorticoids are administered concomitantly.[9] Therapeutically, this is of little importance, since aldosterone is used only for investigational purposes and is usually administered parenterally. However, this fact does help to direct therapy in certain "salt-losing syndromes." The so-called salt-losing syndrome noted in some infants with the adrenogenital syndrome (AGS) may be accompanied by normal aldosterone secretion, but the absence of hydrocortisone nullifies the effectiveness of the salt-retaining steroid. The physician now has oral preparations available which are potent agents for the retention of sodium without the need for concomitant glucocorticoid therapy. The synthetic oral salt-retaining steroid which is most active in the therapy of adrenal insufficiency is fludrocortisone (Florinef).

ACTH Control. ZONA FASCICULATA. *Secretion of Hydrocortisone.* The zona fasciculata and reticularis are both under the control of ACTH (Fig. 419). The zona fasciculata is responsible for the secretion of glucocorticoids (particularly hydrocortisone), and the sex steroids are secreted by the zona reticularis. Hydrocortisone is manufactured by the zona fasciculata in a series of reactions which may start with acetate, which then is converted into cholesterol; or cholesterol itself may be the prime chemical agent.[23] Cholesterol, under the stimulus of ACTH, is taken up by the zona fasciculata and is converted, progressively, into $\triangle$5-pregnenolone$\rightarrow$ progesterone$\rightarrow$ 17-hydroxyprogesterone$\rightarrow$ 11-desoxy-17-hydroxycorticosterone (Compound S)$\rightarrow$ hydrocortisone (Figs. 421 and 422).[4, 25] ACTH also enhances the uptake of glucose as well as increasing the cellular concentrate of adenosine 3' 5' monophosphate (AMP). There is an increase in cellular formation of glucose through the formation of glucose-6-phosphate. This in turn is acted upon

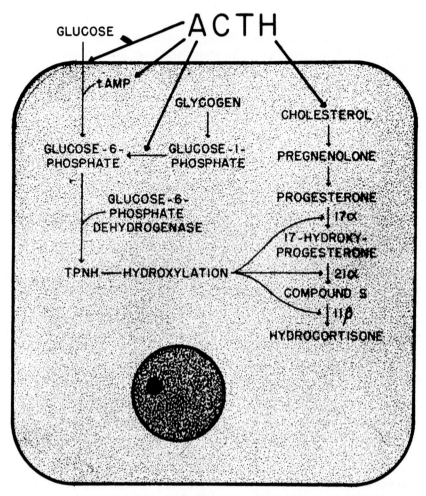

FIG. 421. Diagrammatic presentation of a single adrenal cortical cell with nucleus. ACTH effect on cellular metabolism of the zona fasciculata. It increases accumulation of adenosine 3'5' monophosphate (AMP). This increases intracellular formation of glucose-6-phosphate which in turn is oxidized by its specific dehydrogenase to increase concentration of reduced triphosphopyridine nucleotide (TPNH). TPNH promotes or provides the energy for hydroxylation of the various steroids as shown.

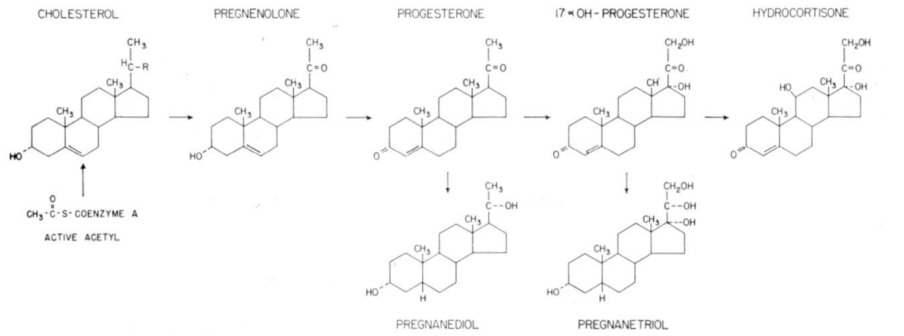

FIG. 422. *Conversion of cholesterol into hydrocortisone showing the intermediate steps and metabolites.*

by the enzyme glucose-6-phosphate dehydrogenase to reduced tri-phosphopyridine nucleotide (TPNH). TPNH provides the energy for the conversion of cholesterol to cortisol through the process of hydroxylation. Hydrocortisone and Compound S are excreted as 17-hydroxysteroids (17-OH) while progesterone and 17-OH progesterone are excreted as pregnanediol and pregnanetriol, respectively.[4] Adult men and women excrete 3 to 9 mg. of 17-OH/24 hours (normal values for our laboratory) and 0 to 1.8 mg. of pregnanetriol/24 hours (normal values for our laboratory.) Women, during the proliferative phase of their menstrual cycle, and men usually excrete less than 0.5 to 1.5 mg. of pregnanediol/24 hours. Women in the ovulatory phase of their cycle will put out 4 to 8 mg. of pregnanediol/24 hours, depending on the stage of their secretory phase and on the activity of the corpora lutea. The 17-OH tend to be elevated during pregnancy and also somewhat more so in the obese individual.[43] This must be considered very carefully in the evaluation of obese patients suspected of having Cushing's disease and in whom there may be a slight elevation of 17-OH. The fact that ACTH promotes an uptake of cholesterol by the adrenal in the formation of glucocorticoids does not mean that this is conducive to lowering of blood cholesterol per se. The amount of cholesterol used is infinitesimal when compared to the cholesterol pool in the body. Indeed, as noted in the previous chapter on hormonology, ACTH may actually elevate blood cholesterol in the normal or adrenalectomized individual.

Another important chemical factor in steroidogenesis in the zona fasciculata is that progesterone plays an essential role in the formation of the different steroid products from all three zone layers of the adrenal cortex. The importance of progesterone in the synthesis of testosterone by the zona reticularis is illustrated in Figure 423. Similarly by the different types of hydroxylation, progesterone can be converted into the principal steroids of the zona glomerulosa and zona fasciculata (Fig. 424). Cortisol, as has been discussed above, is formed from progesterone by 17α-hydroxyla-

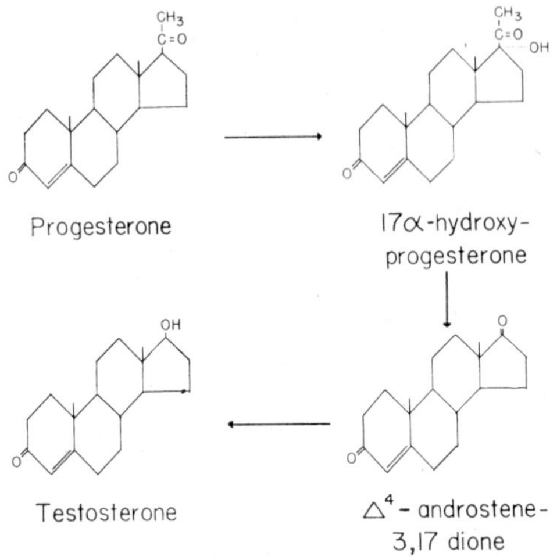

FIG. 423

tion which is the initial step in the hydroxylation of progesterone to cortisol. On the other hand, when progesterone is first subjected to 11β,-21-hydroxylation, then aldosterone is recovered.

Enzymes known as hydroxylases are necessary to change 17-OH progesterone into Compound S and thence into hydrocortisone (Fig. 422). These enzymes are important in bringing about hydroxylation at C-21 and C-11 (Fig. 424).

"Balance of Power." As with other pituitary-end-organ relationships, hydrocortisone, which is controlled or produced under ACTH influence, also has an inhibitory effect on ACTH itself. In other words, when hydrocortisone reaches the necessary or ideal blood level, it inhibits further ACTH secretion. When there is increased tissue utilization so that the hydrocortisone level falls, then ACTH secretion again takes place. This check and balance between hydrocortisone and ACTH may be referred to as the "balance of power" existing between the pituitary tropic hormones and their specific dependent end organs. This balance plays a vital role in the relationship between the two hormones to maintain homeostasis and to prevent either the excessive secretion or production of hydrocortisone and eventual hyperadrenocorticoidism, or secondary hypoadrenocorticoidism when ACTH secretion fails to be adequately maintained in the face of falling glucocorticoid levels. The interrelationship existing between hydrocortisone and ACTH is responsible for creating corticoid homeostasis with a normally functioning gland.

Metyrapone has been made available (Fig. 425) for testing ACTH reserve and secretion. This chemical inhibits hydroxylation at carbon 11. This results in increased ACTH secretion which is followed by enhanced

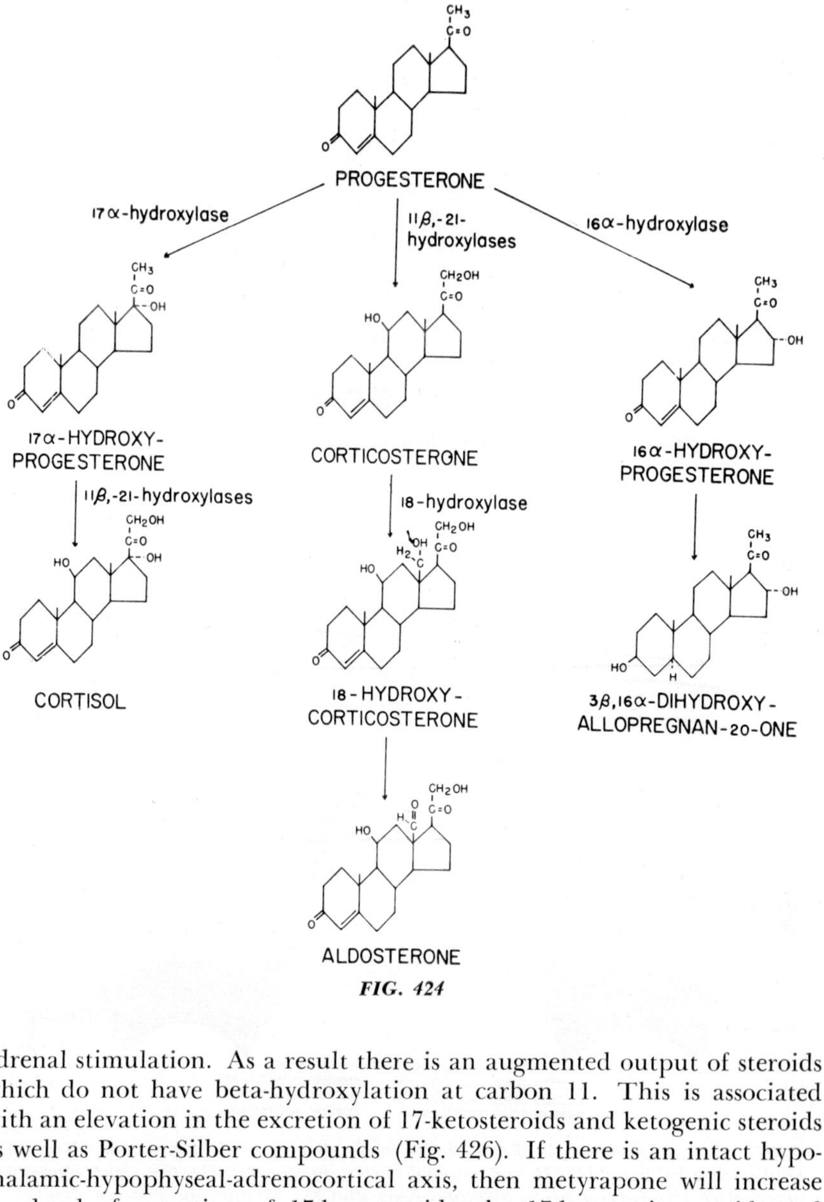

FIG. 424

adrenal stimulation. As a result there is an augmented output of steroids which do not have beta-hydroxylation at carbon 11. This is associated with an elevation in the excretion of 17-ketosteroids and ketogenic steroids as well as Porter-Silber compounds (Fig. 426). If there is an intact hypothalamic-hypophyseal-adrenocortical axis, then metyrapone will increase the level of excretion of 17-ketosteroids, the 17-ketogenic steroids and 17-hydroxysteroids.

ZONA RETICULARIS. *Secretion of Sex Steroids.* ACTH also stimulates and presumably maintains the function of the zona reticularis. This zone layer under ACTH control secretes the sex steroids—androgens,

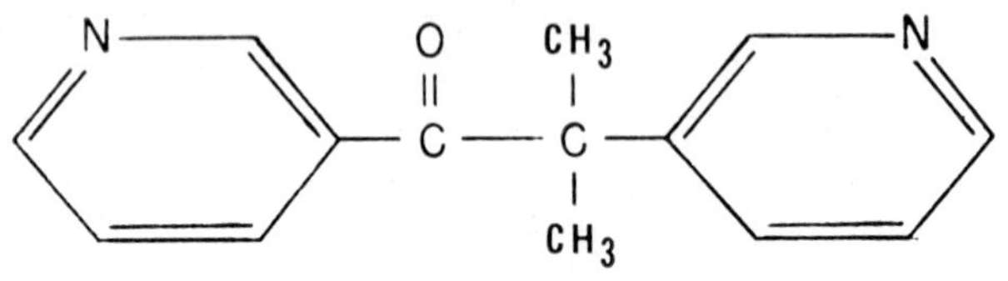

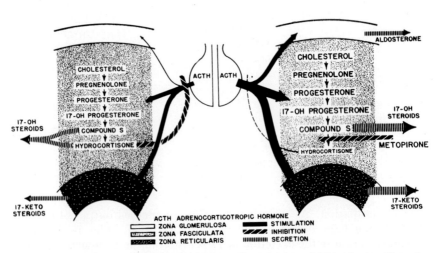

2-methyl-1,2-bis-(3-pyridyl)-1-propanone

SU-4885

FIG. 425. *Metyrapone chemical compound inhibiting beta-hydroxylation at carbon 11.*

FIG. 426. *Diagrammatic sketch shows mode of action of Metopirone. Normal relationship between ACTH and adrenal cortex on the left. On the right, changes noted after Metopirone administration. Note that the Metopirone prevents hydroxylation of Compound S to hydrocortisone, bringing about increased ACTH secretion due to decreased Compound F production. Increased ACTH secretion results in increased 17-KS and 17-OH output.*

estrogens, and progestogens. The androgens are by far the most important clinically, and their excretion product, the neutral 17-ketosteroids (17-KS), is a valuable guide for the laboratory in the diagnosis of adrenal insufficiency. The 17-KS are all derived from the adrenal cortex in the female, while two thirds are from the adrenal and one third is from the testes in the adult male. Estrogens and progestins are produced in much smaller amounts and are excreted as estrogens and pregnanediol, respectively, but the amounts of these excretory products of adrenal origin in the urine of the normal male and female are very small and usually clinically insignificant. Males ordinarily have less than 1.0 to 1.5 mg. of pregnanediol per day, while the estrogen level in males is usually less than 2 to 4 rat units/24 hours. The normal values for the 17-ketosteroid excretion by the method used in our laboratory are as follows:

Sex and Age	*17-KS*
Male—adult	10 to 24 mg./24 hours
Female—adult	8 to 14 mg./24 hours
Children—prior	0.5 to 0.75 mg./24 hours per
to puberty	year of life up to the age
	of 10 to 11 years

Both 17-OH and 17-KS are largely excreted in their conjugated form in the urine, with some being excreted into the biliary tree and discharged into the intestinal tract. Partial reabsorption also occurs from the intestinal tract so that the 17-KS excreted in the urine may represent the steroid excreted directly in the urine as well as that excreted into the urine after reabsorption from the intestinal tract. Occasionally, some of the 17-KS detected in the urine of patients may be due in part to exogenously administered glucocorticoids. This, however, usually represents 5 per cent or less of the exogenously administered corticoids. The reason that the cortisone and cortisol are partly excreted as 17-KS is obvious when we consider Fig. 427 where 17-keto compounds with androgen qualities may be derived from cortisone or cortisol.

The above information is offered in an attempt to provide the physician with a working knowledge of adrenal-pituitary physiology. Further discussion will be concerned with hypoadrenocorticoidism. Many of the observations originally presented by Addison will be enlarged upon herein and discussed in light of modern advances in endocrinology.

Causes of Adrenal Insufficiency. The etiology of primary adrenal insufficiency includes the following: (1) Idiopathic, (2) tuberculosis, (3) iatrogenic disease, and (4) destruction of the adrenal by neoplasm or amyloidosis. In the time of Addison the most common cause of adrenal destruction was neoplastic invasion. In the past two or three decades the great majority of the patients with adrenal insufficiency were shown to have tuberculosis of the adrenal gland, usually secondary to pulmonary tuberculosis. It now appears that spontaneous degeneration of the adren-

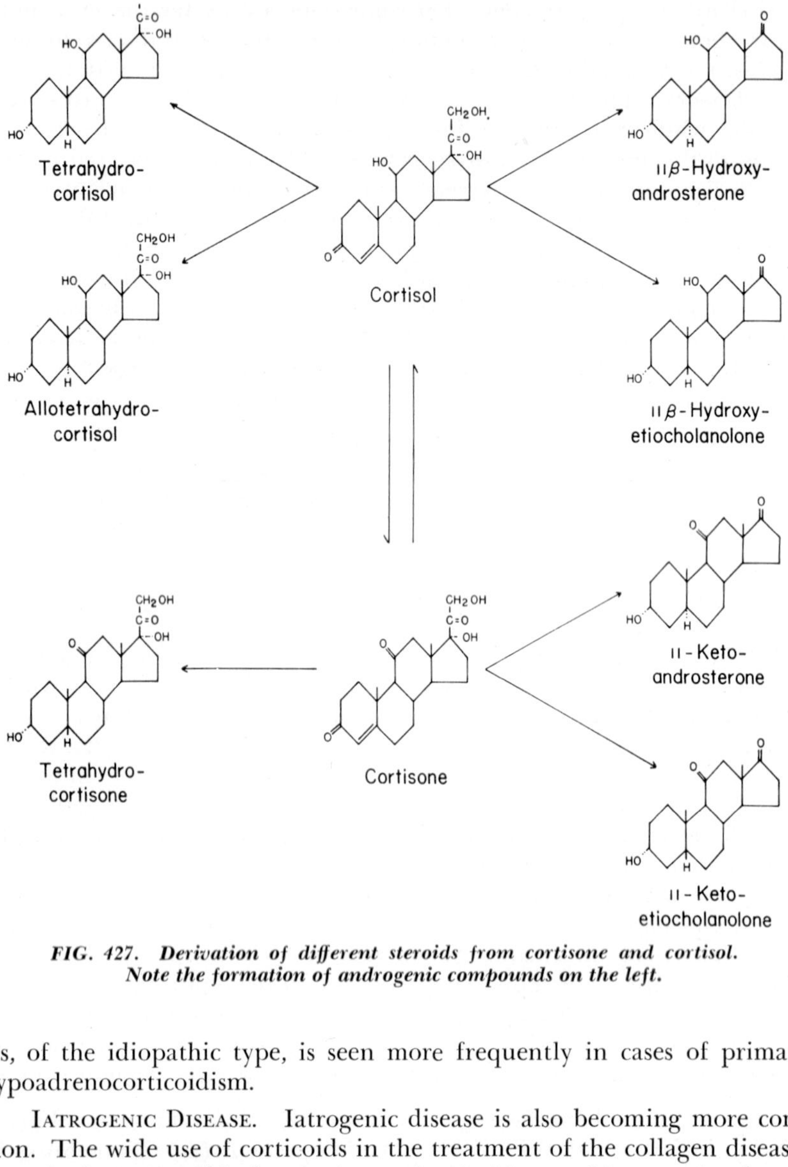

FIG. 427. Derivation of different steroids from cortisone and cortisol.
Note the formation of androgenic compounds on the left.

als, of the idiopathic type, is seen more frequently in cases of primary hypoadrenocorticoidism.

IATROGENIC DISEASE. Iatrogenic disease is also becoming more common. The wide use of corticoids in the treatment of the collagen diseases is no doubt responsible for the increasing incidence of iatrogenic adrenal disease. Corticoids employed in doses greater than 75 mg. of cortisone per day, or its equivalent, have the potential of significantly depressing endogenous adrenal activity by completely inhibiting endogenous ACTH secretion. If such doses of corticoids are administered over a long enough period of time, without the use of concomitant and weekly injections of

ACTH, atrophy of the adrenal glands may be anticipated. Such patients would have iatrogenic hypoadrenocorticoidism as a result of inability of the chronically suppressed gland to respond to either exogenous or endogenous ACTH when the glucocorticoid is stopped. The diagnosis of iatrogenic disease is based on the patient's history and his failure to show an adequate response to exogenous ACTH administration. Adrenal failure may occasionally follow abdominal surgical procedures in the adrenal region where interference with vascular supply to the adrenal may occur.

NEOPLASM OR AMYLOIDOSIS. While Addison, in his classic description, referred to neoplastic invasion of the adrenal glands as an important factor in the development of adrenal insufficiency, it now appears that invasive malignancy of the adrenal gland, bilaterally, is a rare cause of adrenal insufficiency. Nevertheless, it should still be considered, particularly in patients with lymphoblastomas where both adrenals may be destroyed by the primary neoplasm. Amyloidosis is more frequently noted as a cause of adrenal insufficiency than invasive neoplasm, yet it is also uncommon.

Recognizing Adrenal Insufficiency. Diminished adrenal function may be due to either primary (adrenal atrophy or destruction) or secondary (ACTH insufficiency) adrenal failure. The symptoms will be essentially the same in both groups, but the clinical and laboratory findings may differ to some degree. These differences will be elaborated upon after the classic findings and symptomatology are reviewed. Recognizing adrenal insufficiency in the patient with profound hypoadrenocorticoidism requires little in the way of diagnostic acumen. It is the patient with minimal or beginning failure of the adrenals who requires careful consideration and diagnostic awareness for the physician to recognize a disease which may be so insidious in onset as to obscure the basic problem from the eyes of even the expert.

The primary symptom which one sees in the patient with decreased adrenal activity is moderate to profound weakness or asthenia. This may at times be the major reason for the patient to come to the physician. Inasmuch as this complaint is seen in so many other clinical entities, particularly those allied with psychosomatic disorders, it may be difficult to differentiate hypoadrenocorticoidism from other syndromes on the basis of clinical history and physical examination alone. As with all other disease entities involving the adrenal gland, the diagnosis, if suspected from the clinical picture, must be substantiated by modern laboratory procedures. These tests determine with precision the functioning state of the adrenal.

Clinical Findings. Since the clinician should recognize some of the obscure as well as obvious signs of the disease, the following basic symptomatology is presented. This should not imply, however, that all of the clinical findings listed are noted in every Addisonian patient.

WEAKNESS. This is the major complaint and is commonly seen in all patients with Addison's disease. Weakness is out of proportion to exertion and is accentuated together with fatigue during the hot weather when the patient perspires freely, particularly if he does not have adequate salt replacement.

FATIGUE. This must be differentiated from weakness and is ordinarily exhibited in patients who have a low tolerance for their usual daily duties. The fatigue may be so profound as to make the incipient or early Addisonian incapable of completing a physical task to which he has normally been accustomed. Even talking may become an effort. The weakness and easy fatigability of potential, subclinical, or frank Addisonism may result in the clinical diagnosis of neurasthenia due to psychoneurosis. There may also be an associated irritability, nervousness, depression, and insecurity. Consequently, the asthenia of the Addisonian patient should be delineated from the psychological aberration of the patient solely with psychosomatic disease.

TEMPERATURE INTOLERANCE. The Addisonian patient is intolerant of cold temperatures. He also cannot tolerate excessive heat because of his abnormal loss of salt through perspiration. There may be some measure of circulatory failure of the extremities, producing blanching and muscle cramps in cold climates.

WEIGHT LOSS. The patient with Addison's disease invariably shows a decrease in weight which appears to coincide with the onset of his disease and the manifestations of asthenia. Psychoneurotics tend to overeat, but occasionally one sees a weight decrease in these patients. Obesity sometimes obscures the true diagnosis, but even the obese Addisonian still gives a history of weight loss with the onset of his disease.

APPETITE. There is usually some decrease in appetite. However, the Addisonian patient does not have the marked aversion to food noted in patients with anorexia nervosa. The patient with subclinical manifestations of the disease may not show the salt craving described in the classic adrenally insufficient individual. Unlike the adrenalectomized rat who seeks salt, salt craving does not appear to be a common symptom in the Addisonian patient.

BOWEL HABITS. If there is any change in the bowel habits, it generally tends to be toward diarrhea rather than constipation.

BLOOD PRESSURE. Hypotension is usually the rule, but a patient with elevated blood pressure prior to the development of Addison's disease may show a normal blood pressure in the presence of adrenal insufficiency. This normal manometric reading would be hypotensive for him, but this fact would not be recognized unless the past history of hypertension was known.

PIGMENTATION.   Classically, the patient with primary adrenal insufficiency shows increased pigmentation in the pressure areas of the body
(Figs. 428, 429) and in the creases of the palms of the hands and in
other body creases. The alar portion of the nose will also be hyperpig-
mented. Any previously noted pigmented nevi will show an increase in
pigmentation (Fig. 430). Operative scars due to injuries occurring or
surgery performed after the onset of the disease usually will show evidence
of increased pigmentation; however if the injury or surgery was prior to
the onset of the adrenal insufficiency, there will be no evidence of increased pigmentation in the resultant scar (Fig. 432) .

There are also typical pigmentation changes in the mucosal membranes of the mouth and the genital region. The areas showing the
characteristic dark brown to blue-brown pigmentation are usually those
subject to some pressure. Thus, the gums are more apt to be pigmented
than the buccal mucous membranes (Fig. 431).

DIFFERENTIAL DIAGNOSIS OF PIGMENTATION.   Pigmentation of the oral
mucosa can sometimes be attributed to factors other than Addison's
disease. It may occur with poor oral hygiene which is not associated with
adrenal insufficiency particularly where sulfide formation is prone to
occur.

Pigmentation may follow ingestion of heavy metals, such as bismuth,
mercury, silver and lead salts. The pigmentation noted in such cases
is indistinguishable from that observed in Addison's disease, except for
the heavy metal pigmentation being concentrated in the area of the gum
line. It occurs rarely on the mucosal membrane of the cheek or lip. The
external genitalia of the female tend to show increased pigmentation in
the Addisonian patient and a similar increase in pigmentation may be
noted in the perineal region of the male.

Negro Addisonian Patients.   An increase in pigmentation may be
noted in the Negro Addisonian. Many of these patients will complain of
a darkening of their skin, which may be more noticeable to the patient
or his associates than to the physician. On the other hand, oral pigmentation in the Negro or dark-skinned races is of little or no diagnostic
significance. It is not unusual for the healthy, dark-skinned peoples to
show areas of pigmentation of the oral mucosa similar to those seen in
Addison's disease.

Hemochromatosis.   The pigmentation of hemochromatosis is slate-
gray in color, generalized in distribution, not concentrated in certain
areas, and usually associated with some measure of hepatomegaly and
hepatic insufficiency. A diabetic glucose tolerance test with normotensive
or hypertensive blood pressures is a further aid in differentiating the
patient with hemochromatosis from the Addisonian patient.

Melanodermia and Solar Radiation.   Melanodermia due to drug
therapy, solar or x-ray radiation may simulate the skin color seen in
Addison's disease. However, the distribution of color and the history may

help to differentiate these cases from Addison's disease. The history of taking silver salts, for example, together with the ashen gray appearance of the skin, would aid one in establishing the correct diagnosis. Solar radiation tans only the exposed parts of the body. The Addisonian patient tends to show a deeper tan, with a more prolonged retention of the pigment than normally noted after exposure to the sun. Pigmentation of heavy metal poisoning, hemochromatosis, or a reaction to the use of drugs is not accentuated by exposure to the ultraviolet rays of the sun. In contrast, pigmentation of the Addisonian patient shows an unusual degree of accentuation by solar radiation.

Carotenemia. The patient with carotenemia may give a history of excessive ingestion of carrots. The skin pigment is yellowish in color and not particularly noticeable in the pressure areas of the body. The palms of the hands are also yellowish in color, without accentuation of the palmar folds.

Bile Pigment. The deeply jaundiced individual can be delineated from the Addisonian by the fact that the conjunctiva of the Addisonian patient is clear and the pigment associated with jaundice is more yellow or orange in color.

Chloasma of Pregnancy and Amenorrhea. The pigment of chloasma usually has a butterfly distribution over the bridge of the nose and the malar eminences. The face is the only area showing this pigmentation. The rest of the skin remains relatively normal. There is no accentuation of color in the pressure areas of the body. However, the pigmentary changes of chloasma and of the Addisonian patient are indistinguishable in color and shade of pigment and both are accentuated by solar radiation.

Acanthosis Nigricans. Acanthosis nigricans offers no diagnostic problem in differentiation from the pigment of the Addisonian due to the associated dermatologic picture and the velvety feel of the lesions. There is also a tendency for the lesions to be limited to the axillary region of the body. Frequently, they are associated with diabetes mellitus.

Intestinal Polyposis. Oral pigmentation associated with intestinal polyposis is indistinguishable from that noted in the Addisonian. There is no other evidence of increased pigment in these patients, as far as the body is concerned. The history of rectal bleeding and the typical roentgenologic picture by barium enema help to differentiate the two and lead to the diagnosis of the syndrome of Peutz.

Lues and Malaria. In the past, although rarely seen now, hyperpigmentation has been noted in patients with lues and malaria. Here, again, the history of the infection or of therapy helps to establish a correct diagnosis. The pigmentation is of a modest degree and distributed throughout the body with no predilection for a particular site. Such pigmentation is not accentuated by solar radiation.

Pernicious Anemia. The pigmentation of pernicious anemia never presents any specific diagnostic differential problem from the melanin deposition of Addison's disease because of its lemon yellow color, its

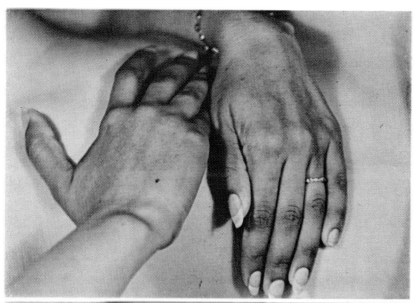

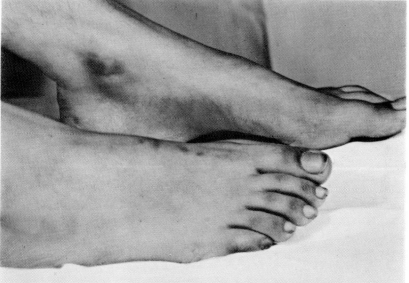

FIG. 428A (upper photograph). Note the increased pigmentation on the extensor surfaces of the knuckles, representing the pressure areas of the hand. Note the increased pigmentation of the exposed part of the hand as compared to the lower portion of the forearm.

FIG. 428B (lower photograph). Note the increased pigmentation in the region of the ankle as well as on the upper portion of the foot, showing hyperpigmentation in the pressure area due to buckles. The toes of the feet, as with the hands, show increased pigmentation at the extensor surfaces of the knuckles.

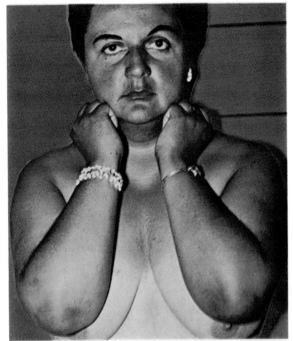

FIG. 429. Note the increased pigmentation on the pressure areas of the elbows and exposed portions of the body.

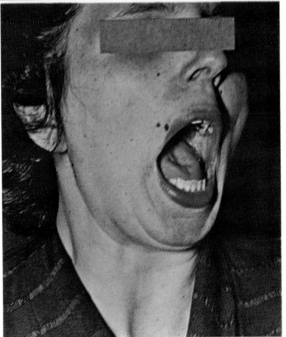

FIG. 430. Note the pigmented nevi as well as accentuated pigmentation of the alar region of the nose.

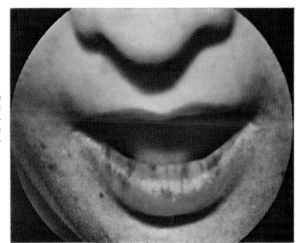

FIG. 431. Pigmentation on the buccal mucosa on the lip showing the typical dark brown changes characteristic of Addison's disease.

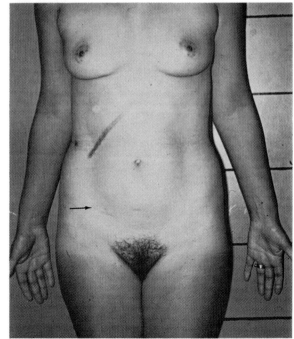

FIG. 432. Abdomen of patient AM with Addison's disease. Highly pigmented gallbladder incision is seen in contrast to the non-pigmented (arrow) appendectomy scar. The cholecystectomy was done shortly after the onset of her adrenal disease.

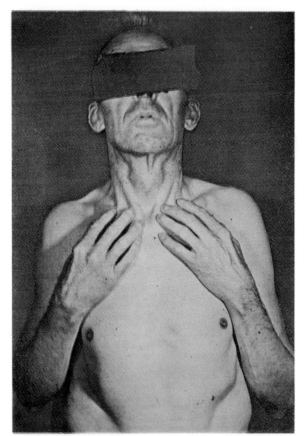

FIG. 433A. Increased pigmentation of the areolae of a normally light-skinned male with Addison's disease of some five years' duration. The pigmentation of the face and arms has persisted for a number of months since exposure to the sun.

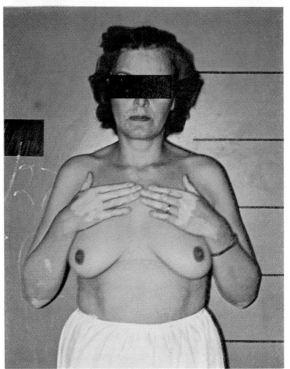

FIG. 433B. Vitiligo associated with hyperpigmentation of Addison's disease.

failure to be accentuated by solar radiation, and its association with a macrocytic, hyperchromic anemia. The anemia originally noted by Addison in his classic description of the disease can perhaps be attributed to inadequate diagnostic techniques. His diagnosis was based empirically on the pallor that his patients presented. The Addisonian patient does not necessarily have an associated anemia.

Increased Melanin in the Nipple.   Characteristically, pigmentation of the Addisonian is associated with an increased melanin deposition in the areola of the nipple (Fig. 433A). This may be so marked that the nipples of both females and males may be pigmented to a degree comparable to that produced in the nipples of patients under treatment with one of the stilbene derivatives.

Vitiligo.   Another feature of the pigmentation seen in the Addisonian is the presence of vitiligo (Fig. 433B). The depigmentation associated with hyperpigmentation may be so pronounced as to provide a striking signpost for the diagnosis of Addison's disease. The vitiligo is sometimes extensive enough to create a picture of depigmentation rather than one of hyperpigmentation, which is the normal finding in Addison's disease. Increased freckle distribution may be noted. Freckles previously present may become darker and appear black in color. Apparently, this is due to accentuation and increase in the amount of melanin already present in the freckled area.

PUBIC AND AXILLARY HAIR.   During the early stages of adrenal insufficiency, there may be slight loss of pubic or axillary hair in the female. The more severe the deficiency, the more profound this becomes. Pubic and axillary hair may diminish very slightly, if at all, in the male Addisonian, particularly if the adrenal insufficiency is mild in nature.

CRAVING FOR SALT.   It is said that Addisonian patients crave salt. In our experience, this has not been the usual finding in most patients with decreased adrenocortical activity. In the markedly salt-depleted state, they are too sick to crave salt. In their compensated state with normally active daily duties, they may use an increased amount of salt in their food but not to the extent that a craving for salt can be detected by their particular dietary habits. Many normal people in our American culture use excessive amounts of salt on their food. It is not unusual at the dinner table to see some people liberally sprinkling salt over their food even before tasting it. It therefore becomes difficult to establish pathologic salt craving in most individuals.

GASTROINTESTINAL SYMPTOMS.   The patient approaching a crisis presents a group of gastrointestinal symptoms worthy of mention. These patients may show marked nausea, vomiting, and diarrhea sufficiently severe to alter the electrolyte findings anticipated in Addison's disease. For example, the loss of fluid via the intestinal tract may result in dehydration and sufficient loss of anions and cations that such patients may appear to have low potassium (due to loss of potassium via the gastrointestinal tract) and normal sodium (due to dehydration). The patients may also have severe gastrointestinal cramps, similar to those in the acute surgical abdomen. The severe pain and cramps have been attributed to sharp alteration in tissue electrolyte contents.

Laboratory Findings.   PROVOCATIVE TESTS.   In the past, two provocative tests were used to establish the potential adrenal reserve in the suspected Addisonian patient. In those patients with subclinical hypoadreno-corticoidism, a diminished adrenal reserve may be demonstrated by tests which exhaust functional capacity of the adrenals. The potassium tolerance test[6] and insulin tolerance test[15, 17, 28] were used prior to the days of steroid analyses to establish a definite diagnosis of adrenal insufficiency.

Potassium Tolerance Test.   The potassium tolerance test is no longer in use because of its potential danger to a patient with adrenal glands incapable of responding to stress. Although an adrenal crisis might be precipitated with the potassium tolerance test, it can now be easily managed with the use of cortisone. The procedure, however, is still not without danger and should be discarded. More precise and less dangerous diagnostic tests are now available.

Insulin Tolerance Test.   The insulin tolerance test may also be placed in the category of a provocative test which bears an inherent danger.[15, 17, 28] This test should also be relegated to the limbo of obsolete diagnostic procedures as far as adrenal insufficiency is concerned and is mentioned here primarily for its historic interest. The risks involved with the use of the insulin tolerance test, nevertheless, are comparatively minimal in view of the availability of intravenous hydrocortisone to counteract the hypoglycemic unresponsiveness that these patients may show. The characteristic insulin tolerance tests are depicted in Figure 434.

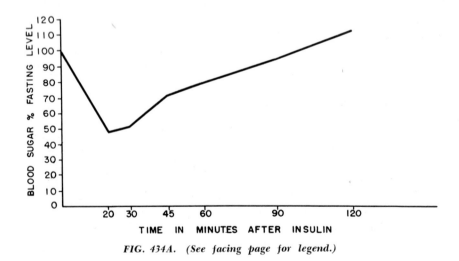

FIG. 434A.   (See facing page for legend.)

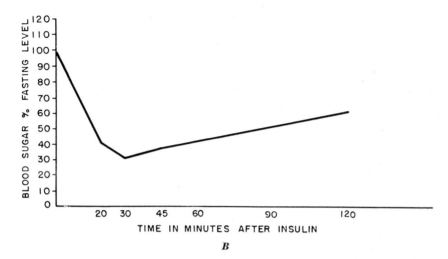

B

PATIENT ___M C___

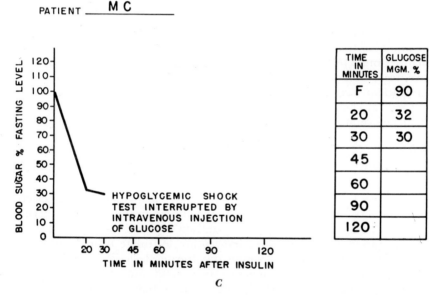

TIME IN MINUTES	GLUCOSE MGM. %
F	90
20	32
30	30
45	
60	
90	
120	

C

FIG. 434. *Insulin tolerance test—a provocative test. When 0.1 unit of regular insulin per kilogram of body weight is injected intravenously and blood is taken at prescribed intervals, the initial drop in blood sugar value is referred to as insulin responsiveness. The rise in blood sugar after its fall is referred to as hypoglycemic responsiveness.*

A, *Normal reaction of patient with normal adrenal function.*

B, *Hypoglycemic unresponsiveness seen in patient with adrenal insufficiency.*

C, *Extreme insulin sensitivity requiring interruption of test in a patient with marked adrenal insufficiency.*

Specific Testing Procedures.   The diagnosis of Addison's disease, while suspected on the basis of the clinical findings, must be confirmed by the performance of one or several of the following laboratory tests.

WATER TOLERANCE TEST.   Hydrocortisone normally inhibits the secretion of antidiuretic hormone (ADH) from the posterior pituitary. In Addisonian patients, diminished hydrocortisone permits excessive or uninhibited secretion of ADH so that there is diminished diuresis after a water-loading procedure.[36]

The water tolerance test may be performed as follows: at 10 P.M. the bladder is emptied and thereafter nothing is taken by mouth. Urine is collected for nine hours from 10 P.M. to 7 A.M. The patient is then given his water load in amounts of 20 cc. per kilogram of body weight. Urine is saved at hourly intervals for the next four hours. The normal patient will excrete a volume of urine during any one of the hourly specimens after hydration greater than the volume of the overnight specimen.

This may be demonstrated in another way. The total volume of urine excreted over a four-hour period is normally 60 per cent or more of the amount ingested. The Addisonian patient is unable to fulfill either of these requirements. This test is a simple screening office procedure. Patients with renal disease, hepatic insufficiency, decreased thyroid function, or cardiovascular disease may be unable to excrete the full volume of liquid so that a positive test reaction in the presence of these abnormalities must be considered as equivocal. Should the test result be negative, regardless of the presence of the above diseases, one can assume that the patient has normal adrenal function. Figure 435 shows, graphically, the radical changes in a water tolerance test in an Addisonian male patient before and after glucocorticoid therapy. It should be noted when the patient was maintained on 9-alpha-fluorohydrocortisone alone, his water tolerance test remained positive despite the fact that he felt well subjectively. When glucocorticoids were added, his water tolerance became negative, i.e., he was then able to handle a water load.

SERUM ELECTROLYTE CONCENTRATIONS.   Changes in serum electrolyte concentrations have been the time-honored procedures for determining the presence or the absence of Addison's disease. However, it should be recognized that detectable changes in electrolyte concentration may be absent in the incipient stages of the disease. Indeed, it would be most unusual for Addisonian patients to show significant alterations in blood sodium and potassium levels during the time that they are not in crisis and are capable of performing their usual activity. At the time of adrenal crisis, the classic changes of hyponatremia and hyperkalemia will often be seen. However, it must be remembered that the patient's sodium and potassium levels will be influenced by the patient's degree of dehydration. If the patient is markedly dehydrated and also has renal failure, the blood electrolyte pattern may be confusing, as there is an apparent hypernatremia as well as a hyperkalemia. The blood electrolytes may represent a

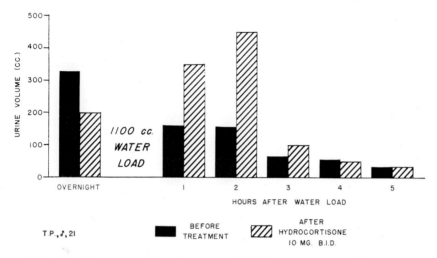

FIG. 435. *Water excretion after a water load in an Addisonian patient before and after glucocorticoid therapy. Mineralocorticoid, alone, failed to induce a normal response to a water load.*

picture of forced maintenance of electrolyte balance at the expense of intracellular changes. In other words, the patient with decreased adrenal activity may have depleted sodium and increased potassium levels within his tissue cells without reflecting these changes in the blood stream. This is another reason why blood or urinary electrolyte studies may be misleading even in patients approaching or in adrenal crisis. At times, the alteration in electrolyte levels may be reflected only in tissue electrolytes. Some evidence of this can be obtained in patients with elevated potassium levels by noting the alteration in the electrocardiogram (ECG). Classically, the ECG in a patient with hyperkalemia and elevated tissue potassium levels may show a high upright T wave with a prolonged P-R and Q-T interval best seen in the precordial leads.[44] A more recent suggestion is that the electrolyte content of the red blood cell may serve as a barometer of comparable sodium and potassium levels in tissue itself.[27]

GLUCOSE TOLERANCE. The glucose tolerance test is an important and simple diagnostic procedure helping to establish the presence or the absence of adrenal insufficiency.

Oral Glucose Tolerance Test. The normal test usually is characterized by an initial rise in blood sugar, followed by a fall. If the decrease in blood sugar is below the euglycemic level, there will then be a rise or a return of the blood sugar to the normal value. The graph of the glucose tolerance test may be somewhat flattened in a patient with adrenal insufficiency. While the initial part of the curve is usually

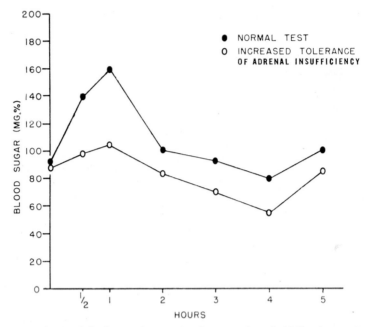

FIG. 436. *Carbohydrate tolerance in the normal and Addisonian patient. Note normal fasting blood glucose level in Addisonian patient with subsequent hypoglycemic level.*

relatively flat in these individuals, there also may be a persistent hypo-glycemic level without sufficient rebound in blood glucose level at the fourth or fifth hour of the test (Fig. 436). If this occurs and the patient is uncomfortable, then the test may be interrupted with intravenous glucocorticoids.

Intravenous Glucose Tolerance Test. This test is much more characteristic and shows a definite hypoglycemic level following the initial rise in the blood sugar. The intravenous glucose tolerance test is performed as follows: ⅓ Gm. of glucose per kilogram of body weight is given intravenously with blood sugars being taken at 0, 15, 30, 45, 60, 90, 120, 150, and 180 minutes after the glucose administration. The hypo-glycemic level represents a rebound phenomenon occurring as a result of the induced hyperglycemia. Hyperglycemia invokes a pouring out of insulin from the pancreas. As there are little or no insulin antag-onists in patients with adrenal insufficiency, a rapid drop in blood sugar to pathologic levels takes place. The normal curve would be characterized by a rapid rise within 30 minutes, followed by a fall in the blood sugar to normal values.

Addison's Disease and Diabetes Mellitus. There appears to be an ever-increasing number of patients with both Addison's disease and diabetes mellitus.[3, 16] The occurrence of the two diseases together appears with greater frequency than anticipated on the basis of chance alone. When Addison's disease appears first and the patients are treated with glucocorticoids, a larger percentage of patients become diabetic than when desoxycorticosterone alone is employed. The coexistence of Addison's disease in a diabetic must be thought of when there is a diminished need for insulin accompanied by hypotension. When this occurs, obviously the glucose tolerance test will not be of great value. A known diabetic in whom the insulin requirements diminished suddenly should be investigated for possible Addison's disease.

There are other clinical entities which may also be associated with some amelioration of diabetes mellitus. These are as follows:

1. Adenoma of islet cells of pancreas,
2. Hepatic failure,
3. Hypopituitarism,
4. Hypothyroidism,
5. Kimmelstiel-Wilson's disease,
6. Caloric intake consisting primarily of protein and amounting to less than 900 calories.

STEROID EXCRETION.   The adrenal gland is the site of production of 17-ketosteroid and 17-hydroxysteroid precursors.

17-Ketosteroids.   In the female, excretion of 17-ketosteroids in less than normal quantities is evidence of decreased adrenocortical activity. In the male, only part of the 17-ketosteroids comes from the adrenal. The remainder comes from the testes. Therefore, the testes must be ruled out as the cause of deficient 17-ketosteroid excretion before the adrenals can be indicted.

Certain other factors affecting steroid output should be considered when urine excretion is below normal. For example, patients with liver disease and gout may have low 17-ketosteroids without evidence of adrenal insufficiency. Those with liver disease are unable to change the 17-ketosteroid precursors into ketosteroids; hence, their low value. For some reason which is not well understood, the patient with gout also has a diminished 17-ketosteroid excretion which is not related to decreased adrenocortical activity.[47] Patients on a starvation diet, particularly those with anorexia nervosa, usually have a low 17-ketosteroid excretion. Before the physician accepts a low 17-ketosteroid as proof of adrenal disease, it is important that he be certain that the patient has been on an adequate protein intake.

The 17-hydroxysteroids are much more specific for evaluation of adrenal function in patients suspected of having decreased adrenal activity. The 17-OH are normal in patients with anorexia nervosa, cirrhosis, or gout; hence, a low 17-hydroxysteroid level is more diagnostic of hypoadrenalism than a low 17-ketosteroid. Therefore, patients who show both diminished 17-hydroxysteroid and 17-ketosteroid excretion levels must be considered as having Addison's disease until proved otherwise.

It is necessary, at times, to determine whether decreased adrenocortical activity is due to primary adrenal failure or to an insufficiency of pituitary ACTH secretion. In order to establish the integrity of the adrenal cortex and rule it in or out as the primary factor in decreased adrenocortical activity, the patient is given either 25 units of ACTH intravenously over an eight-hour period or 40 units of the gel intramuscularly. Urine is collected for four eight-hour periods when the intravenous route is employed; urine collected in the eight-hour period immediately preceding the ACTH administration serves as a control; the urine collected during the eight-hour infusion is a second specimen, and the last two specimens are collected in the two eight-hour periods after the infusion. 17-Ketosteroids and 17-hydroxysteroids are obtained for all four specimens of urine. Failure of the excretion values of these steroids to increase more than 100 per cent in the specimen obtained during the ACTH infusion or for either of the two eight-hour periods after the infusion is evidence of some measure of decreased adrenal response. The absence of a rise in steroid excretion is pathognomonic of Addison's disease due to primary adrenal failure. The patient receiving the gel preparation collects the urine for 24 hours before the injection and for 24 hours after. The same criteria of response are used for the intramuscular as for the intravenous method. A failure of the urinary steroids to increase is evidence of primary adrenal insufficiency.

Blood for 17-hydroxysteroid determinations may also be taken prior to either type of ACTH injection and again eight hours after the intravenous infusion or four hours after the intramuscular injection. Here too, a failure of an increase in blood 17-hydroxysteroids indicates primary adrenal insufficiency.

Secondary Adrenal Insufficiency. If ACTH administration raises steroid excretion by an adequate amount, one must then consider the diagnosis of secondary adrenal insufficiency due to diminished ACTH activity, provided that the control steroid levels, prior to ACTH administration, were low. Secondary adrenal insufficiency may be a manifestation of selective ACTH deficiency due to suppression of endogenous ACTH by exogenous corticoid therapy. There may also be selective ACTH hypofunction as a result of a neurologic disease or neurosurgery involving the midbrain or hypothalamus. One patient in our clinic developed hypoadrenocorticoidism after partial removal of a neoplasm in the area of the midbrain. The patient recovered from her neurosurgical procedure but had a residual ptosis of the right eyelid and paresis and paresthesia (numbness and pin-sticking sensation) of her left arm and left side in general. The patient's evidence of hypoadrenocorticoidism, appearing after surgery, was expressed by hypotension, generalized weakness and asthenia, a low 17-KS and 17-OH, and flat glucose tolerance test with hypoglycemia at the fourth and fifth hours. However, there was normal thyroid function (protein-bound iodine and cholesterol were normal) and normal gonadal function (the patient continued to have regular menstrual periods associated with ovulation). After administration of ACTH, there was the anticipated increase in 17-OH and 17-KS excretion. We believe that this patient represented an example of selective ACTH insufficiency due to disturbances in the hypothalamic-ACTH relationship, as a result of either the neoplasm or the surgery.

The metyrapone test discussed earlier may also be used to differentiate between primary and secondary hypoadrenocorticoidism. If inhibition of 11β-hydroxylation does not cause an increase in 17-KS, 17-OH and/or 17 ketogenic steroids, then the patient may have either primary or secondary adrenal insufficiency. If the same patient shows evidence of a normal response to ACTH, one may then conclude that the patient has hypopituitarism due to failure of release of ACTH. The method involved in performing the test is as follows:

1. A control 24-hour urine is collected for 17-KS, 17-OH and/or 17 ketogenic steroid assay prior to the administration of metyrapone.

2. Metyrapone is then administered in doses of 500 mg. q.i.d. for six doses (i.e., 1½ days).

3. A second 24-hour urine is collected, starting on the morning of the second day of metyrapone therapy.

Steroid excretion is measured in both specimens. If there is a 100 per cent increase in steroid excretion over the control values, one can assume that the patient has an adequate hypothalamic-pituitary-adrenal cortical axis. If the control values, however, are less than 3.0 mg. per 24 hours, obviously a 100 per cent increase in steroid excretion would not be significant. In such patients an elevation of steroid of 4.0 to 5.0 mg. or more would indicate normal functions. If there is little or no increase in steroid excretion after metyrapone, then one must check the integrity of the adrenal cortex by the use of ACTH.

EOSINOPHIL COUNT AND RESPONSE. The eosinophil response to ACTH is no longer considered as reliable a test as the foregoing procedures since its results may be confusing. At times, patients without adrenal disease may not show a drop in eosinophils while, conversely, one who has been adrenalectomized may show evidence of a significant drop in eosinophils, particularly after epinephrine administration. The blood eosinophil response is also inconclusive where the control level of eosinophils is less than 100/cu. mm. It is also unreliable in patients who have a marked eosinophilia related to allergy or to intestinal or systemic parasitism. Observations such as these raise questions as to the validity of this procedure as a whole. Consequently, the blood eosinophil response has been dropped as a significant test for diagnosing Addison's disease.

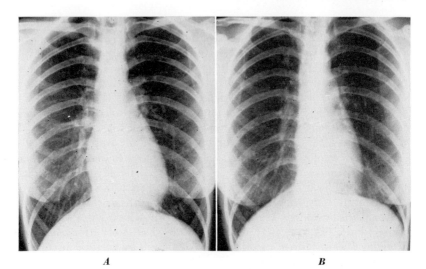

A   B

FIG. 437.   A, Female, age 28 years, one year prior to diagnosis of Addison's disease. Note normal configuration and radiologic appearance of right side of heart.

B, Same patient after diagnosis of Addison's disease. Note the narrowing of the heart with right side of heart being obscured by sternum.

X-Ray.   The use of x-ray in diagnosing adrenal insufficiency may be of some help. This is particularly true where the adrenals have been destroyed by an acid-fast infection and have become calcified. The signs and symptoms of adrenal insufficiency, plus the presence of bilateral suprarenal calcification, would confirm the diagnosis of primary adrenal failure. Serial x-ray pictures of the chest may also give a clue to the diagnosis on the basis of the diminution in heart size. A film taken a year before the patient's illness and again at the time of asthenia, fatigue, etc., would be helpful in establishing the diagnosis of adrenal insufficiency if the follow-up film should show evidence of a significant decrease in heart size (Fig. 437).

Therapy. Sodium Supplementation.   The original observations made by Stewart and Rogoff on the beneficial effects of saline infusion upon the survival of adrenalectomized dogs were responsible for the use of salt in the treatment of patients with Addison's disease.[31, 41] Thus the oldest form of treatment of patients with Addison's disease consisted of the use of sodium supplementation only.[41] High doses of salt, suggested by Robert Loeb, were helpful in the management of some patients with adrenal insufficiency.[31, 32] Before this, there was little that could be offered the Addisonians, and their prognosis was extremely poor. The life expectancy of these patients was still poor with saline replacement. Although it improved their physical stamina at times, it was inadequate in preventing the patients from succumbing to adrenal crises due to any precipitating factor.

ADRENAL CORTICAL EXTRACT.   With the advent of the adrenocortical extracts, the life span of the Addisonian patient was significantly prolonged. Sufficiently potent adrenocortical extracts were prepared almost simultaneously by Swingle[35, 38, 42] and Hartman[20-22] after Rogoff's[37] demonstration that his extracts had some life-maintaining activity in the adrenalectomized rat and the human Addisonian. These extracts offered the Addisonian patient some measure of safety and proved to be lifesaving at times of adrenal crisis. Later, Grollman's charcoal absorbed extract, effective when used orally, also provided some advancement in adrenocortical therapy and permitted a longer and more comfortable life for the Addisonian.[19] While the therapeutic use of the parenteral extracts of either Swingle or Hartman, or the oral preparation of Grollman, represented significant progress in the therapy of Addison's disease, such treatment proved to be exceedingly expensive, and despite it, patients still succumbed in adrenal crisis. Death was caused not by inadequacy of the extracts, but by insufficient amounts being administered to a patient who was also maintained on salt. Consequently, when these patients, in fair control, were in the throes of an adrenal crisis, only poor results could be anticipated from moderately potent adrenocortical extracts. Insufficient supplies may have also played a part in the failures that were observed.

DESOXYCORTICOSTERONE ACETATE.   The problem of maintaining the Addisonian was enormously reduced with the advent of desoxycorticosterone acetate (DCA).[39] This steroid was primarily salt-retaining in activity and when administered intramuscularly in oil solution produced adequate therapeutic effects in patients with adrenal insufficiency. When these patients were subjected to a stressful situation, however, invariably they died unless the aqueous adrenocortical extracts were made available. Shortly thereafter, an amorphous extract of the adrenal cortex, known as lipoadrenal cortex, was developed. This offered the patient some measure of security when he was subjected to a stress situation. The supplementary use of the aqueous and lipoadrenocortical extracts in adequate amounts was sufficient to prevent the death of the Addisonian patient in crisis. Intramuscular DCA appeared on the market and was offered to the patient first as a parenteral oil solution. Later, it was administered orally, in the form of a propylene glycol solution, or by linguet. Subsequently, DCA became available for parenteral pellet implantation.[45] Pellet implantation was extremely convenient and represented the most physiologic approach to the management of the disease up to 1952. The dose of the pellets was usually administered on the basis of the amount of intramuscular DCA required and would provide most patients with effective therapy for six to 12 months. The implantation procedure did not require any unusual preparation and was performed as an office procedure. The dose employed depended upon the patient's maintenance with intramuscular DCA in oil, with one 125 mg. pellet or two 75 mg. pellets being implanted for each 0.5 to 0.75 mg. of DCA required per day. The intramuscular DCA is given together with 3 Gm. of supplementary sodium chloride orally in 1-Gm. enteric coated tablets. This provides a safety factor in preventing overdose with the pellets. Only the 75 mg. pellet is usable by the Kearns Injector, and the mode of implantation is exactly the same as that described for the pellets of estradiol in the female.

DESOXYCORTICOSTERONE TRI-METHYL ACETATE.   The next advance, as far as mineralocorticoid therapy was concerned, was the appearance of desoxycorticosterone tri-methyl acetate (DCTMA).[46] This preparation, an aqueous suspension containing 25 mg. per cc. of the steroid administered intramuscularly in single doses of 25 to 37.5 mg., usually maintained most Addisonian patients in adequate electrolyte control for a period of about four weeks. It certainly represented an advance in convenience over both the pellet implantation and the daily intramuscular use of DCA in oil. It offered the patient a relatively easy way of being maintained in salt and water balance without the necessity of his taking frequent injections of the more rapidly dissipated oil material. DCTMA is more reliable than the DCA linguets. The use of these linguets was convenient but un-predictable because a great deal of their activity was destroyed by faulty absorption and passage of much of the material into the gastrointestinal tract.

ORAL GLUCOCORTICOIDS.   The availability of cortisone and cortisol has simplified the therapeutic management of the Addisonian so that a relatively complex problem may now be effectively controlled by oral therapy. This was particularly true when 9-alpha-fluorohydrocortisone (fludrocortisone), an orally active mineralocorticoid, became available. As a result, both the glucocorticoid and the mineralocorticoid could be administered orally, giving the patient complete replacement therapy with respect to both carbohydrate and electrolyte metabolism.[10, 29] The glucocorticoid is necessary to maintain the patient in a euglycemic phase, to promote hepatic glycogen deposition, and to help combat any stressful situations to which the patient may be exposed. The mineralocorticoid promotes sodium and water retention and prevents dehydration and postural hypotension. The usual doses of the glucocorticoids that may be employed as maintenance therapy in the hypoadrenal individual are as follows:

Cortisone, 12.5 mg.
Hydrocortisone, 10 mg.
Prednisone or prednisolone, 2.5 mg.
6-Methyl prednisolone, 2 mg.
Dexamethasone, 0.375 to 0.5 mg.

Any of these can be administered in the doses indicated two or three times a day along with 9-alpha-fluorohydrocortisone in doses of approximately 0.1 mg. per day. It is rare for glucocorticoids, in the above doses, to create any difficulty in the clinical management of the patient.

Triamcinolone has not been included in this list of glucocorticoids because of its potential effect in causing sodium and/or potassium loss. This peculiar property of triamcinolone has been of therapeutic value in those conditions, other than adrenal insufficiency, where large doses of the glucocorticoids are necessary to suppress inflammatory diseases and to maintain life itself. Where the other corticoids might produce some sodium retention, triamcinolone is less likely to induce this effect, and, indeed, may actually cause sodium loss.

MINERALOCORTICOIDS. If the patient has an associated diabetes mellitus and Addison's disease or develops the former during the presence of the latter, it would be wise to control the adrenal insufficiency with the mineralocorticoids rather than with the glucocorticoids. The mineralocorticoids are less prone than the glucocorticoids to cause decreased carbohydrate tolerance or to induce an anti-insulin effect.

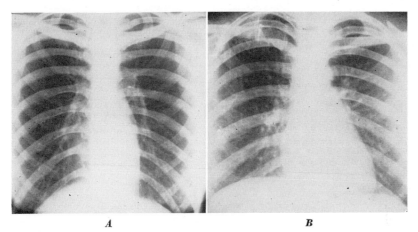

A   B

FIG. 438 A and B. Note excessive increase in heart size with overdosage of (0.2 mg.) 9-alpha-fluorohydrocortisone per day.

Most Frequent Adverse Effects. The mineralocorticoid, if given in excessive doses, may produce some adverse effects, such as: (1) sudden and considerable increase in weight, (2) marked increase in blood pressure, (3) excessive increase in heart size (Fig. 438), (4) peripheral edema, and (5) marked degree of lassitude. These findings illustrate a cardinal principle in endocrinology: at the same dose level, the hypoglandular individual usually is far more sensitive than the normal to the physiologic effects of the particular hormone in which he is deficient. The sodium-retaining qualities of 9-alpha-fluorohydrocortisone may become so marked in the patient with adrenal insufficiency that these adverse effects may occur with doses of the steroid much too small to have any effect in normals. All of these changes are attributed to the retention of sodium, with the resulting hypervolemia producing the increased weight and edema (fluid retention), elevation of blood pressure, and heart size (hypervolemia). The increase in heart size may be particularly dramatic even when comparatively physiologic doses of the corticoids are used. This is emphasized in Figure 439, where the narrow, elongated, small heart of the Addisonian patient rapidly approaches normal size with physiologic doses of the salt-retaining steroid hormone. Some patients may complain of lassitude with this therapy. This is attributed to the hypopotassemia that the mineralocorticoids may induce.

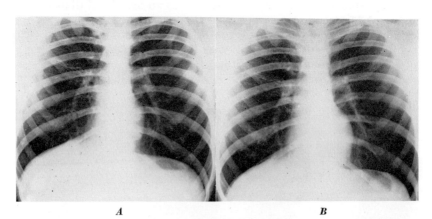

A   B

FIG. 439 A and B. Increase of heart to normal size of Addisonian patient (male, age 20). In November 1958 (A) prior to therapy, patient was admitted in adrenal crisis. After 2 months of therapy with glucocorticoid (hydrocortisone 10 mg. b.i.d.) and 0.1 mg. 9-alpha-fluorohydrocortisone per day, heart became normal in size (B).

Less Frequent Adverse Effects. Other side effects of overdosage with the salt-retaining steroids include headache and accentuation of arthritic complaints. Tendon contractures are occasionally noted. Persistent potassium depletion may lead to sudden, unexplained death in patients who have been over-treated with salt-retaining steroids during adrenal crisis. The acute sodium retention with concomitant increase in blood pressure and hypervolemia may induce cardiac strain. The heart strain can be markedly accentuated by potassium depletion of heart muscle. Unwise use of the corticoid may then be responsible for inducing heart block and/or failure followed by cardiac arrest.

POTASSIUM SUPPLEMENTATION. Hypokalemia is an undesirable side effect or toxic phenomenon which may be rapidly dissipated by discontinuing the 9-alpha-fluorohydrocortisone (9FF) for a period of three to four days. This will usually result in the prompt disappearance of all the adverse effects listed. In addition, the recovery process may be accelerated by potassium supplementation in the form of Kaon Elixir, 15 ml. t.i.d., for the three to four days when off the 9FF therapy. Obviously, if unrestricted Kaon liquid is continued without corticoid therapy, potassium intoxication may develop; hence, potassium supplementation should not be continued in the Addisonian patient without reinitiation of the mineralocorticoid within four to five days. The increased intake of potassium is used in an attempt to overcome the possibility of excessive potassium loss while the patient is on the sodium-retaining steroid. If excessive doses of potassium are used, hyperkalemia may occur, and would be undesirable. This is more prone to take place in patients who have some measure of renal insufficiency. Such patients should be checked carefully and probably not be given any potassium supplementation.

VITAMIN AND ANDROGEN SUPPLEMENTATION. Vitamin supplementation as well as an adequate dietary protein intake will help to restore the patient to a normal clinical state. There is little need for the supplementary use of androgens in female or elderly patients unless a profound degree of muscle wasting is noted together with the adrenal insufficiency.

THE NEED FOR SALT-RETAINING STEROIDS. In discussing therapy of the Addisonian patient, the question always arises of the need, if any, for the salt-retaining steroids. This point appears particularly appropriate when one realizes that most of the undesirable features of adrenocorticoid therapy seem to rest on the adverse effect of overdosage with the mineralocorticoid. If there is no specific indication for the use of such steroids, the management of the Addisonian with physiologic doses of glucocorticoids alone is sufficient, and relatively free of undesirable side effects.

Nevertheless, there are several indications demonstrating the need for combined mineral and glucocorticoids. Combined therapy is warranted when sodium depletion seems to be the predominant feature of the adrenal insufficiency, and the patient shows evidence of hypotension as a result of either primary or secondary hypoadrenocorticoidism. The hypotensive Addisonian provides a specific indication for the administration of the mineralocorticoid along with glucocorticoids, regardless of whether the patient has primary or secondary hypoadrenocorticoidism. Thus if the patient's systolic blood pressure is below 100-105 mm. of Hg, there is a definite need for the use of mineralocorticoid. Apparently, glucocorticoids are needed for the mineralocorticoid (aldosterone) to achieve its specific effect only in the newborn with the adrenogenital syndrome.

Corticoid Central Nervous System Stimulation. There is another untoward effect following glucocorticoid therapy in patients with Addison's disease. During the initial stages of their replacement therapy, the patients may exhibit a marked hyperkinetic state associated with clinical evidence of overactivity, euphoria, and behavior hovering on the border of manic activity. This is due, no doubt, to the central nervous system stimulating effects of corticoids, which may be so marked as to approach abnormal overactivity. Fortunately, tolerance to this effect of the glucocorticoids is achieved rapidly, so that, while the dose of corticoid necessary to achieve an euadrenal state is maintained, the overactive pyschomotor activity will abate with continued use of these physiologic doses of the corticoid. This response of the Addisonian patient to the glucocorticoids is another measure of the sensitivity of the hypoglandular individuals to the hormone in which they are deficient.

Hypoadrenia. The therapeutic management of hypoadrenocorticoidism is dependent on appropriate diagnosis. At times, the physician may be in a dilemma with the patient who presents some of the classic symptoms of hypoadrenocorticoidism but whose laboratory findings are inconclusive or just on the borderline of normality. For example, a patient exhibiting weakness and fatigue of moderate degree associated with mild anorexia, nausea, and weight loss might have some degree of decreased adrenal activity. If these symptoms are accompanied by postural hypotension, diarrhea, and some diminution in degree of axillary and pubic hair growth, the diagnosis might be more apparent. However, if the laboratory data are equivocal, it would then behoove the physician to attempt a therapeutic test with one of the corticoid preparations.

THERAPEUTIC TRIALS IN DIAGNOSIS. Therapeutic trials in cases where the diagnosis may not be too apparent is an accepted procedure in medicine. For example, a therapeutic trial with digitalis with a good response may be diagnostic in indecisive cases of congestive heart failure. Trials with a positive effect of the nitrite drugs may give a definite clue to the presence of angina caused by relative coronary insufficiency.

Corticoids. Similar justification may be offered for therapeutic trials with corticoids in the patient with diagnostically indecisive hypoadrenocorticoidism, referred to by the older clinician as hypoadrenia. A patient who fails to show the specific laboratory findings of adrenal insufficiency must be considered as one with hypoadrenia if corticoids in the same doses recommended above for Addison's disease produce a dramatic therapeutic change. Findings such as these warrant continued treatment with corticoid therapy.

Placebo. Obviously, one must check the validity of the therapeutic test with the use of a placebo. If the patient fails to show an adequate response with a placebo but does well on corticoids, provided, of course, that the patient has no knowledge of the fact that a placebo had been substituted for the active compounds, one must consider this as confirmatory evidence for the presence of hypoadrenia.

Water Tolerance Test. The most consistent, positive, objective finding in patients with hypoadrenia has been a positive water tolerance test—i. e., the patients fail to show a normal response to a water loading test (they cannot excrete a volume of urine in any one hour after hydration which is greater than the total volume of the overnight specimen). However, water intolerance may persist in some patients with hypoadrenia whether or not they are maintained on corticoid therapy. In contrast, it is indeed rare for the frank Addisonian patient not to show a correction of the water intolerance when placed on adequate corticoid medication. Thus, despite the clinical improvement in both categories of patients, only the frank Addisonian will show a reversal of his water intolerance. While water intolerance may suggest hypoadrenia, other factors may also be responsible for the disturbance in water tolerance.

It has been suggested that the effect of glucocorticoids in reversing the abnormal water tolerance test (inability to handle a water load) to normal is achieved by the corticoids by inhibiting endogenous antidiuretic hormone (ADH) secretion. ADH secretion presumably is uninhibited in patients with primary hypoadrenocorticoidism. Corticoids may improve water excretion by increasing glomerular filtration and by antagonizing the effect of ADH at the tubular level—that is, at the distal convoluted tubule. These are alternate theoretic pathways for the action of corticoids on water excretion and cannot be denied or affirmed at the present time.

POSSIBLE ADVERSE EFFECTS OF CORTICOID THERAPY. Glucocorticoid therapy may theoretically have adverse effects by causing a flare-up of a latent acid-fast infection. However, since the doses of glucocorticoids used are physiologic, and since the amount does not exceed that estimated as produced by the normal adrenal, it is unlikely that such corticoid therapy would have an adverse effect on any type of tuberculous infection. If the patient is considered as being potentially in danger of gross infection, it would be wise to institute appropriate antimicrobial therapy. The glucocorticoid should be continued in the recommended doses whether or not antibiotics are added.

Peptic Ulcer. Another problem must also be considered in the same light; i. e., the problem of peptic ulcer. The untreated Addisonian patient rarely, if ever, shows clinical manifestations of gastrointestinal ulceration. However, we have seen a peptic ulcer occur in a Negro Addisonian maintained on glucocorticoid therapy. It seems that the treated patient maintained on the recommended regimen is as prone to peptic ulcer as anyone in the general population. However, we have seen only this one patient develop an ulcer, an incidence actually lower than one would expect on the basis of chance alone.

Treatment of Adrenal Crisis. Treatment of adrenal crisis was once as difficult to manage as bacterial lobar pneumonia and, as with pneumonia, modern therapeutics has offered the physician an easy and successful method of treating acute hypoadrenocorticoidism or adrenal failure, provided that the diagnosis is suspected and early therapy is instituted.

INTRAVENOUS GLUCOCORTICOIDS. There is a definite urgency for the use of intravenous glucocorticoids in these patients. Adverse effects due to overdosage are rare in intravenous therapy despite the fact that pharmacologic activity of this preparation is achieved rapidly. A hemisuccinate derivative of either prednisone, 6-methyl prednisolone, or hydrocortisone is readily soluble in water and is available as an aqueous solution for intravenous administration.

In the acute shock phase associated with adrenal insufficiency, the following procedures should be used: infusion of either 100 mg. of hydrocortisone hemisuccinate, or 25 mg. of prednisone or 6-methyl prednisolone hemisuccinate, plus the addition of 5 mg. of 9-alpha-fluorohydrocortisone hemisuccinate.

The infusion is usually made in 500 cc. of physiologic glucose and saline with the addition of 40 to 60 mEq. of potassium salts, provided that there is no evidence of renal failure. The purpose of the potassium is to prevent the signs and symptoms of hypokalemia that may be induced with the intravenous corticoid therapy. The hemisuccinate of 9-alpha-fluorohydrocortisone is administered intravenously to achieve a rapid correction of any abnormality of electrolyte metabolism. DCA may be given intramuscularly in doses of 10 mg. as the initial dose, with 5 mg. administered on the second day. Further dosage is dependent on control of the adrenal crisis. The patient may also be started on the intramuscular administration of either 50 mg. of cortisone or 10 mg. of prednisone or 8 mg. of 6-methyl prednisolone. Either is given twice per day on the first day, and one half the amount of either preparation is administered twice per day on the second day. If the patient is progressing satisfactorily, the dose may then be reduced to 2.5 mg. of the prednisone t.i.d. or 2 mg. of 6-methyl prednisolone or 10 mg. of hydrocortisone t.i.d. orally. Oral therapy with 9-alpha-fluorohydrocortisone should be instituted at this time, together with the glucocorticoid of choice.

Supplementary Therapy. During the time of administration of the high doses of parenteral glucocorticoid, the patient should also receive an effective, broad-spectrum parenteral antibiotic in adequate doses as prophylaxis against the spread of any intercurrent infection. The antibiotic should be maintained for as long a period of time as infection appears to threaten, or as long as the patient is on the relatively high doses of corticoid. Adequate vitamin substitution therapy either orally or parenterally also should be given.

One may use 40 to 50 mg. of mephentermine sulfate (Wyamine) intramuscularly or intravenously if the patient's blood pressure stays at a particularly low or unresponsive level despite steroid therapy in the above dosage. This dose of the pressor amine may be repeated as necessary if the blood pressure is not sustained, and continued until a stable blood pressure is achieved as a result of corticoid therapy. Norepinephrine may also be employed as the sympathomimetic amine to raise the blood pressure above shock levels. The danger with norepinephrine is sloughing if infiltration should take place outside the vein. Occasionally, similar effects may be observed, even when excessive amounts of norepinephrine are used without extravasation. The average dose should not exceed 1 to 2 mg. every eight to 10 hours. A recent report suggests that these adverse effects of norepinephrine may be nullified by adding a sympatholytic agent. The addition of 5 mg. of phentolamine (Regitine) intravenously together with the sympathicomimetic amine will combat norepinephrine's propensity to induce sloughing without diminishing its pressor effect.[48] If these observations are substantiated, much of the adverse effects of norepinephrine will be nullified.

ORAL THERAPY. After the manifestations of dehydration and the signs and symptoms of the adrenal crisis are under control, the intravenous route of drug administration can be discontinued and the patient maintained adequately on oral therapy. This should still include potassium supplementation for the first week of oral therapy. The parenteral regimen may be discontinued as soon as the patient is able to feed himself and provided, of course, that mineralocorticoid therapy is also maintained.

The treatment outlined for adrenal crisis or adrenal insufficiency should be used regardless of the etiology of the disease, whether it is primarily of adrenal origin or secondarily due to pituitary ACTH insufficiency.

DIFFERENTIAL DIAGNOSIS. Before treatment is started for an acute adrenal crisis and/or chronic adrenocorticoid insufficiency, it is necessary for the physician to exclude the possibility of neurasthenia, chronic infection (tuberculosis or brucellosis), chronic gastrointestinal disturbances, myasthenia gravis, as well as hyperthyroidism. Hypoparathyroidism and spontaneous hypoglycemia are sometimes confused with decreased adrenal function. The salt-losing syndrome noted in the newborn infant is another type of adrenal insufficiency due to an error in metabolism. Paradoxically, these infants have adequate aldosterone secretion but lack hydrocortisone. They have hyperadrenocorticoidism, with excessive 17-ketosteroid precursors present and despite their salt-losing syndrome they will require only glucocorticoid therapy. Pertinent laboratory data are required to differentiate the above clinical entities from true hypoadrenocorticoidism.

Adrenal Surgery. Adrenal insufficiency can be induced by surgical removal of the adrenal glands. Correct preparation of the patient for therapeutic bilateral total adrenalectomy is just as important as his correct maintenance after surgery.

SURGICAL PREPARATION. The preparation of the patient for adrenal surgery requires the following:

1. Two days before surgery in the evening the patient should receive 50 mg. of cortisone or hydrocortisone intramuscularly.

2. The day before surgery the patient should receive 50 mg. of cortisone or any equivalent preparation in the morning and evening and another 50 mg. on the morning of surgery.

3. On the day of surgery prior to the surgical procedure, the patient should receive an intravenous infusion containing 100 mg. of hydrocortisone hemisuccinate or 20 mg. of prednisone hemisuccinate. Additional treatment depends on the patient's reaction during the removal of both adrenal glands. Mephentermine or norepinephrine is used to maintain systolic blood pressure at a minimum of 90 to 100 mm. Hg or more. (Postoperatively, the patient receives the same treatment regimen recommended for adrenal crisis, including adequate replacement with potassium salts.)

Secondary Adrenal Insufficiency. Adrenal insufficiency may be secondary to pituitary failure, which could result from hypophysectomy, a tumor, panhypopituitarism, or selective ACTH failure. The diagnosis of adrenal insufficiency secondary to pituitary insufficiency is anticipated in the hypophysectomized patient. It may be identified by noting the patient's response to ACTH and metyrapone as previously described. If the patient has adequate adrenal function after, but not before ACTH, and no evidence of adrenal stimulation after metyrapone, the diagnosis of secondary adrenal insufficiency is then established. Another important clinical sign is the presence or absence of pigmentation. Pigmentary changes are normally absent in the patient with secondary adrenal insufficiency. However, these patients have all of the other clinical and chemical stigmata of primary adrenal insufficiency and will show all of the biochemical stigmata listed for primary hypoadrenocorticoidism. Rarely will the water tolerance test results be negative except in those patients where the posterior lobe is also removed or damaged together with the anterior lobe. Even these patients may have a positive reaction to the water tolerance test.

While replacement therapy with the adrenocorticotropic hormone might appear to be the most logical approach, such therapy is impractical and expensive. ACTH therapy is more feasible than other pituitary tropic hormone therapy as, theoretically, antihormone formation would not take place in the human receiving ACTH of animal origin. This too may be open to question, as recent studies have demonstrated antigenicity to ACTH in animals when certain techniques of injections are used.[14] These patients are maintained, therefore, on precisely the same preparations as those with primary adrenal failure. In these patients, 9-alpha-fluorohydrocortisone is used if their blood pressure is below 100 mm. Hg. Therapeutic response is excellent, provided that corticoids are continued indefinitely.

It now appears that Addison's disease, which once required all the skills and efforts of the physician to maintain the life of the patient on an even keel, has become a more readily correctable disease. Moreover, the life expectancy of the correctly treated Addisonian patient need be no less than that of the euadrenal individual.

References

1. ADDISON, T.: On the constitutional and local effects of disease of the suprarenal capsules. D. Highey, London, 1855.

2. ARNOLD, J.: Ein beitrag zu der feineren structur und dem chemismus der nebennieren. Virchow's Arch. Pathol. Anat. 35:64-107, 1866.

3. BEAVEN, D. W., NELSON, D. H., RENOLD, A. E., AND THORN, G. W.: Diabetes mellitus and Addison's disease. New Engl. J. Med. 261:443-454, 1959.

4. BONGIOVANNI, A. M.: The detection of pregnandiol and pregnantriol in the urine of patients with adrenal hyperplasia. Suppression with cortisone; preliminary report. Bull. Johns Hopkins Hosp. 92:244-251, 1953.

5. CRABBÉ, J., REDDY, W. J., ROSS, E. J., AND THORN, G. W.: Stimulation of aldosterone secretion by adrenocorticotropic hormone (ACTH). J. Clin. Endocr. 19:1185-1191, 1959.

6. CUTLER, H. H., POWER, M. H., AND WILDER, R. M.: Concentrations of chloride, sodium and potassium in urine and blood. The diagnostic significance in adrenal insufficiency. J.A.M.A. 111:117-122, 1938.

7. DEANE, H. W., AND GREEP, R. O.: A morphological and histochemical study of the rat's adrenal cortex after hypophysectomy, with comments on the liver. Amer. J. Anat. 79:117-146, 1946.

8. DEANE, H. W., SHAW, J. H., AND GREEP, R. O. The effect of altered sodium or potassium intake on the width and cytochemistry of the zona glomerulosa of the rat's adrenal cortex. Endocrinology 43:133-153, 1948.

9. EBERLEIN, W. R., AND BONGIOVANNI, A. M.: Steroid metabolism in the "salt-losing" form of congenital adrenal hyperplasia. J. Clin. Invest. 37:889-890, 1958.

10. EPSTEIN, J. A., AND KUPPERMAN, H. S.: Management of chronic adrenocortical insufficiency with oral replacement therapy. J. Amer. Geriat. Soc. 5:117-121, 1957.

11. FARRELL, G.: Steroidogenic properties of extracts of beef diencephalon. Endocrinology 65:29-33, 1959.

12. FARRELL, G.: Glomerulotropic activity of an acetone extract of pineal tissue. Endocrinology 65:239-241, 1959.

13. FINE, D., MEISELAS, L. E., AND AUERBACH, T.: The effect of acute hypovolemia on the release of "aldosterone" and renal excretion of sodium. J. Clin. Invest. 37:232-243, 1958.

14. FISHMAN, J., MCGARRY E. F., AND BECK, J. C.: Studies using anterior pituitary hormones as antigens. Proc. Soc. Exp. Biol. Med. 102:446-447, 1959.

15. FRASER, R. W., ALBRIGHT, F., AND SMITH, P. H.: The value of the glucose tolerance, the insulin tolerance test and the glucose-insulin tolerance test in the diagnosis of endocrinologic disorders of glucose metabolism. J. Clin. Endocr. 1:297-306, 1941.

16. GITTLER, R. D., FAJANS, S. S., AND CONN, J. W.: Coexistence of Addison's disease and diabetes mellitus: Report of three cases with a discussion of metabolic interrelationships. J. Clin. Endocr. 19:797-804, 1959.

17. GREENBLATT, R. B., AND KUPPERMAN, H. S.: Diagnostic value of the glucose tolerance and insulin tolerance tests in endocrine disorders. Southern Med. J. 40:737-744, 1947.

18. GREEP, R. O., AND DEANE, H. W.: Cytochemical evidence for the cessation of hormone production in the zona glomerulosa of the rat's adrenal cortex after prolonged treatment with desoxycorticosterone acetate. Endocrinology 40:417-425, 1947.

19. GROLLMAN, A., FIROR, W. M., AND GROLLMAN, E.: Studies on the adrenal. VIII. A simple preparation of the adrenal cortical hormone suitable for oral administration. J. Biol. Chem. 109:189-200, 1935.

20. HARTMAN, F. A., AARON, H., AND CULP, J. E.: The use of cortin in Addison's disease. Endocrinology 14:438-442, 1930.

21. HARTMAN, F. A., AND BROWNELL, K. A.: The hormone of the adrenal cortex. Science 72:76, 1930.

22. HARTMAN, F. A., MACARTHUR, C. G., AND HARTMAN, W. E.: A substance which prolongs the life of adrenalectomized cats. Proc. Soc. Exp. Biol. Med. 25:69-70, 1927.

23. HECHTER, O., ZAFFARONI, A., JACOBSEN, R. P., LEVY, H., JEANLOZ, R. W., SCHENKER, V., AND PINCUS, G.: The nature and biogenesis of the adrenal secretory product. Recent Progr. Hormone Res. 6:215-241, 1951.

24. HOWARD-MILLER, E.: A transitory zone in the adrenal cortex which shows age and sex relationships. Amer. J. Anat. 40:251-293, 1927.

25. JAILER, J. W., GOLD, J. J., VANDE WIELE, R., AND LIEBERMAN, S.: 17-Alpha-hydroxy-progesterone and 21-desoxyhydrocortisone: their metabolism and possible role in congenital adrenal virilism. J. Clin. Invest. 34:1639-1646, 1955.

26. JONES, I. C., AND WRIGHT, A.: Some aspects of zonation and function of the adrenal cortex. IV. The histology of the adrenal in rats with diabetes insipidus. J. Endocr. 10:266-272, 1954.

27. KANOSKY, S. A., BOUTWELL, J. H., AND SALOFF, L. O.: Relationship of the electrocardiogram to the potassium content of red blood cells. Presented at American Heart Association Meeting in Philadelphia, October, 1959.

28. KUPPERMAN, H. S.: Extrapancreatic factors in diabetes mellitus. Postgrad. Med. 20:151-159, 1956.

29. KUPPERMAN, H. S., AND EPSTEIN, J. A.: Oral therapy of adrenal cortical hypofunction. J.A.M.A. 159:1447-1449, 1955.

30. LANMAN, J. T.: The adrenal fetal zone: its occurrence in primates and a possible relationship to chorionic gonadotropin. Endocrinology 61:684-691, 1957.

31. LOEB, R. F.: Chemical changes in the blood in Addison's disease. Science 76:420-421, 1932.

32. LOEB, R. F.: Effect of sodium chloride in treatment of a patient with Addison's disease. Proc. Soc. Exp. Biol. Med. 30:808-812, 1933.

33. LUETSCHER, J. A., JR., AND AXELRAD, B. J.: Increased aldosterone output during sodium deprivation in normal man. Proc. Soc. Exp. Biol. Med. 87:650-653, 1954.

34. LUETSCHER, J. A., JR., AND AXELRAD, B. J.: Sodium-retaining corticoid in the urine of normal children and adults and of patients with hypoadrenalism or hypopituitarism. J. Clin. Endocr. 14:1086-1089, 1954.

35. PFIFFNER, J. J., AND SWINGLE, W. W.: The preparation of an active extract of the suprarenal cortex. Anat. Rec. 44:225, 1929.

36. ROBINSON, F. J., POWER, M. H., AND KEPLER, E. J.: Two new procedures to assist in the recognition and exclusion of Addison's disease: A preliminary report. Proc. Mayo Clin. 16:577-583, 1941.

37. ROGOFF, J. M., AND STEWART, G. N.: Suprarenal cortical extracts in suprarenal insufficiency. J.A.M.A. 92:1569-1571, 1929.

38. ROUNTREE, L. J., GREENE, P. H., SWINGLE, W. W., AND PFIFFNER, J. J.: Addison's disease: Experience in treatment with various suprarenal preparations. J.A.M.A. 96:231-235, 1931.

39. SIMPSON, S. L.: The use of synthetic desoxycorticosterone acetate in Addison's disease. Lancet 235:557-558, 1938.

40. STARKEY, W. F., AND SCHMIDT, E. C. H., JR.: The effect of testosterone-propionate on the X-zone of the mouse adrenal. Endocrinology 23:339-344, 1938.

41. STEWART, G. N., AND ROGOFF, J. M.: Studies on adrenal insufficiency. Proc. Soc. Exp. Biol. Med. 22:394-397, 1925.

42. SWINGLE, W. W., AND PFIFFNER, J. J.: The revival of comatose adrenalectomized cats with an extract of the suprarenal cortex. Science 72:75-76, 1930.

43. SZENAS, P., AND PATTEE, C. J.: Studies of adrenocortical function in obesity. J. Clin. Endocr. 19:344-350, 1959.

44. THORN, G. W., DORRANCE, S. S., AND DAY, E.: Addison's disease, evaluation of synthetic desoxycorticosterone therapy in 158 patients. Ann. Int. Med. 16:1053-1096, 1942.

45. THORN, G. W., HOWARD, R. P., EMERSON, K., JR., AND FIROR, W. M.: Treatment of Addison's disease with pellets of crystalline adrenal cortical hormone (synthetic desoxy-corticosterone acetate) implanted subcutaneously. Bull. Johns Hopkins Hosp. 64:339-365, 1939.

46. THORN, G. W., JENKINS, D., ARONS, W. L., AND FRAWLEY, T. F.: Use of desoxy-corticosterone trimethylacetate in the treatment of Addison's disease. J. Clin. Endocr. 13:957-973, 1953.

47. WOLFSON, W. Q., GUTERMAN, H. S., LEVINE, R., COHN, C., HUNT, H. D., AND ROSENBERG, E. F.: An endocrine finding apparently characteristic of gout: very low urinary 17-ketosteroid excretion with clinically normal androgenic function. J. Clin. Endocr. 9:497-513, 1949.

48. ZUCKER, G., EISINGER, R. P., FLOCH, M. H., AND SINGER, M. M.: Prevention of ischemic necrosis by use of levarterenol-phentolamine mixtures in treatment of shock. Circulation 20:789, 1959.

chapter 20

Until the last decade, adrenal cortical hyperplasia of the classic adrenogenital type, while readily recognized, was managed only by surgical removal of the offending organs. As a result of incomplete knowledge of adrenal physiology and lack of effective adrenal cortical preparations, bilateral adrenalectomy was necessary to control the excessive masculinization in patients with the congenital adrenogenital syndrome (AGS) or pseudohermaphroditism. It sometimes appeared that the cure was worse than the disease itself. The subclinical variants of the syndrome were unrecognized at that time.

Corticoid Synthesis in the Adrenal Gland. The entire picture changed when the biochemical and enzymatic mechanisms involved in the synthesis of hydrocortisone were understood. The elucidation of the basic principles provided one of the major advances in endocrinology in the past decade.[12, 31-33] The discovery of these basic processes demonstrated the interrelation existing between the adrenal cortex, the pituitary, and the gonads. It has led to the demonstration of the specific biochemical defect concerned with the adrenogenital syndrome which was shown to play the key role in the etiology of adrenal hyperplasia.[3, 4]

It now appears that there is a relatively high incidence of adrenal disease of the adrenogenital type stemming from defective metabolic pathways in the conversion of the basic cyclopentenophenanthrene (cho-

Hyperadrenal Corticoidism – I. The Adrenogenital Syndrome

lesterol) steroids into adrenal hormones. Today the adrenogenital syndrome is no longer considered to be a relatively rare phenomenon. This increase in incidence may be due to a more frequent occurrence of adrenal hyperplasia per se, or it may be attributed, in part, to a greater diagnostic ability in detecting these cases, particularly in patients lacking the typical or classic stigmata of the disease.

Adrenal Cortical-Pituitary Interrelationships.   In discussing the adrenogenital syndrome (AGS), the physician should have a basic comprehension of the physiologic interrelationship existing between the pituitary and the adrenal cortex. A description of the adrenal cortical-pituitary-gonadal interdependence will clarify some of these mechanisms. Only those factors concerned with the AGS will be emphasized here. The adrenal cortex is divided into three parts, but only the zona fasciculata and reticularis will be discussed at this point since these are the two zone layers involved in the adrenogenital syndrome (Fig. 440). The zona glomerulosa is concerned with the elaboration of aldosterone and does not appear to play an integral role in the etiology or management of the AGS except for those infants with the salt-losing syndrome. The level of aldosterone secretion in these infants will be discussed later when the congenital AGS in the newborn is considered.

ADRENOGENITAL SYNDROME

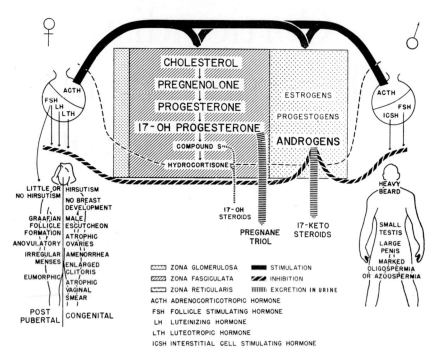

FIG. 440. *Diagrammatic presentation of the relationship between the pituitary, adrenal cortex, and gonads. As a result of a deficiency of hydroxylase, incomplete production of hydrocortisone takes place bringing about an increased secretion of ACTH. Masculinization and/or gonadal inhibition take place as a result of excessive stimulation by ACTH of the zona reticularis to secrete increased amounts of androgenic precursors.*

Zona Fasciculata. The zona fasciculata, which is dependent on ACTH for its function, plays a major role in adrenal corticoid homeostasis and is responsible for the elaboration of glucocorticoids.

CONVERSION OF CHOLESTEROL TO HYDROCORTISONE. It is from this layer that hydrocortisone is secreted. Presumably, hydrocortisone (compound F) is synthesized in the zona fasciculata under the stimulus of ACTH through a progression of chemical reactions that may start with acetate or cholesterol.[3, 4, 12, 14] ACTH stimulates the zona fasciculata to take up cholesterol from the blood stream and converts it in stepwise progression into pregnenolone, to progesterone, and then to 17-hydroxyprogesterone. By a process of hydroxylation, 17-hydroxyprogesterone is converted into compound S and eventually into hydrocortisone (see Fig. 422). The intracellular factors as well as the stepwise progression of cholesterol to cortisol are implicated and have been considered in more detail in Figures 419, 421, and 422. These will not be elaborated upon here but will be referred to again when pertinent to the present discussion.

INTERMEDIARY EXCRETORY PRODUCTS. The metabolic breakdown products of hydrocortisone's intermediary metabolites are excreted into the urine, together with the usually anticipated 17-ketosteroids. For example, progesterone is excreted as a pregnanediol, 17-hydroxyprogesterone is excreted as pregnanetriol, and compound S and hydrocortisone are both excreted as Porter-Silber steroids or hydroxycorticoids.[3, 4, 14] Normally, the pregnanetriol levels are low (0 to 1.8 mg./24 hours) while the glucocorticoids or Porter-Silber positive material is usually found in the urine in relatively larger amounts so that the normal male or female will excrete 3 to 9 mg./24 hours.

Hydroxylation and Hydroxylase. The process of hydroxylation depending on the enzyme hydroxylase is the terminal event in the sequential production of hydrocortisone from its precursors. Experimental evidence has demonstrated that, if hydroxylation occurs at carbon 11 before it takes place at carbon 17 or carbon 21, it will then be almost impossible for hydroxylation to take place at these latter carbon atoms. However, if hydroxylation occurs first at carbon 17, then steroid synthesis will progress, with hydroxylation at carbon 21 and carbon 11 occurring in appropriate sequence.

The process of hydroxylation (specifically of carbon 21 and carbon 11), while under the control of an enzymatic system known as hydroxylase, is no doubt dependent on other systems necessary to complete the glucocorticoid synthesis (Figs. 419, 421, 422). This may include some participation of the desoxyribonucleic acid and ribonucleic acid systems in the adrenal cortex as a prerequisite for the production of hydrocortisone. As mentioned in Chapter 19, adenosine monophosphate and TPNH (Fig. 422) also play vital roles in the process of hydroxylation. However, the mechanism is not known specifically at the present time and the role of these basic nuclear requirements in the biosynthesis of hydrocortisone must still be elucidated.

Regardless of the process necessary for the synthesis of hydrocortisone by the normal adrenal, it now appears that an *enzymatic deficiency of hydroxylase* exists in the adrenal cortex of the patients with the classic adrenogenital syndrome (Fig. 440).[2-4, 12, 14, 32] It is the resultant abnormality which initiates the series of events responsible for the clinical manifestation of the AGS. It is important that these abnormalities be understood in order to achieve a rational approach to the problem of diagnosis and therapy of the AGS.

CONTROL OF ACTH SECRETION RATE. Enzymatic defects are the basis for the underlying disturbances in adrenal homeostasis resulting in the AGS. Consequently an inadequate supply of hydrocortisone is released from the zona fasciculata and is responsible for increased secretion of ACTH. The increased ACTH secretion is due to the principle of endo-

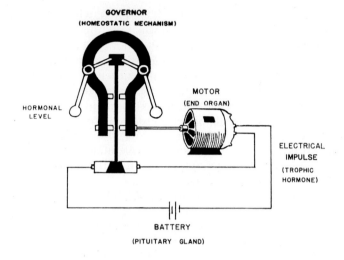

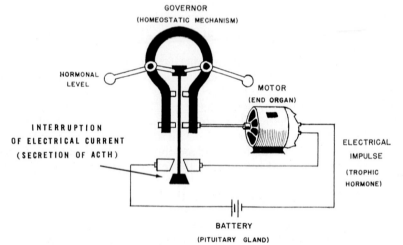

FIG. 441. *Top, Hormone level of end organ (centrifugal arms of governor) is low—hence no interruption of pituitary (source of energy) end-organ (motor) stimulation.*

Bottom, End organ (motor) has reached maximal speed (homeostatic level) raising the centrifugal arms, thereby breaking the circuit and interrupting further stimulus of end organ (motor) by the electrical current (tropic hormone) from the battery (pituitary) so that the homeostatic level is not exceeded.

crinology which states that end-organ hormone (hydrocortisone) controls the secretion of the pituitary tropic hormone (ACTH).

This system is akin to the centrifugal governor on a machine exhibited in Figure 441. When the speed of the machine exceeds the normal (homeostatic) level, the centripetal forces elevate the arms of the governor and reduce or cut off the source of fuel supply (tropic principle) to the mechanical parts (endocrine end organ), resulting in a diminution of speed (rate of secretion). When this secretion falls below the necessary levels, the arms of the governor fall and fuel again enters the system, maintaining the necessary speed. Specifically, whenever blood hydrocortisone, which is produced by the zona fasciculata under the influence of ACTH secretion, reaches the homeostatic or physiologic level, it will tend to inhibit further secretion of ACTH. If the blood level of hydrocortisone remains low, there is inadequate inhibition of ACTH. As a consequence of uninhibited ACTH secretion, there will be excessive stimulation or hyperplasia of those portions of the adrenal cortex ordinarily responsive to ACTH—i.e., not only the zona fasciculata, but also the zona reticularis.

Zona Reticularis. The zona reticularis, while under the control of ACTH much in the same manner as the fasciculata, is responsible for the secretion of sex steroids which are three in number—androgens, estrogens, and progestogens. The androgens excreted in the urine as 17-ketosteroids are by far the most important substances secreted as far as diagnosis and clinical effects are concerned. It is the increased level of the androgens which is responsible for inducing the widespread clinical manifestations or aberrations of the adrenogenital syndrome.

Suppression of Pituitary Gonadotropic Hormone Secretion. Since the major hormone of the adrenal cortex is hydrocortisone, the sex steroids produced by the zona reticularis are, in a sense, a by-product of the ACTH-adrenal axis and have little or no influence on the regulatory mechanism controlling the secretion of ACTH itself. Despite the fact that these sex steroids are of adrenal origin, they are still, biologically speaking, gonadal steroids, and when present in adequate amounts they will suppress pituitary gonadotropic hormone secretion. The gonadotropic hormones are responsible for stimulating the gonads to secrete the sex steroids necessary for normal sexual function and development. These steroids, in turn, are the physiologic regulators of pituitary gonadotropic hormone secretion in much the same manner that hydrocortisone or glucocorticoids are the physiologic regulators of ACTH. Therefore, the sex steroids of adrenal origin, when present in adequate amounts, despite their dependency on ACTH secretion, will partially or completely suppress the gonadotropic triad of hormones [follicle-stimulating hormone (FSH), luteinizing hormone (LH), and luteotropic hormone (LUTH)].

Gonadotropic Inhibition by 17-Ketosteroid Precursors. The presenting clinical picture of the AGS primarily due to the excessive secretion of adrenal androgens will vary, depending on the relative degree of deficiency of the 11β-hydroxylase of the adrenal cortex. Early in the development of the adrenogenital syndrome, when only a slight to moderate increase in 17-ketosteroid precursors is present, gonadotropin inhibition may be limited to only the luteinizing hormone and thereby interfere primarily with ovulation.[10, 15] This obviously will result in infertility but not necessarily in defeminization or excessive degree of hair growth. If increased amounts of 17-ketosteroid precursors are elaborated from the zona reticularis, complete inhibition of all of the above modalities of gonadotropic secretion will take place. In the female, this results in complete absence of ovarian activity accompanied by defeminization and excessive hirsutism.[2, 13, 16, 32] If these changes in the adrenal cortex occur prepubertally, the consequence may be afeminization. If a marked increase in 17-ketosteroid precursors occurs postpubertally, the result may be defeminization. The hirsutism is due primarily to the androgenic potential of the 17-ketosteroid precursors, and the defeminization is related to the fact that endogenous estrogenic activity of the ovary is absent as a result of the total inhibition of FSH and LH.

The same process may occur in the male where complete inhibition of the pituitary gonadotropic complex will result in azoospermia, well-developed phallus and usually small testes. Excessive androgen stimulation would not produce any gross somatic changes which would give the clinician a clue as to the basic disturbance except for a well-developed phallus but small testes.

Congenital AGS in Females.   The adrenogenital syndrome must be considered as being one of two related clinical entities: (1) the prepubertal or congenital type and (2) the postpubertal or acquired type. The congenital type shows all the classic stigmata of the syndrome, characterized by many of the anticipated features of pseudohermaphroditism. The postpubertal or acquired AGS may range from the female with a moderate degree of masculinization (never to the degree depicted in the congenital variant) to the eumorphic well-formed female with or without significant hirsutism but with anovulatory menses usually irregular in nature.

BLOCKAGE OF ENZYMATIC PROCESS.   In the congenital type, the basic disturbance apparently lies in a deficiency of the enzyme responsible for hydroxylation in converting 17-hydroxyprogesterone into compound S or compound S to hydrocortisone. As a result of the partial or total deficiency of this particular enzyme, the zona fasciculata is unable to form hydrocortisone in adequate amounts (Fig. 440). If the block is complete, then obviously no hydrocortisone is formed and all the stigmata of acute adrenal insufficiency may be seen in the newborn child. Frequently, the untreated AGS infant may die in Addisonian crisis during the neonatal period unless appropriate corticoid therapy is instituted.

INCREASED PREGNANETRIOL EXCRETION.   In partial or complete inhibition of 11β- or 21α-hydroxylation, one would expect the following series of events to occur in sequential order: since 17-hydroxyprogesterone is not being entirely converted into hydrocortisone, it is present in increased amounts. The enhanced 17-hydroxyprogesterone levels will be associated with an inordinately high pregnanetriol output.[3] The pregnanetriol ex-

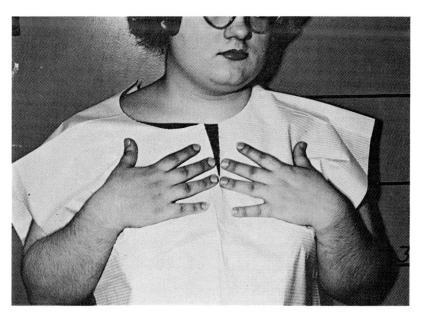

FIG. 442.   Patient PF, female, age 18 years, with congenital adrenogenital syndrome. She is poorly controlled with corticoid. An increased pigmentation of pressure areas of knuckles was noted and presumably was due to enhanced melanophoric-stimulating activity associated with increased release of ACTH.

cretion may be of such magnitude in some patients as to exceed in amount the excretion of 17-ketosteroids on a milligram-per-24-hour excretion basis.

ELEVATION IN ACTH SECRETION RATE. As a result of the decreased rate of conversion of 17-hydroxyprogesterone into hydrocortisone, the control of ACTH secretion by the diminished glucocorticoid secretion is ineffective so that increased ACTH elaboration is noted (Fig. 440). Elevated blood ACTH levels have been reported in a number of patients with the congenital adrenogenital syndrome.[28]

Pigmentation. Further signs of enhanced ACTH secretion in these patients is evidenced by the accentuation of the pigmentation of the skin on the extensor surfaces of the body. This pigmentation is similar to that of the Addisonian with primary adrenal failure due in part to the melanophoric stimulating moiety (MSH) associated with ACTH. Figure 442 demonstrates increased pigmentation of the knuckles of a poorly controlled adrenogenital syndrome patient.

VIRILISM DUE TO RETICULARIS HYPERPLASIA. The increased ACTH secretion causes excessive stimulation of the zona reticularis and the zona fasciculata. This brings about the prevalent anatomic finding of adrenal cortical hyperplasia and hypertrophy. Depending on the degree of enzymatic defect, the excessive ACTH stimulation of the zona fasciculata may achieve some measure of hydrocortisone production. However, the zona reticularis is also stimulated excessively by the elevated ACTH levels, and a significant increase in level of secretion of androgenic steroids takes place from this zone layer. These steroids, being primarily sex steroids in character, will have the potential effect of inhibiting completely or partially all modalities of pituitary gonadotropic secretion (Fig. 440). The 17-ketosteroid precursors are the principal steroids produced by the zona reticularis and these substances, because of their potential androgenic effect, will induce a marked arrhenomimetic effect resulting in the typical masculinizing picture of the congenital adrenogenital syndrome (Figs. 443 and 444).

Pituitary-Gonadal Disturbances. Because of the deficient corticoid production, the pituitary gland is compelled to maintain increased and uninhibited secretion of ACTH.[11]

ACTH OVERPRODUCTION. It has been suggested that the excessive activity (ACTH hypersecretion) causes amenorrhea and other basic disturbances in pituitary gonadal function. It is presumed that the elevated ACTH secretion occurs at the expense of secretion or production of the other pituitary tropic hormones, particularly the gonadotropic principle. In other words, this concept suggests that the pituitary cells are "so busy manufacturing ACTH" that there is little or no time for production of FSH, and consequently gonadal function is held in abeyance.[11]

Comparison with the Addisonian Patient. There are obvious flaws in such reasoning. For example, in the days before cortisone, Addisonian patients were maintained on desoxycorticosterone acetate (DCA) without alteration or disturbance in genital function. In these patients

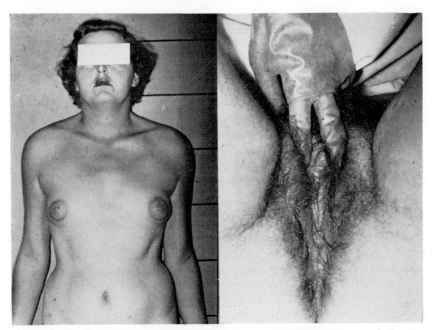

FIG. 443. *Patient EK, female, age 26 years, having classic adrenogenital syndrome with markedly elevated 17-ketosteroids (57.4 mg. per 24 hours). Note broad shoulders and poor female secondary sexual development plus the presence of an enlarged clitoris.*

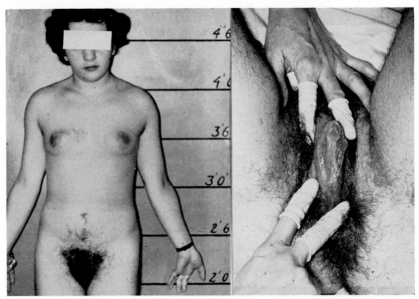

FIG. 444. *Patient EC, female, age 26 years, having classic adrenogenital syndrome with elevated 17-ketosteroids (26.8 mg. per 24 hours), showing the typical masculine body build—broad shoulders and narrow hips associated with significant clitoral enlargement, marked oligomenorrhea without therapy but regular menses with glucocorticoid.*

with primary hypoadrenocorticoidism, ACTH secretion was increased. These patients always exhibited a marked increase in pigmentation despite the fact that their electrolyte disturbances were well regulated. In addition, we now know that the doses of DCA employed were not capable of suppressing endogenous ACTH activity. Normal menstrual function, however, was noted in many of these patients and pregnancies occurred. This indicates that normal gonadotropic excretion existed. These data offer evidence against the theory of the limited capacity of the pituitary gland to produce the various tropic hormones. It appears that the amenorrhea or allied disturbances in menstrual function are due not to ACTH excess per se, but to the gonadotropin inhibitory effect of the elevated level of androgenic steroids. This effect is secondary to the increased ACTH levels causing the excessive stimulation of the zona reticularis.[2, 18, 19, 28, 32, 33]

Finally, if the theory that overproduction of one tropic hormone takes place at the expense of secretion of another tropic hormone were a valid concept, in addition to the gonadotropic lack, one would uniformly expect diminished secretion of TSH. However, it is indeed rare for any patients with the adrenogenital syndrome to show evidence of decreased thyroid function. This is another indication that the all-or-none concept of secretion of pituitary tropic hormones is probably not the mechanism of action responsible for the depressed gonadotropic secretion in the adrenogenital syndrome.

DIAGNOSIS. The congenital adrenogenital syndrome due to a defect in adrenal cortical hydroxylation presents no problem in diagnosis on the basis of the clinical picture alone.

Clinical Findings. These patients invariably will show the following clinical stigmata:

1. Increased hirsutism of a marked degree will be noted early in life. As the female patient approaches adulthood, male-like recession of the hairline in the temporal regions may occur.

2. Patients will usually show evidence of premature acneform eruption of the skin of the face and the back, with some extension to the chest. The acne is premature as far as the chronologic age of the patient is concerned.

3. The skin is tough, thick, and masculine-like in texture.

4. Patients will show clinical evidence of defeminization or afeminization, depending on the age at which the disease originates.

5. There is invariably an accentuated masculine type of body build associated with broad shoulders and narrow hips (Fig. 445A).

6. The muscular strength of these patients is considerably increased.

7. There is no evidence of striae or areas of ecchymosis.

8. The clitoris may be slightly or enormously enlarged (Figs. 445B-449). It may be associated with different phases of labial-vulvar fusion, ranging from one of almost imperceptible degree to one of such magnitude that the external genitalia appear to be essentially those of a male, usually with a third-degree hypospadias and a scrotum devoid of testicular organs (Fig. 449).

9. Pelvic examination will reveal a marked hypoplasia of the fundus and cervix with a normal or markedly abbreviated or even absent vaginal tract.

10. The voice of the patient, if a child, is husky and mature, while in late adolescence or early adulthood the voice is characterized by a bass and coarse quality.

11. Increased height will be noted as a child, but the patient will become a short adult due to accelerated epiphyseal closure.

Laboratory Findings. The following laboratory findings are noted:

1. A moderate to marked elevation of 17-ketosteroid is present.

2. Patients will usually show no significant to a marked elevation of the pregnanetriol.

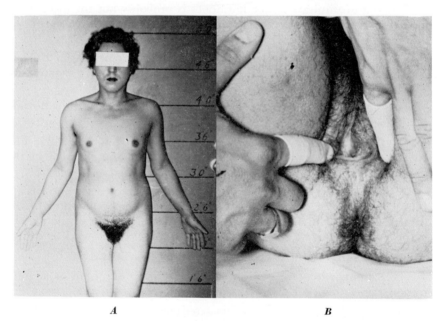

A   B

FIG. 445. *Patient IC, female, age 24 years, showing the typical adrenogenital-syndrome physiognomy (narrow hips and wide shoulders) with moderately elevated 17-ketosteroids (28.3 mg. per 24 hours) and enormously high pregnanetriol (32.7 mg.). Primary amenorrhea prior to glucocorticoid therapy, with menses following adequate control with corticoid steroid.*

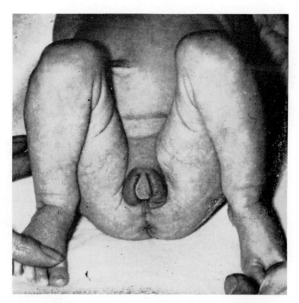

FIG. 446. *Patient MC, age 19 days, having congenital adreno-genital syndrome. Infant with positive chromatin pattern who is markedly dehydrated and who has shown no weight gain since her birth. Note the marked enlargement of the clitoris, the obvious evidence of dehydration, and the pigmentation of the labial folds and clitoris. 17-Ketosteroids were 5.2 mg. per 24 hours; pregnanetriol 0.4 mg. This infant is one in whom the adrenogenital syndrome is associated with a metabolic defect at the 3β position where a deficiency of 3β-hydroxy dehydrogenase occurs and is characterized by a salt-losing syndrome. Her control has been difficult, as has been reported, but was successfully accomplished by the parenteral use of glucocorticoids plus desoxycorticosterone triphenylacetate.*

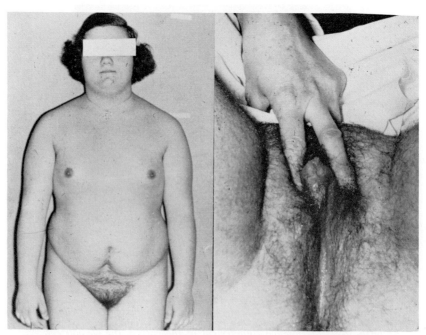

FIG. 447. Patient PF, female, age 13 years, with primary amenorrhea, greatly elevated 17-ketosteroids (69.0 mg. per 24 hours), and enlarged clitoris. Excellent control with corticoids with regular catamenia occurring. Patient had been operated on prior to the availability of corticoid therapy and had one adrenal removed because of virilization.

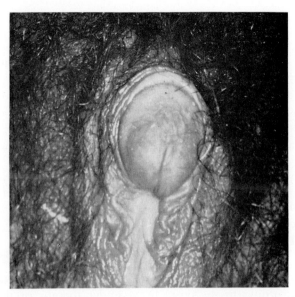

FIG. 448. Patient GO, female, age 28 years, having an enormous clitoris with 17-ketosteroids above 80 mg. per 24 hours. Excellent control with corticoids, followed by three pregnancies.

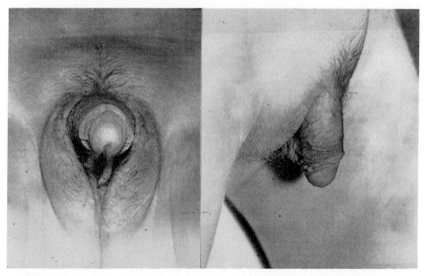

FIG. 449. Patient LS, female, age 9 years, untreated congenital adrenogenital syndrome. Note markedly enlarged clitoris with third degree hypospadias. 17-Ketosteroids exceeded 60 mg. per 24 hours. A plastic operation was done to remove the clitoris. The patient was placed on glucocorticoids with excellent results (Fig. 464) in that regular, ovulatory menstrual cycles resulted when she began to menstruate.

3. The 17-hydroxysteroid excretion may be low-normal or almost absent.

4. The glucose tolerance test may be characterized by a hypogly-cemic level at the fourth or fifth hour because of the diminished hydro-cortisone secretion level in these patients (Fig. 450).

5. Patients may also show some degree of insulin sensitivity, as well as a tendency for decreased hypoglycemic responsiveness.

6. There will be no evidence of osteoporosis.

7. An atrophic vaginal smear is present and associated with uterine hypoplasia.

8. Only those infants with the salt-losing syndrome with almost a total deficiency in enzymatic hydroxylation will show evidence of hypo-natremia and hyperkalemia.

9. Aldosterone excretion is usually normal.

10. ACTH levels are elevated.

FUNCTIONAL TESTS. *Therapeutic Test with Corticoids.* The diag-nosis of the AGS is established by noting the patient's response to oral corticoids according to the doses listed under therapy or more acutely after intravenous administration of 5 mg. of 9-alpha-fluorohydrocortisone

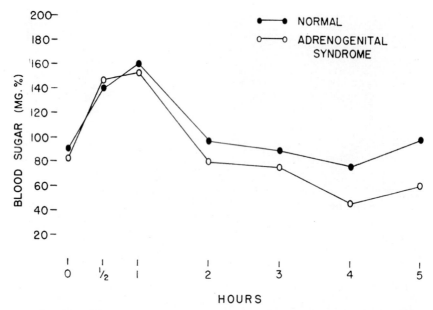

FIG. 450. *Glucose tolerance test of patient with the adrenogenital syndrome. Note the hypoglycemic response at the fourth hour as compared to the glucose tolerance test in the normal individual.*

TREATED ADRENOGENITAL SYNDROME

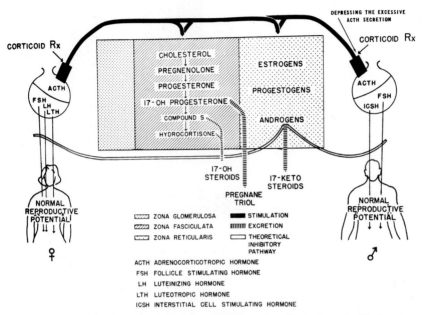

FIG. 451. *Diagrammatic presentation showing the effect of corticoid therapy upon suppression of excessive ACTH secretion in the adrenogenital-syndrome patient. The resultant effect upon diminution of secretion of the androgenic precursors from the zona reticularis brings about release of gonadotropins with normal gonadal function.*

or 100 mg. of hydrocortisone hemisuccinate in 500 cc. of a solution of 5 per cent glucose and 0.9 per cent saline (Fig. 451). The rationale for the use of glucocorticoids in the adrenogenital syndrome to inhibit the excessive secretion of endogenous ACTH is depicted in Figure 451. The corticoids may be administered intravenously to achieve a rapid effect or orally to accomplish a somewhat slower but less variable response. The infusion may consist of any one of the following corticoids: (a) 100 mg. hydrocortisone hemisuccinate; (b) 5 mg. 9α-fludrocortisone hemisuccinate; (c) 25 mg. prednisolone hemisuccinate. Urine is collected for several eight-hour periods: eight hours before the infusion, eight hours during the infusion, and two eight-hour post-infusion periods. Prompt and rapid drop in 17-ketosteroid and pregnanetriol levels during and immediately after the infusion is indicative of adrenal cortical hyperplasia (Fig. 452).[2-4, 16, 20, 27, 30-32]

The response to oral corticoids takes one to two weeks before a significant drop in steroid level is obtained.

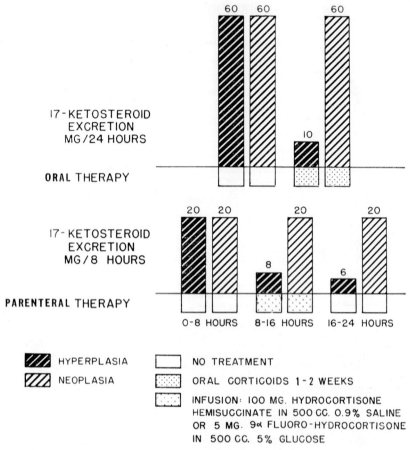

17-KETOSTEROID
EXCRETION
MG/24 HOURS

ORAL THERAPY

17-KETOSTEROID
EXCRETION
MG/8 HOURS

PARENTERAL THERAPY

0-8 HOURS   8-16 HOURS   16-24 HOURS

HYPERPLASIA   NO TREATMENT
NEOPLASIA   ORAL CORTICOIDS 1-2 WEEKS
                     INFUSION: 100 MG. HYDROCORTISONE
                     HEMISUCCINATE IN 500 CC. 0.9% SALINE
                     OR 5 MG. 9α FLUORO-HYDROCORTISONE
                     IN 500 CC. 5% GLUCOSE

FIG. 452. *Corticoid depression test in the differentiation between hyperplasia and neoplasia in the etiology of the adrenogenital syndrome. Note that oral or intravenous corticoids will suppress the elevated 17-ketosteroid in hyperplasia of the adrenal cortex, while there will be little or no depression of this steroid in neoplasia.*

Provocative Test with ACTH. A significantly increased level of secretion of 17-ketosteroid and pregnanetriol after ACTH without a comparative increase in 17-hydroxysteroid levels would be indicative of the AGS associated with adrenal hyperplasia (Fig. 453).[2, 14, 22] ACTH, 25 u., is infused intravenously in 500 cc. of saline over an eight-hour interval. Urine is collected for the eight-hour periods before the infusion, during the infusion, and post-infusion. A marked increase in 17-KS and pregnanetriol of 150 to 300 per cent over the control level during the infusion and the eight-hour period post-infusion would point to adrenal hyperplasia. No change in 17-OH would be anticipated. The provocative test with ACTH could also be accomplished with the zinc or gel preparation. A control urine for 17-KS, pregnanetriol and 17-OH is collected for the 24-hour period preceding the ACTH injection and again for the 24-hour period following the injection. An increase of 17-KS and pregnanetriol of 200 per cent or more with no significant change in 17-OH is indicative of hyperplasia. An increase of all the steroids of less than 100 per cent would point to neoplasia if the 17-KS level is high and if the pregnanetriol and 17-OH levels, previous to ACTH injection, are normal.

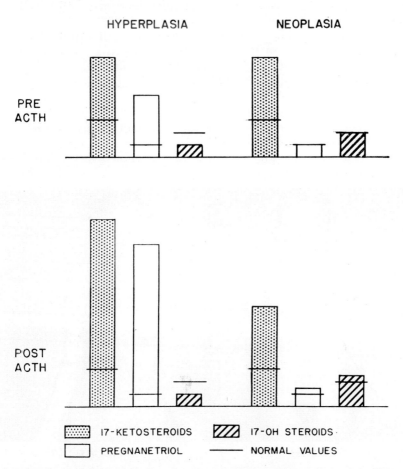

FIG. 453. *ACTH provocative test in the differentiation between hyperplasia and neoplasia in the etiology of the adrenogenital syndrome. In patients with hyperplasia, ACTH significantly increases elevated 17-ketosteroid and pregnanetriol but has little effect upon 17-hydroxysteroid levels. In contrast, patients with neoplasia show only a modest or slight increase in the urine excretory products similar to the level expected in the normal individual.*

Postpubertal AGS in Females. The second type of adrenogenital syndrome patient is one who develops the disease in the postpubertal phase of her life.

CLINICAL FEATURES. Frequently she may not be recognized by the anticipated clinical stigmata alone. Many times these patients fail to show evidence of excessive hirsutism and may be looked upon as eumorphic females with a characteristically feminine body build (Figs. 454, 455).[13, 15, 19] Others, as would be anticipated on the basis of biologic variation alone, may exhibit some of the physical findings anticipated in the congenital adrenogenital syndrome; they may show excessive hirsutism plus signs of defeminization (Figs 456, 457). However, many of the postpubertal patients are of normal or tall stature (Figs. 456, 457). The patient may or may not have clitoral enlargement. Pelvic examination is usually devoid of specific abnormal findings.

LABORATORY FINDINGS. Laboratory data reveal the ketosteroids to be slightly to moderately elevated, and the pregnanetriols may be normal or only slightly elevated. The patient will usually show no evidence of ovulation or only intermittent ovulation at the best. Tests for luteinizing hormone activity will show decreased levels. FSH secretion may be normal or depressed. The glucose tolerance may show hypoglycemic levels

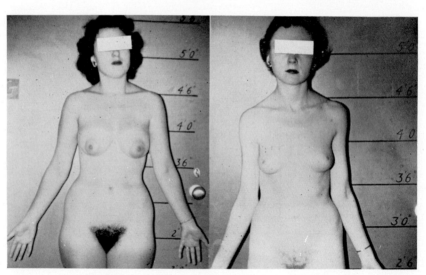

FIG. 454   FIG. 455

FIG. 454. Patient HF, age 24 years. Normal eumorphic female with the adrenogenital syndrome showing no evidence of virilism yet with elevated 17-ketosteroid (26.4 mg. per 24 hours) and irregular menses.

FIG. 455. Patient MMcG, age 25 years. Diagnosis of adrenogenital syndrome made on basis of elevated 17-ketosteroid and irregular, anovulatory menses in a normal, eumorphic patient without evidence of virilism.

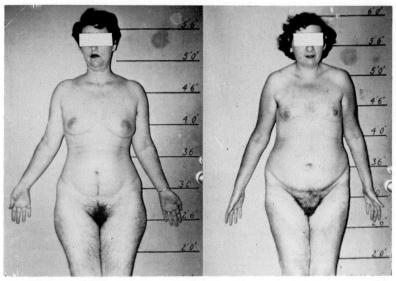

FIG. 456   FIG. 457

FIG. 456. *Patient MM, female, age 37 years. There is marked increase in facial hirsutism plus excessive hirsutism on thighs and lower abdomen. This female is a relatively tall patient with the adrenogenital syndrome. 17-Keto-steroid, 22.4 mg. per 24 hours.*

FIG. 457. *Patient SF, female, age 34 years. Tall, moderately obese, hirsute female in whom the diagnosis of adrenogenital syndrome was based upon her elevated 17-ketosteroids (40 mg. per 24 hours) and totally irregular menstrual periods characterized by hypo- and oligomenorrhea. Corticoids induced normal, regular, ovulatory menses. Pregnancy resulted.*

at the fourth or fifth hour.[8] There is usually no sign of abnormal insulin responsiveness or hypoglycemic unresponsiveness.

INTERPRETATION OF THE 17-KETOSTEROID LEVEL. The critical diagnostic test in these patients is to determine whether or not the level of 17-ketosteroid excretion is elevated. One must be aware, of course, of the normal variation for these values in the particular laboratory doing the procedure. It is important to elaborate upon the significance of a specific reading, particularly if this level is at the upper limits of normal or slightly above.

Significance of 17-Ketosteroid Levels. The importance of even a minimal degree of elevation becomes apparent if we draw an analogy between the 17-ketosteroid values and the readings occasionally noted in patients subjected to basal metabolic tests. For example, if we were to do a basal metabolic test on a patient and note a minus 10 BMR, one could not definitely state that thyroid disease was present on the basis of this laboratory procedure alone. However, one year from now, if the patient were to show an increase in 20 points and have a plus 10 BMR, one would still adhere to the accepted variation of the norm and not consider the patient as one with thyroid dysfunction on the basis of this reading alone.

Let us consider another patient in whom the BMR is first reported as being a plus 10. Later, as in the preceding example, his BMR increases 20 points and is now read as being plus 30. In this case we would certainly suspect the diagnosis of hyperthyroidism. In other words, a patient having an increase of 20 points in the basal metabolic rate, but starting out with a level at the higher limit of normal, definitely would be suspected of hyperthyroidism, and if clinical stigmata were present, the diagnosis would be placed on a firmer footing. On the other hand, in the first example, a change from the lower limit of normal to the higher limit, despite the 20 point increase, would be disregarded since both values are considered to be within the limits of normal variation.

17-Ketosteroid Suppression with Corticoids. Similar logic may be considered in the interpretation of 17-ketosteroid levels when these values are at the upper limit of normal. The same analogy drawn for the BMR applies to the clinical significance of these 17-ketosteroid determinations. The normal 17-ketosteroid value in our laboratory for the adult female may range from 8 to 14 mg./24 hours. If a patient now has a 17-ketosteroid excretion of 14 mg./24 hours, this figure would not appear to be abnormal. However, it may be clinically significant, as in the patient with the BMR tests, if one year ago the 17-ketosteroid level had been only 8 mg./24 hours. Since both figures are within the limits of normality, one would be reluctant to institute the corticoid therapy for an androgenital syndrome unless clinical signs were present. However, if a patient has had a 17-ketosteroid excretion of 14 mg. which then goes up to 20 mg., also a difference of 6 mg., we certainly would entertain the diagnosis of the adrenogenital syndrome based on a significantly elevated 17-ketosteroid level. This would be almost mandatory if the patient showed some of the clinical stigmata of the disease. In other words, a 17-ketosteroid level at the upper limit of normal, or slightly above, may be of some clinical importance, particularly if the patient has an abnormality of the menstrual cycle and shows signs of increased hirsutism and there are no findings pointing toward the ovaries as a site of the possible endocrine disturbance or androgenic production.

THERAPEUTIC TEST USING CORTICOIDS. A therapeutic test with corticoids may be used in these patients to establish whether or not there is an adrenogenital syndrome. The diagnosis is confirmed or denied by determining whether or not there is a depression of the 17-ketosteroid levels following corticoid therapy. If the borderline 17-ketosteroid value is depressed by the recommended doses of corticoids, then such a patient must be considered as having the adrenogenital syndrome and must be maintained on corticoid therapy until the anticipated therapeutic response is achieved. It is of utmost importance to recheck the initial steroid level in menstruating females since they tend to show *cyclic variation* in excretion of 17-ketosteroids—their highest levels being obtained during the premenstrual phase. If these variables have been checked and the 17-ketosteroids are still elevated, then the diagnosis of the postpubertal adrenogenital syndrome may be established on the basis of a positive therapeutic test—i.e., a drop in 17-ketosteroid level after an appropriate course of corticoid therapy. To repeat: a significant decrease in 17-ketosteroid levels, from a value at the upper limit of normal to one just at or below the lower limit of normal, would confirm the presence of the androgenital syndrome (Figs. 458, 459), despite the normal eumorphic appearance of the patients. Many of these patients are moderately or markedly hirsute. Corticoids in the doses recommended will usually not suppress the 17-ketosteroids in patients with normal adrenal function, as the doses are considered to be physiologic and equivalent to those secreted normally by the adrenal cortex.

PREGNANETRIOL VERSUS 17-KETOSTEROID LEVELS. There is another diagnostic point that must be emphasized. There are patients with the postpubertal type of AGS who exhibit a dichotomy between their level of excretion of 17-ketosteroid and pregnanetriol. Such patients may show

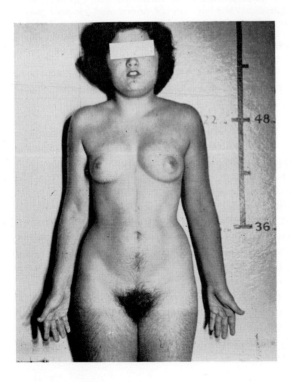

FIG. 458. Patient AD, female, age 21 years. In this patient the diagnosis of adrenogenital syndrome was based upon hirsutism, elevated 17-ketosteroids (16 mg. per 24 hours), and irregular menstrual periods. Note the normal eumorphic female, who is very feminine in appearance.

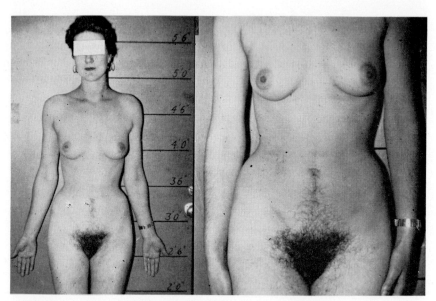

FIG. 459. Patient PT, age 24 years with adrenogenital syndrome. This patient is a tall, shapely female with moderate degree of hirsutism. The diagnosis was based upon elevated 17-ketosteroids (39.8 mg. per 24 hours) and elevated pregnanetriol (7.7 mg. per 24 hours). Patient had irregular anovulatory periods. Steroid pattern became normal and was associated with ovulatory regular menses when patient was placed upon corticoid therapy.

a greatly increased pregnanetriol output while their 17-ketosteroid excretion levels are relatively normal so that there is a proportionately higher excretion of pregnanetriol than of 17-ketosteroids. Normally, the pregnanetriol levels may vary between 0 to 1.8 mg./24 hours. However, patients with this dichotomy of steroid excretion may have a pregnanetriol in the range of 5 to 7 mg., representing an enormous elevation, while there is little, if any, significant elevation in 17-ketosteroid excretion. This discrepancy has been noted in one elderly patient and also in a young child where a ketosteroid determination alone may have been insufficient to establish the presence of the adrenogenital syndrome. In these patients, the significantly elevated pregnanetriol offered the necessary laboratory clue to establish the diagnosis of the AGS. In addition, administration of ACTH to one of these patients caused a profound increase in pregnanetriol with only slight elevation of her 17-ketosteroid.

A dichotomy is also noticed following the discontinuance of corticoid therapy in patients with the congenital adrenogenital syndrome who had been appropriately controlled with adequate corticoid suppressive treatment. Prior to therapy, these patients usually have astronomically elevated 17-ketosteroid levels with comparative (but lower) elevation of pregnanetriol. However, when the treatment is stopped, the ketosteroid excretion usually never returns to the original pretreatment levels. On the other hand, the pregnanetriol excretion in these patients may rise to amounts considerably higher than those of the pretreatment level and may exceed in milligrams/24 hours the output of 17-ketosteroid. The ketosteroid excretion will never approach the unusually high values seen during the control period but the pregnanetriol level may even exceed the original control reading.

Therapy. ORAL DOSES OF CORTICOIDS. Therapy of the adrenogenital syndrome requires the use of glucocorticoids in doses sufficient to suppress the excessive ACTH secretion responsible for the elevated 17-ketosteroid excretion (Fig. 451). The following doses of the different corticoids are the average that may be employed and will be equivalent in their effect.[9, 15, 17-21] However, in discussing average doses, one must realize that individual patients may require less or more than the so-called recommended regimen:

Cortisone, 12.5 mg. t.i.d.

Hydrocortisone, 10 mg. t.i.d.

Prednisone or prednisolone (Meticorten or Meticortelone), 2.5 mg. t.i.d.

6-Methyl prednisolone (Medrol), 2 mg. t.i.d.

Triamcinolone (Aristocort, Kenacort), 2 to 3 mg. t.i.d.

Dexamethasone (Decadron, Deronil), 0.375 mg. t.i.d.

Betamethasone (Celestone), 0.3 mg. t.i.d.

Fluprednisolone (Alphadrol), 0.75 mg. t.i.d.

Paramethasone acetate (Haldrone), 1.0 mg. t.i.d.

The above medication is administered orally and approximately at eight-hour intervals. Excellent control may be achieved. There is usually no need for the parenteral use of corticoids in these patients since the oral route offers an effective means of therapy. Occasionally, the parenteral use of long-acting corticoids may be a convenient form of therapy in adults or children with the AGS in whom it is difficult to maintain the appropriate and necessary oral regimen. In these patients, the intramuscular administration of 40 mg. of 6-methylprednisolone acetate-aqueous suspension (Depo-Medrol) once every 10 to 14 days usually achieves adequate control and satisfactory 17-ketosteroid levels. The doses advised are in the physiologic range, so there is no necessity to impose any type of dietary restriction on the patient; nor must one use potassium supplementation. The patient may be permitted to take salt ad libitum.[9, 17, 21] This is in contrast to the patient who is receiving pharmacologic doses of corticoids, usually for their anti-inflammatory effects, where excessive amounts of the corticoids are necessary. In this latter group, restricted intake of sodium and carbohydrate plus potassium supplementation may be necessary to prevent the adverse effects of the corticoids on electrolyte balance and carbohydrate metabolism.

The steroid, 9-alphafluorohydrocortisone, was purposely omitted in the above discussion on the treatment of the AGS. It is a potent pituitary inhibitor of ACTH. When 2 to 3 mg. per day is given to the AGS patient, prompt suppression of the elevated 17-ketosteroid and pregnanetriol excretion occurs. However, this dose level will also produce profound sodium retention, causing significant edema. It is for this reason that this steroid is contraindicated for the treatment of the patient with the AGS.

The dose of corticoid necessary to control the patient with the adrenogenital syndrome is judged to a certain extent by the level of 17-ketosteroid and pregnanetriol that is achieved with therapy. The effect of different doses of corticoids on 17-ketosteroid excretion is depicted in Figure 460 where the comparative activity of the steroids is measured by the resultant 17-ketosteroid level. One should maintain the 17-ketosteroid excretion level at 10 mg./24 hours or below and/or keep the pregnanetriol level below 1.8 mg./24 hours. If these levels are achieved readily, the amount of corticoids administered may then be diminished to a lower dose which must still maintain the 17-ketosteroid excretion at the desired point.

LEVEL OF 17-KETOSTEROID AND CORTICOID DOSAGE. Frequently there may be patients with the classic adrenogenital syndrome where the initial levels of 17-ketosteroids and pregnanetriol are unusually high. This does not mean that they will require higher doses of corticoids than do patients with lower control values since prompt suppression of the precursors of these steroids, regardless of the amounts excreted, may be achieved by the use of the average corticoid doses listed above and graphically presented in Figure 460. There is no correlation between the pretreatment elevation of 17-ketosteroids and the dose of glucocorticoids necessary for its suppression to normal values. Subsequently, the corticoid doses may be diminished and still maintain the same level of steroid excretion. As a result, these patients may be controlled adequately for years on corticoids in amounts one half to one third of that required originally. Conversely, there have been occasional patients in whom a previously effective dose had to be increased by one third or more.

While the corticoid dose is an individual one, it should be emphasized that the maintenance dose, after initial suppression is achieved, is fairly constant as the years go by. Usually one rechecks the urinary steroid excretion levels of the patient approximately three to four weeks after therapy has been instituted to permit an appropriate period of time for corticoid suppression to have taken place (Fig. 460).

DISCONTINUING CORTICOID THERAPY. How long will the patient with the AGS have to be maintained on corticoid therapy? When corticoids are discontinued after several months of treatment in the postpubertal adrenogenital syndrome, the patient's abnormal pattern of steroid excretion

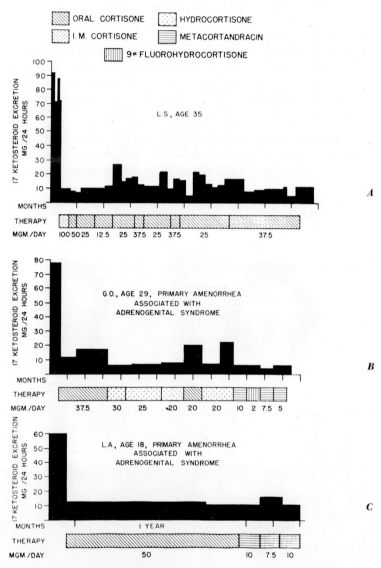

FIG. 460. *The 17-ketosteroid levels in three classic adrenogenital syndrome patients. The changes in steroid excretion are based upon the dose of corticoid administered. The changes correlate well quantitatively with the amount of corticoid ingested.*

may never revert back to the level noted prior to instituting corticoid therapy. Hence, the postpubertal patient with the adrenogenital syndrome may not have to continue therapy with adrenocortical preparations for the rest of her life. In contrast, our experience to date indicates that an abnormal pattern of steroid excretion recurs promptly after discontinuing corticoid therapy in patients with the congenital adrenogenital syndrome. This is characterized by marked elevation of pregnanetriol but with less of a rebound increase in 17-ketosteroid, never approaching the initially high level noted during the pretreatment phase. The marked increase in pregnanetriol and modest elevation of 17-ketosteroid occurs promptly after discontinuing corticoid therapy in the congenital adrenogenital syndrome patients. They must, therefore, be maintained on glucocorticoid therapy continuously for the rest of their lives if normal adrenal function is desired.

SEQUENCE OF CHANGES RELATED TO CORTICOID THERAPY.   When one uses corticoids in the pre- or postpubertal adrenogenital syndrome, what

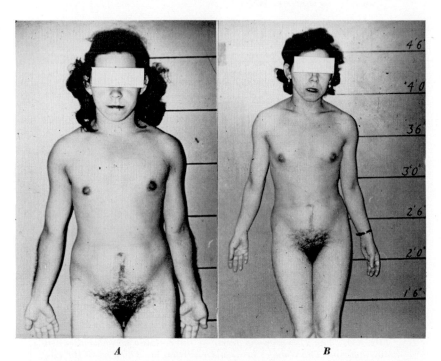

A   B

FIG. 461. Patient GR, female, age 19 years, with classic adrenogenital syndrome with control 17-ketosteroids above 80 mg. per 24 hours, pregnanetriols
48.7 mg. per 24 hours. Before therapy (A), note the masculinized female showing
no evidence of feminization. After corticoid therapy (B) there is a tendency for
some loss of masculinizing musculature and beginning breast development, plus
minimal female fat deposition.

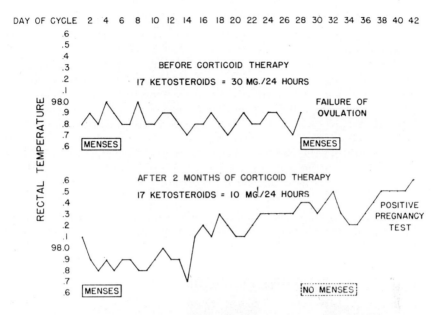

FIG. 462. *The elevation in basal body temperature indicated ovulation after the patient had been placed upon corticoid therapy. Pregnancy occurred.*

is the sequential series of events that take place in the female patient with ovulatory defects, abnormal menstrual function, elevated steroid excretion patterns, and increased hirsutism?

The following sequence of changes related to therapy can be anticipated:

Correction of the Elevated Steroid Excretion. The earliest response of the patient to corticoid therapy is the decline of the elevated urinary 17-ketosteroid and pregnanetriol levels to normal. This may be observed as early as seven to 14 days after the initiation of oral therapy or within hours after intravenous infusion of the steroids. Figure 460A demonstrates the prompt fall in 17-ketosteroid levels after parenteral corticoids. The only reason the cortisone was administered intramuscularly was that this patient was the first one studied by us in 1951 and 1952 and only parenteral cortisone was available then.

Release of FSH Secretion. The next response is the release of the secretion of FSH. If FSH secretion is suppressed in the patient with the adrenogenital syndrome at an age when the menarche should normally be expected, its release is manifested by the beginning of development of secondary sexual characteristics, increased maturation of the vaginal smear, and appearance of menstruation (Fig. 461).

Correction of Ovulatory Defects. The third phenomenon is the initiation of ovulatory cycles. The release of FSH secretion will occur as early as three to four weeks after initiating the appropriate therapy, and ovulatory effects with normal menstrual cycles will be observed as early as seven to nine weeks. The correction of ovulatory defects in infertile patients has been one of the most gratifying effects noted following appropriate corticoid therapy in patients with mildly to markedly elevated 17-ketosteroids (Fig. 462). If ovulation occurs while the patient is on corticoid therapy, and if the 17-ketosteroids are depressed to physiologic levels or below, we then have confirmatory evidence of the accuracy of the diagnosis and the need for such treatment. When the crown of pregnancy is given to the previously barren patient, the ultimate of a therapeutic triumph has been achieved (Fig. 463).

Corticoid Therapy During Pregnancy. If pregnancy occurs while the patient is on corticoid therapy, is continued medication required? Since the placenta is known to produce increased amounts of corticoids and ACTH, we believe that all exogenous corticoids may be discontinued

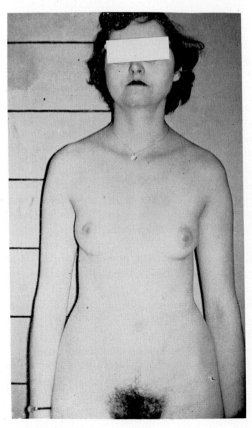

FIG. 463. Patient EB, female, age 25 years, with adrenogenital syndrome without evidence of virilization. Her temperature chart was anovulatory until she received corticoid therapy (Fig. 462). The control 17-ketosteroids were 22 mg. per 24 hours.

once pregnancy takes place and adequate placental function is established (by the sixth to eighth week). Discontinuing corticoid therapy, whether abruptly or slowly, has no adverse effects on either the progress or the outcome of the pregnancy.

Normal Spermatogenesis. In the male AGS, spermatogenesis may approach anticipated normal values after two to three months' therapy.

Diminution of Hirsutism. Many patients seek therapy only because of concern over their excessive hirsutism. Can one assure those patients who are candidates for corticoid treatment that the hirsutism will be significantly diminished? Patients should be advised that the decrease in hirsutism, if it occurs at all, may not be seen until after nine months of continuous corticoid therapy. It should be emphasized that decreased hair growth may not be visible grossly. Even after nine months of corticoid therapy, the changes may be so imperceptible that the only decrease in the rate of hair growth that can be demonstrated is the slower rate of regrowth of hair after its removal by electrolysis. Unfortunately, in our experience, the effect of corticoids on diminishing the excessive hirsutism in these patients has not been so dramatic as that described by others.

Loss of Turgidity in the Clitoris. The enlarged clitoris of the patients with the adrenogenital syndrome may never show any dramatic decrease in size. However, there will be some loss of turgidity, giving the appearance at times of some diminution in size. If the clitoris has approached grotesque proportions prior to corticoid therapy, then a satisfactory cosmetic effect can be achieved only by clitorectomy. Clitoral amputation should be performed in such a manner as to preserve the prepuce and the nerve supply to the glans. Some patients have noted a loss of libido when the operation is performed with no attempt being made to preserve the vascular and neurogenic supply to the glans. Careful maintenance of the normal anatomic relationships of the nerve supply after clitoral amputation offers the patient the chance of adequate libido after completion of the surgical procedure.

Feminization. Feminization of the body of the female (enlargement of the breast, loss of masculine muscle deposition and increased trochanteric fat deposition) with development of female contours may take as long as 12 to 15 months of continuous corticoid therapy (Fig. 464).

Clinical Management of Congenital AGS Infants. The clinical management of the classic adrenogenital syndrome at birth is somewhat different from the problem seen in the more mature congenital case. The undifferentiated state of the external genitalia may lead to a possible error in establishing the correct anatomic sex of the individual. The infant may show relatively indifferent genitalia due to the presence of an enlarged clitoris associated with partial or complete labial fusion. Every possible means available to the physician should be used to establish the correct sex, from both the phenotypic and the genotypic points of view.

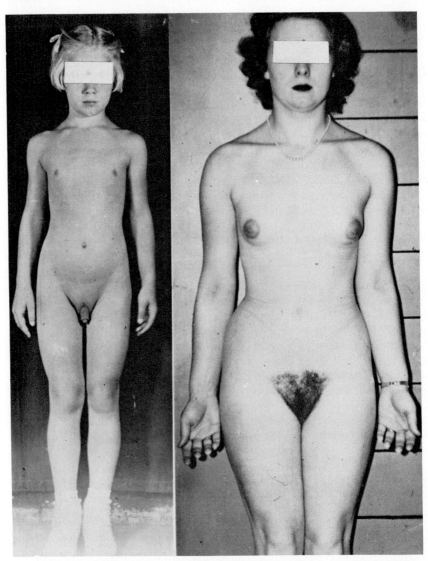

FIG. 464. Patient LS, female, age 22 years. A, Before corticoid therapy, age 9.
B, After corticoid therapy, age 22. Patient placed upon corticoid therapy at
age 18. Control steroid excretion: 17-ketosteroid 60 mg. per 24 hours, pregnanetriol
not obtained. The patient developed excellent feminization and female fat
deposition on corticoid therapy. Her clitoris was amputated as a child.

One should suspect the presence of the adrenogenital syndrome in an infant with partially fused labia, an enlarged clitoris, and a positive chromatin pattern. The syndrome should also be suspected in any infant who appears to have the external genitalia of a male but without palpable testes in the presence of a well-developed scrotum and phallus and who shows signs of dehydration and increased pigmentation of the external genitalia.

Hypospadias may or may not be present and may vary from minimal or first-degree to marked or third-degree (see Fig. 237). The most common defect is the third-degree hypospadias in masculinized females. One's suspicions should be directed toward the adrenogenital syndrome if, in addition to the above findings, the infant has some evidence of increased pigmentation in the area of the scrotum and the perineum (Figs. 465, 466). When these findings are associated with clinical evidence of hypoadremia, then a more solid basis for the diagnosis is established.

DIAGNOSTIC PROCEDURES. Three important diagnostic procedures also must be performed: (1) examination of tissue and blood to establish the nuclear chromatin patterns of the child, (2) determination of 17-ketosteroid and pregnanetriol excretion levels, and (3) determination of the skeletal bone age. Both 17-ketosteroids and pregnanetriol are markedly elevated in hyperplasia, but only the 17-ketosteroids are notably increased in adrenal neoplasm. The values for 17-ketosteroids in hyper-

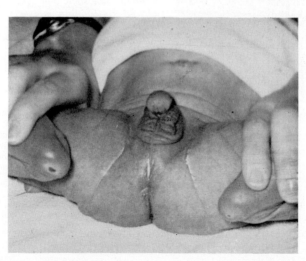

FIG. 465. Patient RS, age 2 weeks. Control 17-ketosteroid 6.8 mg. per 24 hours; after corticoid treatment, 2.2 mg. Chromatin pattern positive (female). Patient christened a male, but after the diagnosis of adrenogenital syndrome was made the child was considered to be a female. The patient died due to inadequate corticoid therapy. Autopsy showed complete normal female genitalia.

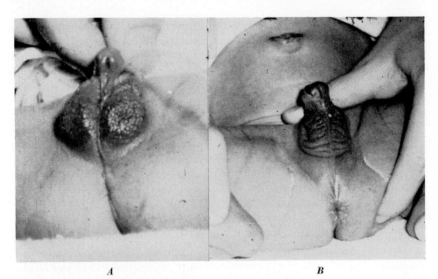

A   B

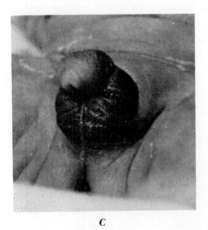

C

FIG. 466. *Three patients with congenital adrenogenital syndrome and female chromatin pattern. All had complete fusion of scrotum and elevated 17-ketosteroid and pregnanetriol values. There was marked increase in pigmentation of scrotum in these children with signs and symptoms of hypoadrenal corticoidism and a salt-losing syndrome.*

A, Patient RW, a newborn infant. Before treatment, 17-ketosteroid and pregnanetriol values were 9.7 and 4.7 mg. per 24 hours respectively; after corticoid treatment they were 1.8 and 1.9 mg.

B, Patient JS, a newborn infant. Before treatment the 17-ketosteroid value was 6.8 mg. per 24 hours and the pregnanetriol, 7.0. After treatment with corticoid the 17-ketosteroids were 2.2 mg. per 24 hours.

C, Patient G, an infant. In this child, high 17-ketosteroid and pregnanetriol values decreased following corticoid therapy.

plasia or neoplasia are usually above 5 to 7 mg./24 hours, while the pregnanetriols are elevated to comparable levels. The patient may be "chromatin positive" and yet the external genitalia may range in appearance from that of a typical female with an enlarged clitoris to an apparently well-developed male with bilateral cryptorchidism. A positive chromatin pattern with abnormal steroid excretion is helpful in establishing a correct diagnosis and preventing a genotypic female, potentially fertile, from going through life as a sterile phenotypic male. If the congenital adrenogenital infant has a "negative chromatin" pattern and exhibits considerable enlargement of the phallus plus a well-developed scrotum, usually with bilaterally descended testicles which are smaller than normal in size, one must consider the child as a potentially normal male. While there would be no doubt as to the true nature of the anatomic sex of such an individual, 17-ketosteroid and pregnanetriol levels establish the diagnosis of the adrenogenital syndrome.

The pregnanetriol may not always be elevated in the adrenogenital syndrome. Bongiovanni has described infants with a profound "salt-losing" syndrome in whom a normal pregnanetriol was noted.[4] This was attributed to a deficiency of 3β-hydroxy dehydrogenase. These children would succumb if mineralocorticoids were not administered. They are usually markedly dehydrated when initially seen.

A significant advance in bone age in an infant with the clinical stigmata previously noted would favor the diagnosis of the adrenogenital syndrome. The increased secretion of androgens *in utero* in these patients is responsible for the acceleration of bone age. If the adrenal hyperplasia continues unabated during infancy and childhood, premature closure of the epiphyses may occur, producing an adult of short, stocky stature.

ACUTE ADRENAL CORTICAL INSUFFICIENCY. Early diagnosis in neonatal AGS is important so that prompt administration of corticoids may prevent excessive masculinization in a genetic female and be lifesaving in those infants with concomitant acute adrenal cortical insufficiency. When this insufficiency occurs, the infants usually exhibit the biologic and biochemical findings typical of a patient with an acute salt-losing syndrome. The question arises as to whether or not these infants with the congenital adrenogenital syndrome are actually secreting a specific steroid responsible for salt depletion. In all probability, there is no such endogenously secreted steroid. It is now believed that the salt-losing syndrome is purely a manifestation of extreme hypoadrenocorticoidism with almost total absence of hydrocortisone production. In other words, as a result of total or complete enzymatic blockage of hydroxylation in the zona fasciculata, no hydrocortisone is elaborated.

ALDOSTERONE SECRETION. Aldosterone secretion, however, appears to be perfectly normal, as evidenced by studies on aldosterone excretion levels in such salt-losing infants.[7] Since aldosterone appears to require the permissive effects of hydrocortisone to achieve sodium retention, the normal aldosterone secretion is ineffective in bringing about sodium retention necessary for these patients to maintain electrolytic homeostasis and life itself. The sodium loss which occurs is profound in these patients not because of a specific salt-losing effect of any new steroid being excreted, but rather because of the inability of aldosterone secretion to achieve a positive salt-retaining effect in the absence of hydrocortisone. This phenomenon is well exhibited in adrenalectomized dogs where, after adrenalectomy, aldosterone alone may not be sufficient to maintain appropriate sodium retention. However, when hydrocortisone is administered in small amounts to these animals, the permissive activity of this steroid comes into effect in allowing aldosterone to achieve some measure of sodium retention. A similar dependency of aldosterone on hydrocortisone[7] appears to exist in the human. Paradoxically, it is the lack of hydrocortisone production from the hyperplastic adrenals, and not lack of aldosterone, which is undoubtedly the factor responsible for the sudden and early death of these infants.

DIAGNOSIS OF ADRENAL INSUFFICIENCY. The clinical evidence of adrenal insufficiency in these infants, however, may be masked by a picture of dehydration with an infectious overlay associated with diarrhea, anorexia, and hemoconcentration. Their poor appetite, diarrhea, and accompanying fluid loss mimic an infectious process with an elevation of the white cell count (due to dehydration) but usually without a shift toward the left. While antibiotics are used and may prevent intercurrent infection, the infant will survive only if placed on adequate corticoid dosage as promptly as possible. As soon as the diagnosis of the adrenogenital syndrome is established by finding elevated 17-ketosteroid and pregnanetriol levels in the urine, initiation of appropriate corticoid therapy may be life saving and will reverse the phenomena noted above.

Corticoid Dosage. The dose of corticoids to be employed should be the same as the adult dose and not proportional to the weight of the infant. The corticoids may be given in the dietary fluids. If fluids cannot be taken orally, then the steroid selected may be administered parenterally, preferably in the form of an aqueous suspension of the water-insoluble form of cortisone or hydrocortisone in daily doses of 37.5 to 50 mg., respectively. Sodium retaining steroids as DCA, 5 mg. IM every day, or DCTMA, 25 mg. IM every 3 to 4 weeks, may be injected conjointly with the glucocorticoid to combat sodium loss.

It is important for the parents of these children to realize that these infants lead a very precarious existence in the early postnatal period, even with the institution of appropriate corticoid therapy. If the infants show any signs of infection, nausea, emesis, or dehydration, they should be hospitalized to assure adequate fluid replacement and to prevent the irreversible changes of extreme dehydration. Despite adequate corticoid therapy, any slight deviation in the homeostatic state due to the above-mentioned entities may precipitate a crisis requiring all of the skill of the attending pediatrician to prevent the infant from succumbing. One should remember to add potassium supplementation in the management of the crisis so that profound hypopotassemia with the resultant adverse effects does not occur.

LACK OF ADRENAL ENZYME HYDROXYLASE. Before the appearance of cortisone, many of the congenital AGS infants survived because of the mild nature of their salt-losing phase of infancy. They developed into typically short, broad-shouldered, muscular, adrenogenital females, never showing clinical stigmata of adrenal insufficiency. In other words, the congenital AGS is not always associated with an acute salt-losing syndrome because there may not be a complete block of hydroxylation at C 21 and C 11 in the adrenal cortex. Those infants, however, who completely lack the adrenal enzyme hydroxylase are the ones who would be expected to expire due to irreversible salt loss unless appropriate corticoid therapy is instituted.

NEED FOR THERAPY. Treatment of the patient with the congenital adrenogenital syndrome is necessary not only to maintain life itself but also to prevent the evidence of masculinization in a feminine individual or the onset of sexual precocity in a chromatin negative child. In addition, by depressing endogenous androgen hypersecretion from the adrenal cortex, corticoid therapy will prevent the premature closure of the epiphyses and thereby avoid the stunted growth these patients present as adults. In the early stages of the disease, congenital adrenogenital syndrome patients appear somewhat taller and better developed than the normal individual of the same age (Figs. 467, 468). However, the accelerated epiphyseal closure eventually produces a short, stocky individual who is considerably shorter than the normal adult when he reaches maturity (Fig. 469). The early administration of corticoids will prevent excessive stimulation of bone growth and epiphyseal closure by the sex steroids. The best response with respect to adequate future growth potential is achieved if corticoid therapy is started as early as possible in the neonatal period.

GENETIC TRANSMISSION. Mothers giving birth to children with the congenital adrenogenital syndrome must be suspected of a possible genetic transmission of this condition. It is not unusual for more than one infant with the adrenogenital syndrome to appear in the same family. If an infant died in the early postnatal period, and there were abnormal or indifferent genitalia, one should suspect the possibility of the adrenogenital syndrome in the sibling who has similar genital abnormalities. Thus, appropriate corticoid therapy may be instituted immediately after the necessary laboratory procedures have been obtained in an infant showing evidence of androgenicity, especially when there has been a family history of a similar condition in an older sibling.

Adrenogenital Syndrome in the Male. The adrenogenital syndrome may play as important a role in fertility and gonadal abnormalities in the adult male as it does in the adult female. Oligospermia or azoospermia are to be anticipated as the end result of the syndrome in the male.

CLINICAL FINDINGS. On casual inspection, it would be difficult to recognize the adrenogenital syndrome in the male by clinical signs alone. How can one determine whether a male is more masculine than he should be? The answer becomes more apparent if we consider the fact that there are several cardinal clinical signs that should be looked for in

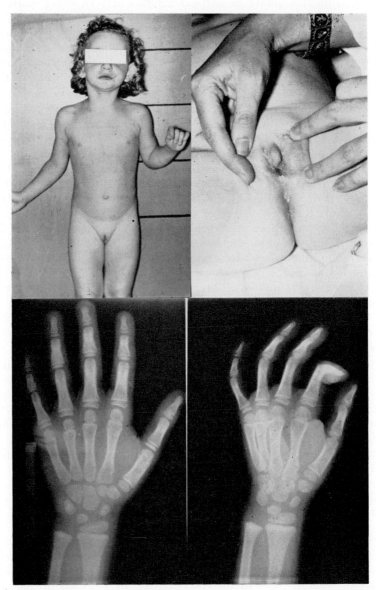

FIG. 467.   Patient DL, female, age 3 years, with classic adrenogenital syndrome.   17-Ketosteroids, 10.2 mg.; pregnanetriol, 24.4 mg.   Note enlarged clitoris.
Patient 37½ inches tall; this represents a significant increase over the average
height of a child of this age.   X-rays of the hands and wrist show considerable
advancement of the bone age in this child.

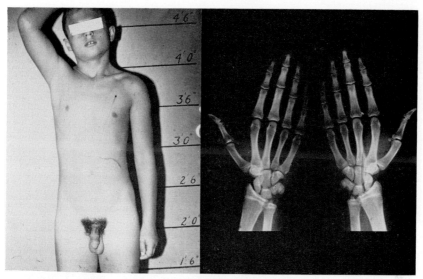

FIG. 468. Patient GG, male, age 8 years, with extraordinarily well-developed genitalia and testes. Control 17-ketosteroid 20 mg. per 24 hours. X-ray showed a considerable advancement of bone age. Steroids were adequately depressed with appropriate corticoid therapy.

establishing the diagnosis of the adrenogenital syndrome in the male. These may be listed as follows:

1. The presence of an unusually well-developed and large phallus (Fig. 470).

2. A well-developed scrotum.

3. A firm prostate of good size.

4. Testes that are rather small, soft, and flabby, and certainly not commensurate in size and turgidity with the rest of the secondary sexual development.

LABORATORY FINDINGS.   In order to establish the diagnosis from the laboratory point of view, these males should show:

1. Elevated 17-ketosteroid.

2. Elevation of pregnanetriol. This would be expected in the congenital adrenogenital syndrome, although the pregnanetriol levels may be normal in most patients with the postpubertal adrenogenital syndrome.

If the steroid excretory products are higher than normal (namely, over 24 mg./24 hours for the 17-ketosteroid and over 2 mg. for the pregnanetriol), one has concrete evidence for the support of the diagnosis of the adrenogenital syndrome.

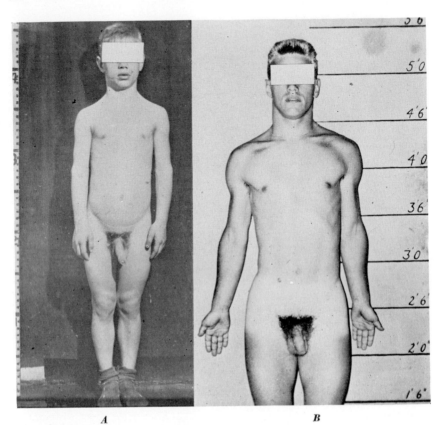

A   *B*

FIG. 469. Patient FF. A, Age 5 years. 17-Ketosteroid 17.3 mg. per 24 hours. Height, 55 inches. The patient is excessively tall for his age. His phallus is enormous; his testes, however, are small.

B, Age 15½ years, height 62¾ inches. Epiphyses are all closed. The patient now is a short adult. His genital development is excellent. Testes developed adequately under corticoid therapy.

3. Sperm count. The patient may exhibit either necrospermia with marked oligospermia, or azoospermia.

To make the picture more confusing, one must remember that complete suppression of FSH by androgenic substances from the zona reticularis may not always result in azoospermia. For example, the seminiferous tubule in the hypophysectomized animal may be maintained by endogenously (other than gonadal) secreted or exogenously administered androgen.[5, 6, 25, 29] It may be possible, then, that the excessive production of androgens by the adrenal cortex may have a slight or significant gametogenic effect despite the fact that suppression of the gonadotropins by the androgen would be expected so that azoospermia would be present.

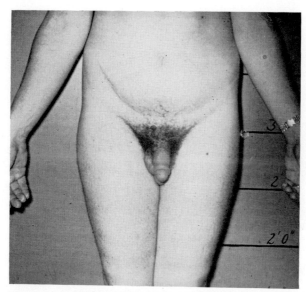

FIG. 470. Patient HJ, age 27 years. The phallus is well developed; the testes are small. 17-Ketosteroid 38-40 mg. per 24 hours. Marked oligospermia. The 17-ketosteroids were depressed and sperm count improved following corticoid therapy.

Indeed, the testes may even be enlarged due to occasional neoplastic formation noted in the testes of the adrenogenital patient[30] (usually children) not treated with corticoids when adrenal cortical hyperplasia is present.

As the adrenogenital male is usually found during a routine sterility work-up of an infertile couple, it would be helpful to subject these individuals with diminished sperm count and elevated 17-ketosteroid excretion to corticoid therapy to increase their sperm production. Several such patients have been seen in our clinics and their response has been gratifying. Normal spermatogenic activity has been achieved with precisely the same corticoid regimen recommended for the female and in most of these patients has resulted in a fertile outcome.

Neoplasia and the Adrenogenital Syndrome. Up to the present point in this discussion, only adrenal hyperplasia has been considered as the etiologic factor in the adrenogenital syndrome. However, the differential diagnosis between neoplasia and hyperplasia has been considered in the cases discussed earlier (Figs. 452, 453). One must never overlook the possibility that adrenal and/or gonadal neoplasia may produce the identical clinical findings of the adrenogenital syndrome due to adrenal hyperplasia. Neoplasia is not associated with any defect in hydroxylation, so there is no disturbance in the conversion of cholesterol into hydrocortisone, nor is there any increase in ACTH secretion. Pregnanetriol

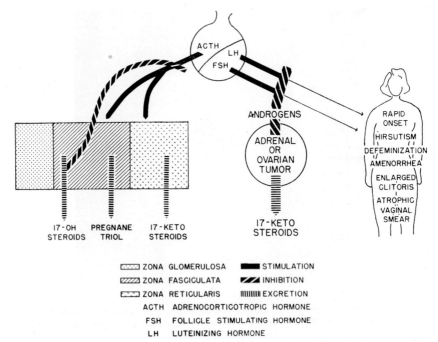

ZONA GLOMERULOSA ▪▪▪ STIMULATION
ZONA FASCICULATA ▨▨ INHIBITION
ZONA RETICULARIS ‖‖‖‖ EXCRETION
ACTH ADRENOCORTICOTROPIC HORMONE
FSH FOLLICLE STIMULATING HORMONE
LH LUTEINIZING HORMONE

FIG. 471. *Neoplasia causing adrenogenital syndrome. The pituitary-gonadal interrelationship is interrupted by excessive androgen production by the neoplasm. Pituitary-adrenal cortical relationship as well as the 17-hydroxysteroid and pregnanetriol excretions are normal.*

excretion is invariably normal. Basically normal adrenal-pituitary interrelationship exists (Fig. 471). The androgenic steroids produced by the neoplasm primarily affect the gonadal-gonadotropic system.

CLINICAL FINDINGS. Neoplasia should be suspected in any patient showing the following findings and history:

1. A sudden onset of the signs of virilism or defeminization in a female, including: (a) increased degree of hirsutism, (b) deepening of voice, (c) the presence of acne, (d) decrease in breast size.

2. Sudden irregularity of menstrual periods which previously had been regular, plus change of cycles from ovulatory to anovulatory and eventually terminating in prolonged secondary amenorrhea.

3. A sudden increase in body growth, weight, and size of the phallus in a young male not showing any evidence of testicular tumor.

The final diagnosis as to etiology, however, must await the results of specific laboratory data.

LABORATORY FINDINGS. The following laboratory findings would point toward the presence of a tumor with an androgenic potential rather than toward adrenal hyperplasia:

1. While the level of excretion of 17-ketosteroids is usually of prime diagnostic importance, the proportion of alpha to beta 17-ketosteroids is diagnostic inasmuch as a relative increase in dehydroepiandrosterone (β-17-ketosteroids) occurs in the urine in those patients with a tumor. Normally, in the euadrenal state as well as in patients with adrenal hyperplasia, the percentage of dehydroepiandrosterone excreted is relatively low (less than 10 to 15 per cent). A reversal of the normal proportions of the total 17-ketosteroid and dehydroepiandrosterone excreted would imply the presence of a neoplasm. Excessive amounts of dehydroepiandrosterone can be detected by a positive Allen reaction (violet-blue fluorescent color when sulfuric acid is added to the dried 17-ketosteroid extract prior to the development of the normal color reaction) and would point toward the presence of a neoplasm.[1]

2. Normal or very modestly elevated pregnanetriol levels in a patient with a markedly elevated 17-ketosteroid would also indicate the presence of an adrenal or gonadal neoplasm (Fig. 471).

3. Failure to note depression of excessive steroid excretion by appropriate corticoid therapy. Normally, the patient with hyperplasia will show a decreased level of the elevated 17-ketosteroids after either oral or intravenous infusion with appropriate doses of corticoids (Fig. 452). If a neoplasm is suspected, one can determine the sensitivity of the neoplasm to oral corticoids as evidenced by their ability to depress the elevated excretion of 17-ketosteroids. The dose of corticoids to be used is some 33 to 50 per cent larger than the amounts advised for the treatment of the adrenogenital syndrome due to adrenal hyperplasia (Fig. 460).[13, 14, 16, 27] If there is no significant depression of steroid excretion after one to two weeks of such therapy, one should suspect the presence of an autogenously functioning neoplasm. The same information can be obtained more rapidly by the use of intravenous corticoids administered over a period of six to eight hours (Fig. 452). The suppressive procedure may be performed as follows: either 5 mg. of 9-alpha-fluorohydrocortisone hemisuccinate or 100 mg. of hydrocortisone hemisuccinate is administered by infusion in glucose or saline, respectively. Glucose is used as a vehicle with 9-alpha-fluorohydrocortisone because of the steroid's sodium-retaining potential, while saline is employed with the hydrocortisone because of the possible adverse effect this steroid may have on carbohydrate metabolism. Urine is collected at eight-hour intervals: starting eight hours before the corticoid infusion, during the eight hours of the infusion, and then for two eight-hour periods after the completion of the infusion. Patients with adrenal hyperplasia invariably will show depression of the elevated 17-ketosteroid excretion in contrast to a failure of suppression to occur in patients with adrenal neoplasia (Fig. 452). Normally, the 17-ketosteroids would be depressed to 50 per cent or more of the control level during the period of corticoid administration as well as during the first eight-hour post-infusion interval. Occasionally, a patient with an adenoma will show some measure

of suppression after these doses of corticoids. However, the decrease will never be of the magnitude noted with hyperplasia. As a rule, patients with carcinoma will rarely show any significant alteration in steroid excretion with the procedures recommended above.

4. The 17-hydroxysteroid levels will usually be normal in neoplasia or occasionally elevated if there is a mixed tumor present. In contrast, the congenital adrenogenital syndrome with hyperplasia will usually show a low 17-hydroxysteroid which would be diminished further when the 9-alpha fluorinated preparation is used in the suppressive studies.

5. Glucose tolerance is usually normal and the patients will fail to show a hypoglycemic level at the fourth or fifth hour.

6. ACTH provocative procedure (ACTH challenge). Intramuscular administration of 40 mg. of ACTH gel or zinc ACTH will normally be followed by a modest increase (50 per cent) in 17-ketosteroid, pregnanetriol, as well as 17-hydroxysteroid levels.[2, 13, 16, 22] In contrast, patients with adrenal cortical hyperplasia of the adrenogenital type will show a decided increase in 17-ketosteroid and pregnanetriol excretion, with little or no increase in hydroxysteroids, after ACTH administration (Fig. 453). Occasionally, a patient with an adenoma will show some moderate increase in urine 17-ketosteroid excretion. Those with carcinoma fail to show any significant increase in 17-ketosteroid or pregnanetriol excretion after ACTH. An infusion with 25 units of ACTH for eight hours may also be used as a diagnostic provocative procedure; urine being collected for the eight-hour interval before the infusion, during the infusion, and for the two eight-hour periods post-infusion. After intramuscular ACTH, patients with hyperplasia and occasionally those with adenomatous changes but never those with carcinoma will show marked increases in levels of 17-ketosteroid or pregnanetriol with little change in hydroxysteroid output (Fig. 453).

7. X-ray aids. An intravenous pyelogram or perirenal air insufflation is of debatable help in diagnosis in adrenal hyperplasia or neoplasia. Frequently, no tumor is seen when these procedures are used; or, on the other hand, a tumor may be demonstrated on x-ray, yet none is found when surgical exploration is accomplished (the so-called phantom tumor of insufflation). X-ray may be used to confirm but not to establish the diagnosis.

Case Reports. Case 1. A typical case of adrenal neoplasm is that of the young male patient, MS, who at the age of two showed marked acceleration of bone age, enlarged phallus, small to normal-sized testes, and a generalized acceleration of somatic development (Fig. 472). His 17-ketosteroids were markedly elevated for his age (53.6 mg./24 hours) while there was no significant increase in pregnanetriol (0.1 mg./24 hours). A suppression test with corticoid suggested a possible tumor, as significant depression of 17-ketosteroid was not achieved after either

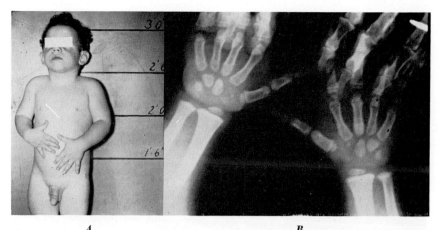

A   B

FIG. 472 (A and B). Patient MS, age 2 years, height 37 inches, weight 38 pounds; 17-ketosteroids 53.6 mg. per 24 hours; pregnanetriol 0.1 mg. per 24 hours. The ketosteroids were not depressed with corticoids. Diagnosis: AGS due to adrenal neoplasm. Laparotomy revealed adrenal carcinoma. There is considerable advancement in bone age.

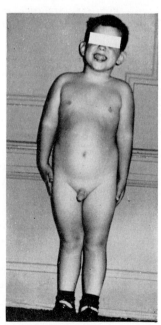

FIG. 472C. Patient MS, age 3¾ years, one and one-quarter years following surgery. Note regression of penis and normal general body configuration. His postoperative 17-KS levels have been less than 2.6 mg./24 hours.

C

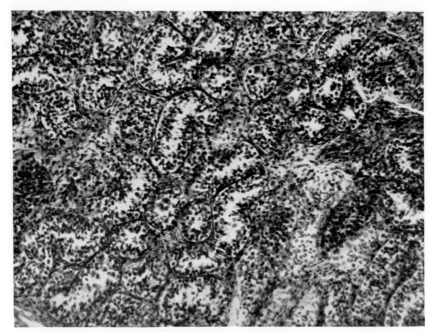

*FIG. 473. MS (Fig. 472). Testicular biopsy shows some moderate
advance in the histologic picture.*

parenteral or oral corticoid dosage. Testicular biopsy revealed a slight
acceleration of testicular morphology for the patient's age (Fig. 473).
Intravenous pyelogram was reported as normal and failed to demonstrate
the presence or absence of any suprarenal mass. Surgery was advised and
performed. The operative specimen consisted of a well-encapsulated
adrenal carcinoma (Fig. 474). Fortunately, it did not show any evidence
of metastatic spread. The adrenal on the side of the anaplastic tissue
was normal in size and morphology, indicating an absence of any suppression of endogenous ACTH by the products of secretion of the
neoplasm (Fig. 475).

Immediately after surgery and one year later, the patient's
17-ketosteroids were again at normal levels for a boy of his age. Postoperative x-ray therapy was deferred in this case because prophylactic x-ray
treatment in a child so young might induce extensive damage to the adjacent vital organs (kidney, etc.) Anti-carcinogenic doses of x-ray might
also affect some of the growth centers of the spinal column in the adjacent
areas. This would induce significant alteration in growth and maturation,
with bizarre growth effects eventuating if the child remained free of the
neoplasia and lived. If there was no metastasis, x-ray treatment obviously
was not necessary. Should metastases have been present, then even x-ray

therapy would have been of doubtful value in arresting the spread of the carcinoma. It should also be emphasized that in the boy, MS, the abdominal surgical approach was the procedure of choice because the localization and extent of his disease were not known preoperatively.

The postoperative management of this patient presented no clinical problem since his intact adrenal was not suppressed (as was anticipated from the normal 17-hydroxysteroid excretion and adrenal morphology, Fig. 474) and the patient's endogenous corticoid excretion carried him through his postoperative period.

The possible presence of future metastasis will be noted readily if and when the patient's 17-ketosteroid excretion shows an inordinate increase. The determination of these steroids periodically (every three to four months) offers the physician an accurate index of the presence or absence of metastatic spread of the disease.

There is one other aspect that must be mentioned concerning the testicular morphology noted in this patient. The moderate advancement in the morphologic picture that was found would not be anticipated in

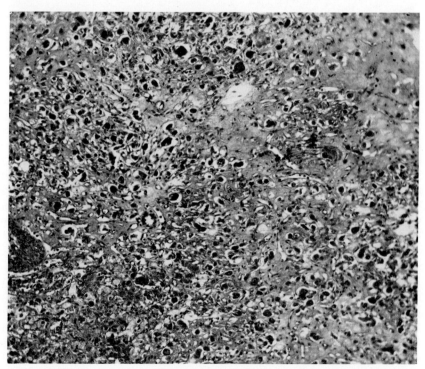

FIG. 474.   MS (Fig. 472). Adrenal neoplasm showing typical, highly malignant, carcinomatous changes with nuclear anaplasia and pleomorphism.

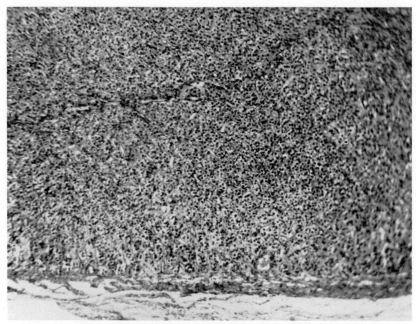

*FIG. 475. MS (Fig. 472). Normal adrenal indicating that the
neoplasm did not suppress endogenous ACTH.*

patients with excessive gonadal hormone secretion due to adrenal neoplasia or hyperplasia (Fig. 473). The sex steroids in such cases would be
expected to suppress endogenous gonadotropic secretion and thereby
cause testicular atrophy. However, the surprising stimulation may be
explained by the role that androgens have in maintaining or stimulating
gametogenesis. In addition, it has been shown that estrogens and
androgens may cause gonadal hypertrophy in the immature female and
male rat, respectively.[5, 6, 23-26, 29, 34] These experimental data may then
explain the reason why the patient's testes showed evidence of stimulation rather than inhibition.

CASE 2. A second patient demonstrates the difficulty in differentiating between adrenal hyperplasia and adrenal or ovarian neoplasia.
In addition, this patient emphasizes the advantage of the abdominal
approach as compared to the dorsal lateral technique when adrenal
surgery is being considered.

The patient, a 34-year-old female, showed a fairly rapid onset of an
arrhenomimetic phenomenon after a history of normal regular menses
and three normal pregnancies (Fig. 476). The patient complained of an
increased degree of facial acne and hirsutism of the face and the body.
This occurred some time after her last delivery and had gradually

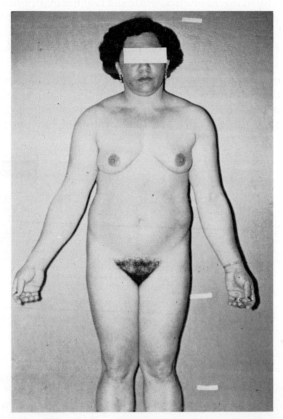

FIG. 476. Patient CE, female, age 34 years. 17-Ketosteroids 31.2 and 51.0 mg. per 24 hours; 17-hydroxysteroid, normal. Rapid onset of virilization with recent period of amenorrhea of 6 months' duration. Steroids were not suppressed with corticoids. Laparotomy revealed adrenal rest tumor of the ovary.

progressed over a period of six to eight months until it reached the
marked degree present at the time she was first seen. Her menses, which
had occurred spontaneously postpartum after the usual anticipated
interval, had become less in amount and finally stopped completely. The
patient showed an increase in excretion of 17-ketosteroids to levels ranging between 28 to 40 mg./24 hours, while she had normal 17-hydroxysteroid
output and normal glucose tolerance. There was no depression of
17-ketosteroid excretion after either oral or parenteral administration of
corticoids. The pregnanetriol determination was not available at that
time.

   In view of the rather sudden onset of the patient's symptoms and
amenorrhea, the elevated 17-ketosteroid excretion pattern after corticoid
administration, and the relatively normal pelvic findings, an adrenal
neoplasm was considered the most likely cause of her amenorrhea and

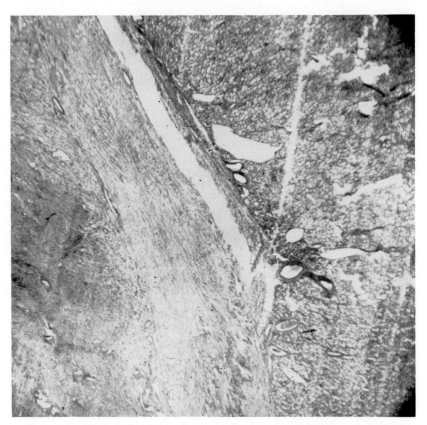

FIG. 477. Section of adrenal rest tumor of patient CE (Fig. 476). On left side,
ovarian tissue; on right side, neoplastic tissue.

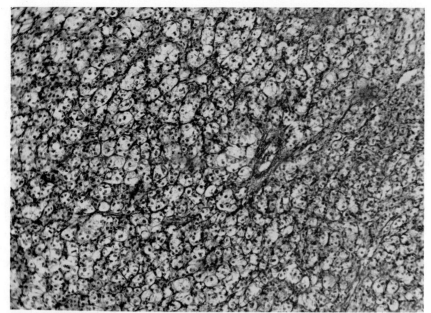

FIG. 478. Patient CE (Fig. 476) with adrenal rest tumor. High-power view showing typical morphology of adrenal rest tumor.

masculinization. However, because of insistence that the abdominal approach be used to check both adrenals simultaneously, the surgeon was able to evaluate the status of the ovaries at the time of surgery. This was indeed a fortunate step, for it was shown upon inspection and section that the left ovary was almost completely replaced by a circumscribed yellow tumor. The adrenal glands were examined and found normal. The ovarian tumor was the source of the endocrine disturbance, since with its removal her 17-ketosteroids promptly fell to normal values and spontaneous regular menses occurred followed by a fourth, uneventful pregnancy. The tumor was shown histologically to be an adrenal rest tumor of the ovary and extracts of the tumor revealed a considerable amount of 17-ketosteroid material per gram of ovarian tissue (Figs. 477, 478).

In this case, the use of the abdominal approach to investigate the cause of the patient's androgenic phenomenon permitted complete abdominal exploration and localization of the tumor site with relative ease. Had the dorsolateral approach been used, the tumor undoubtedly would have been missed and multiple surgery would have been necessary to correct this patient's symptomatology.

CASE 3. Another patient with an adrenal carcinoma also demonstrates the various points emphasized above as well as other pertinent findings. The patient had gone on a self-imposed diet which resulted in profound weight loss and irregular menstrual periods. In addition, the patient also noted an increase in amount of hirsutism which was more pronounced about her face (Fig. 479). A chance 17-ketosteroid showed an enormous elevation which was not suppressed with corticoids. A large mass was demonstrated by a barium enema, where depression and compression of the splenic flexure of the large intestine was noted. Surgery was performed and an encapsulated adrenal carcinoma was removed (Fig. 480).

Conclusions. Enormous strides have been made in endocrinology by an understanding of the physiopathology of the adrenogenital syndrome. Knowledge of the basic biochemical disturbance has elucidated the mechanism of steroidogenesis by the adrenal cortex and eliminated the need for surgical ablation of adrenal glands since the AGS can be controlled by appropriate corticoid therapy. The principles and procedures which indicate the need for corticoid therapy have provided the physician with diagnostic measures which permit him to recognize and differentiate

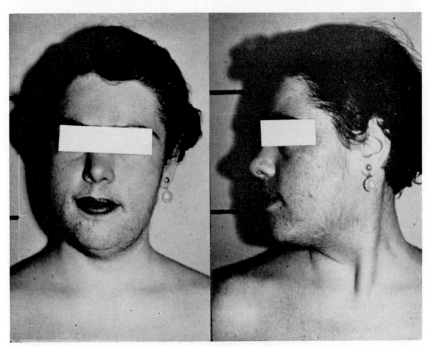

FIG. 479. *Patient EF, age 25 years. Recent onset of facial hirsutism; menses comparatively regular although diminished in amount. 17-Ketosteroids elevated, not depressed with corticoids. On exploratory operation, an adrenal carcinoma was found.*

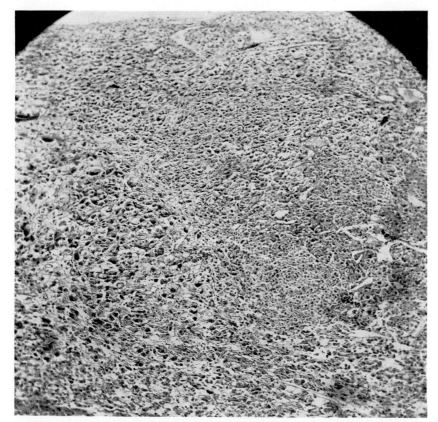

FIG. 480. *Adrenal carcinoma of patient EF (Fig. 479). Note the completely disoriented cyto-architecture of the adrenal carcinoma.*

neoplasia from hyperplasia. This diagnostic methodology has advanced to the stage where patients may be spared unnecessary surgery. However, if adrenal surgery is needed, modern medicine has greatly reduced the morbidity of the procedure.

References

1. ALLEN, W. M., HAYWARD, S. J., AND PINTO, A.: A color test for dehydroisoandrosterone and closely related steroids, of use in the diagnosis of adrenocortical tumors. J. Clin. Endocr. 10:54-70, 1950.

2. BARTTER, F. C., ALBRIGHT, F., FORBES, A. P., LEAF, A., DEMPSEY, E., AND CARROLL, E.: The effects of adrenocorticotropic hormone and cortisone in the adrenogenital syndrome associated with congenital adrenal hyperplasia: an attempt to explain and correct its disordered hormonal pattern. J. Clin. Invest. 30:237-251, 1951.

3. BONGIOVANNI, A. M.: The detection of pregnanediol and pregnanetriol in the urine of patients with adrenal hyperplasia: suppression with cortisone. Bull. Johns Hopkins Hosp. 92:244-251, 1953.

4. BONGIOVANNI, A. M.: Unusual steroid pattern in congenital adrenal hyperplasia. Deficiency of 3β-hydroxy dehydrogenase. J. Clin. Endocr. 21:860-862, 1961.

5. DVOSKIN, S.: Local maintenance of spermatogenesis by intratesticular implanted pellets of testosterone in hypophysectomized rats. Amer. J. Anat. 75:289-328, 1944.

6. DVOSKIN, S.: Reinitiation of spermatogenesis by pellets of testosterone and its esters in hypophysectomized rats. Anat. Rec. 99:329, 1947.

7. EBERLEIN, W. R., AND BONGIOVANNI, A. M.: Steroid metabolism in the "saltlosing" form of congenital adrenal hyperplasia. J. Clin. Invest. 37:889-890, 1958.

8. EPSTEIN, J. A., AND KUPPERMAN, H. S.: Alteration of carbohydrate metabolism in the adrenogenital syndrome. J. Clin. Endocr. 16:985-986, 1956.

9. EPSTEIN, J. A., AND KUPPERMAN, H. S.: Dexamethasone therapy in the adrenogenital syndrome—a comparative study. J. Clin. Endocr. 19:1503-1506, 1959.

10. GREENBLATT, R. B.: Cortisone in the treatment of the hirsute woman. Amer. J. Obstet. Gynec. 66:700-710, 1953.

11. GREENBLATT, R. B.: The adenohypophysis and ovulation. Fertil. Steril. 8:537-546, 1957.

12. HECHTER, O., ZAFFARONI, A., JACOBSEN, R. P., LEVY, H., JEANLOZ, R. W., SCHENKER, V., AND PINCUS, G.: The nature and biogenesis of the adrenal secretory product. Recent Progr. Hormone Res. 6:215-241, 1951.

13. JAILER, J. W.: Virilism. Bull. N. Y. Acad. Med. 29:377-394, 1953.

14. JAILER, J. W., GOLD, J. J., VANDE WIELE, R., AND LIEBERMAN, S.: 17-Alpha-hydroxy-progesterone and 21-desoxyhydrocortisone; their metabolism and possible role in congenital adrenal virilism. J. Clin. Invest. 34:1639-1646, 1955.

15. JONES, G. E. S., HOWARD, J. E., AND LANGFORD, H.: Use of cortisone in follicular phase disturbances. Fertil. Steril. 4:49-59, 1953.

16. KELLEY, V. C., ELY, R. S., AND RAILE, R. B.: Metabolic studies in patients with congenital adrenal hyperplasia. Effects of cortisone therapy. J. Clin. Endocr. 12:1140-1162, 1952.

17. KUPPERMAN, H. S.: The treatment of endocrine causes of sterility in the female. Clin. Obstet. Gynec. 2:808-825, 1959.

18. KUPPERMAN, H. S., BLATT, M. H. G., VESELL, M., GAGLIANI, J., WIESBADER, H., AND VOSBURGH, L.: The comparative effects of metacortandracin, 9-alpha-fluorohydrocortisone and hydrocortisone upon ACTH secretion in man. J. Clin. Endocr. 15:911-922, 1955.

19. KUPPERMAN, H. S., AND EPSTEIN, J. A.: Endocrine therapy of sterility. Amer. Pract. 9:547-563, 1958.

20. KUPPERMAN, H. S., FINKLER, R., AND BURGER, J.: Quantitative effect of cortisone upon ketosteroid excretion and clinical picture of the adrenogenital syndrome. J. Clin. Endocr. 13:1109-1117, 1953.

21. KUPPERMAN, H. S., AND STUDDIFORD, W. E.: Endocrine therapy in gynecologic disorders. Postgrad. Med. 14:410-425, 1953.

22. LEWIS, R. A., AND WILKINS, L.: The effect of adrenocorticotrophic hormone in congenital adrenal hyperplasia with virilism and in Cushing's syndrome treated with methyl testosterone. J. Clin. Invest. 28:394-400, 1949.

23. MAZER, C., ISRAEL, S. I., AND ALPEN, B. J.: The time element in the pituitary-ovarian response to large doses of the estrogenic hormone. Endocrinology 20:753-761, 1936.

24. MEYER, J. E., AND BRADBURY, J. T.: Influence of stilbestrol on the immature rat ovary and its response to gonadotrophin. Endocrinology 66:121-128, 1960.

25. NELSON, W. O., AND GALLAGHER, T. F.: Some effects of androgenic substances in the rat. Science 84:230-232, 1936.

26. PAYNE, R. W., AND HELLBAUM, A. A.: The effect of estrogens on the ovary of the hypophysectomized rat. Endocrinology 57:193-199, 1955.

27. SEGALOFF, A., GORDON, D., HORWITT, B. N., AND WEED, J. C.: Differential diagnosis of virilism. J. Clin. Endocr. 15:142-147, 1955.

28. SYDNOR, K. L., KELLEY, V. C., RAILE, R. B., ELY, R. S., AND SAYERS, G.: Blood adrenocorticotrophin in children with congenital adrenal hyperplasia. Proc. Soc. Exp. Biol. Med. 82:695-697, 1953.

29. WALSH, E. L., CUYLER, W. K., AND McCULLAGH, D. R.: Physiologic maintenance of male sex glands: effect of androtin on hypophysectomized rats. Amer. J. Physiol. 107:508-512, 1934.

30. WILKINS, L., FLEISCHMANN, W., AND HOWARD, J. E.: Macrogenitosomia precox associated with hyperplasia of the androgenic tissue of the adrenal and death from corticoadrenal insufficiency. Endocrinology 26:385-395, 1940.

31. WILKINS, L., GARDNER, L. I., CRIGLER, J. F., JR., SILVERMAN, S. H., AND MIGEON, C. J.: Further studies on the treatment of congenital adrenal hyperplasia with cortisone. I. Comparison of oral and intramuscular administration of cortisone, with a note on the suppressive action of compounds F and B on the adrenal. J. Clin. Endocr. 12:257-276, 1952.

32. WILKINS, L., LEWIS, R. A., KLEIN, R., GARDNER, L. I., CRIGLER, J. F., JR., ROSEMBERG, E., AND MIGEON, C. J.: Treatment of congenital adrenal hyperplasia with cortisone. J. Clin. Endocr. 11:1-25, 1951.

33. WILKINS, L., LEWIS, R. A., KLEIN, R., AND ROSEMBERG, E.: The suppression of androgen secretion by cortisone in a case of congenital adrenal hyperplasia. Bull. Johns Hopkins Hosp. 86:249-252, 1950.

34. WILLIAMS, P. C.: Effect of stilboestrol on the ovaries of hypophysectomized rats. Nature 145:388-389, 1940.

chapter 21

DIAGNOSIS

Recognition of Cushing's disease in a patient with the classic, fully developed syndrome needs little in the way of diagnostic tests. Nevertheless, because a great variety of clinical manifestations may obscure recognition of the syndrome, it would be worth while to review the physical findings and laboratory aberrations one can expect to find in the patient with the classic Cushing's syndrome or disease. The patient with *Cushing's disease* has the classic features of the syndrome (to be described) plus pituitary basophilism in the form of hyperplasia, adenoma, or carcinoma. *Cushing's syndrome* is characterized by all the clinical stigmata noted in the following paragraphs but with no evidence of pituitary basophilism.

Clinical Picture. The important clinical features of Cushing's disease or syndrome are presented below. It must not be considered that the findings which are enumerated are seen invariably in all patients with the disease. It is indeed rare to find all of them in any one patient. Some patients may present only one or two of the clinical stigmata noted and still be considered to have typical Cushing's syndrome.

OBESITY. Characteristically, the obesity in patients with Cushing's syndrome is centripetal in nature. The patient has relatively thin arms and legs in contrast to a heavy trunk with a protuberant abdomen (Fig. 481). There also may be certain areas, such as the dorsal cervical region, with a propensity for fat deposition resulting in a fat hump not

Hyperadrenal Corticoidism – II. Cushing's Syndrome

unlike that noted in the American buffalo, thus providing the basis for the term "buffalo obesity" (Figs. 482, 483). Chemical constituents of the dorsal cervical fat are no different from those of fat elsewhere in the body.

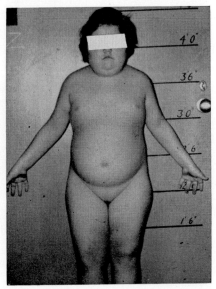

FIG. 481. Patient TZ, age 9 years, with typical Cushing obesity and the "fish-mouth" frequently seen in Cushing's syndrome. Patient has retinitis pigmentosa.

747

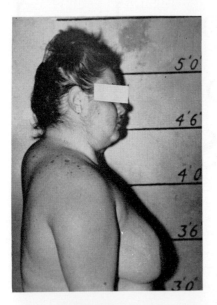

FIG. 482. Patient YS, age 28 years. Note the marked accentuation of the dorsal cervical fat pad, rather striking in this patient who has frank evidence of Cushing's syndrome. The patient's 17-hydroxysteroids were significantly elevated and her glucose tolerance test showed a minimal decreased tolerance. Some measure of insulin resistance was observed. Lanugo-like hair was present on the lateral aspects of her face.

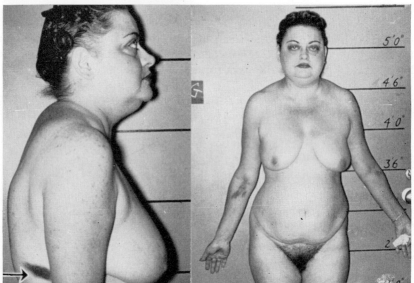

FIG. 483. Patient MG, 39 years of age, with marked centripetal obesity, whose 17-hydroxysteroid was elevated to 21 mg. per 24 hours. She showed a considerable increase in 17-hydroxysteroid excretion after a provocative test with ACTH. Note the presence of the dorsal cervical fat hump and the tendency for the arms and legs to be relatively thin compared to the size of the trunk. The patient had periorbital edema and her eyes had a staring-like quality. Ecchymosis occurred rather spontaneously without any history of trauma (note arrow). The full-face view tends to obscure the patient's ears owing to the supramalar fat deposition on the cheek bones.

The cervical fat, however, does have a tendency to increase in mass with glucocorticoids.

Despite their unusually obese appearance, many of these patients do not exhibit the typical history of weight gain that one expects in an individual of comparable size. Their weight is deceptively less than anticipated. Usually, there is also an increased degree of facial roundness with fat deposition over the malar eminences and cheeks. The fat depots may be so heavy and prominent in these areas that, when the patient is viewed from a full-face aspect, the ear lobes may not be visible (Fig. 483). The mouth may be shaped as a "fish mouth" with corners being depressed when the patient is obese (Figs. 481, 484). At other times, the patient's obesity may be unremarkable and may only lead one to suspect Cushing's syndrome because of the dorsal cervical fat hump (Fig. 484). The patient may show evidence of marked supraclavicular fullness giving the appearance of a thick, short neck (Figs. 481-486).

MUSCULAR STRENGTH.   The patients with Cushing's syndrome, unlike those with hyperadrenocorticoidism of the adrenogenital type, show a definite decrease in muscular strength and work ability. Moreover, this

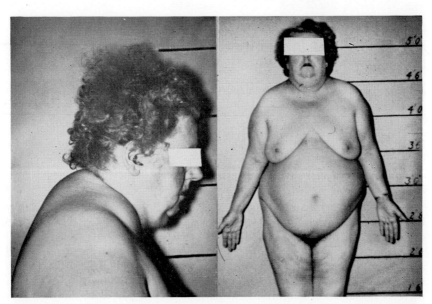

FIG. 484. Patient MW, age 47 years. This patient showed the typical steroid pattern of excretion of Cushing's syndrome, but the physiognomy of the patient was not classically characteristic of the disease. Her dorsal cervical fat pad was greatly accentuated, her arms and legs were relatively thin, although her picture is not unlike that seen in some cases of obesity. However, the provocative test with ACTH plus the elevated 17-hydroxysteroid levels revealed an unequivocal diagnosis of Cushing's syndrome due to adrenal hyperplasia. This was confirmed by surgical laparotomy.

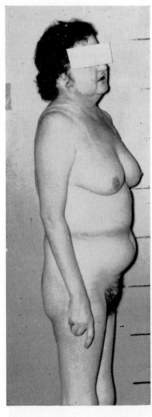

FIG. 485. Patient KK, age 34 years. The hair on the lateral aspect of her face extends down to the submental region but there is no evidence of excessive amounts of hair on her body. This type of hair and its distribution is not unusual in patients with Cushing's syndrome.

loss of muscle strength invariably is associated with a definite decrease in actual muscle mass, particularly of the striated muscle groups. This accounts for the relatively thin arms and legs depicted by the patients in Figs. 485 and 486.

HIRSUTISM. Hirsutism in the patient with Cushing's syndrome may be minimal in amount. When present, it consists primarily of the lanugo type of hair growth on the sides of the face and extends down toward the submental region (Figs. 482, 485). There may also be an increased amount of lanugo hair growth on the abdomen and the back. Obviously, there may be many variations of hair growth and distribution so that there is no constant picture. One patient may differ from another very widely in the degree of hair amount and distribution. While lanugo hair growth may be characteristic of Cushing's syndrome, patients with more extensive growth of coarse hair are reminiscent of those with the adreno-genital syndrome.

STRIAE. The patient with Cushing's syndrome frequently exhibits purple striae. The striae may be minimal or extensive in distribution.

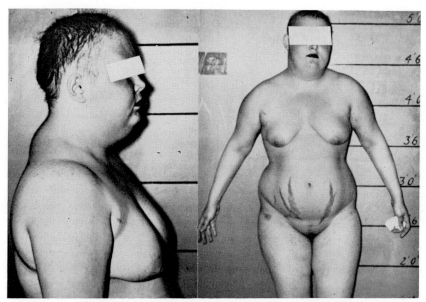

FIG. 486. Patient MM, age 20 years, with the typical physiognomy of Cushing's syndrome. Note the dorsal cervical fat hump, the very definite centripetal obesity, and the unusually large striae which radiate toward the pelvic area.

They are located characteristically on the lateral aspect of the lower protuberant abdomen. Sometimes they radiate peripherally from each axillary region and laterally and medially from the areolae of the breasts (Figs. 486, 487). These striae, in contrast to the pearl-gray stretch marks of the obese or pregnant person, are characteristically depressed, giving a broad, furrowed effect.

Typical violaceous striae are seen occasionally in individuals without any manifestation of Cushing's syndrome. Striae may be noted on the rapidly growing breasts of either the pubescent girl or the adolescent boy with gynecomastia. Characteristic purple striae may also be detected on the abdomen of the young male going through puberty (Fig. 488). When striae appear suddenly, however, in a mature individual or in a young child, they must be considered as pathognomonic of Cushing's syndrome until proved otherwise.

SKIN. The skin will bruise easily. Numerous areas of ecchymosis frequently appear without significant trauma (Fig. 483, at arrow). The skin of patients with Cushing's disease usually lacks the coarse, tough, male-like skin characteristically seen in the adrenogenital syndrome. A mild acneform type of eruption and facial plethora are common and offer a clue to the presence of the disease. Occasionally, the plethoric facies is associated also with redness and erythema of the anterior chest wall.

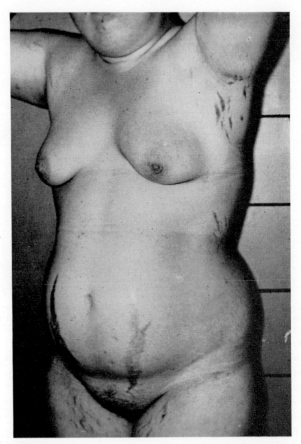

FIG. 487. *A close-up of patient MM (Fig. 486) showing the striae in the axillary region radiating from the axillary area down toward the lateral aspect of the body. Striae are on the anterior abdominal wall as well as on the upper thighs.*

The decreased muscular strength, striae and skin changes (ecchymosis, plethora) are probably all due to one common factor which is a part of the syndrome's pathophysiology: protein catabolic effects of the increased output of glucocorticoids from the adrenal cortex (Fig. 489). These steroids are catabolic in the sense that they promote a significant degree of protein wasting via the process of gluconeogenesis (Fig. 489). The breakdown of protein to form glucose is at the expense of a considerable destruction or reduction of muscle mass, with resultant loss of muscular strength. Similar catabolism and breakdown of the protein matrix of the skin thins this organ so that the underlying capillaries are readily visible. This seems to be the major cause for the formation of the purple striae and one of the factors leading to plethora. Basically, the violaceous striae are not a result of increased skin tension, as is commonly seen in normal obesity with the formation of stretch marks, but are an expression of thinning of the skin. In addition, the reduction of the protein matrix of the skin results in less support for the under-lying capillaries so that even minor trauma results in their rupture. This event is manifested grossly by the appearance of ecchymoses.

CLITORIS. The clitoris of the patient with "pure" Cushing's syn-drome is usually not enlarged. This is in contrast to the patient with the adrenogenital syndrome whose clitoris may attain gigantic proportions.

MENSTRUATION. As a rule, the patient with Cushing's syndrome will be amenorrheic during the active phase of her disease. Once the disease has been controlled, regular and spontaneous menses will resume. If the syndrome occurs prior to the menarche, menstruation will most likely

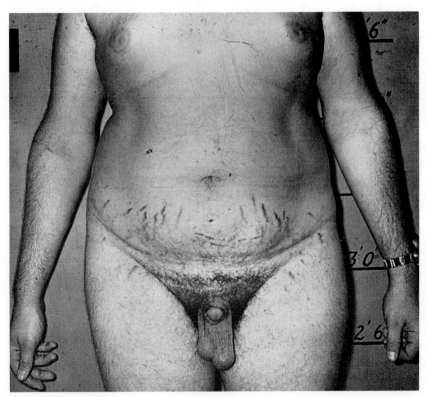

FIG. 488. Patient PE, age 20 years. The patient was first seen in the clinic because of the presence of significant striae on the lower abdomen; however, he showed no evidence of Cushing's syndrome. Striae such as these are occa-sionally seen in the adolescent child.

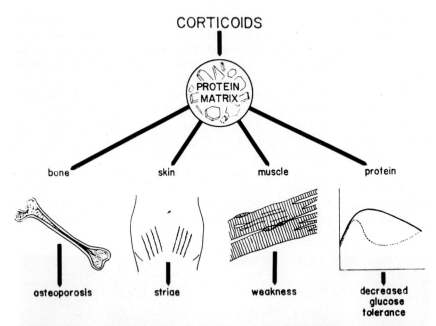

FIG. 489. *A diagrammatic presentation of the multiplicity of action of corticoids on bone, skin, and muscle protein producing the various manifestations of Cushing's syndrome.*

not begin until the basic disturbance of increased corticoid production is alleviated. The vaginal smear in such patients will usually show a mild to marked estrogenic deficiency. Sections of the ovaries of these patients appear fibrotic throughout and are associated with a diminution of ovarian activity (Fig. 490).

GROWTH. If Cushing's syndrome appears during the period of active growth in a preadolescent patient, a definite retardation of growth occurs. It would seem that excess glucocorticoids have an inhibitory effect on secretion or production of hypophyseal growth hormone. Children placed on high doses of corticoids have similar inhibition of growth.[4] However, when the effect of excessive exogenous corticoids is discontinued, there will usually be a growth spurt so that the eventual height achieved will be equal to the height normally expected in the patient.

On the other hand, if the patient with endogenous Cushing's syndrome has been treated effectively and shortly thereafter experiences menarche, the patient's growth potential is diminished. In other words, Cushing's disease deprives the patient of the usual preadolescent growth spurt, and when menstruation begins after the disease has been eliminated, acceleration of epiphyseal closure due to beginning gonadal function will occur so that the anticipated growth can never be achieved. The short stature of these individuals is similar to that seen in children with precocious sexual maturity. Here, too, the time for the usual "agonadal growth spurt" is cut short by the premature appearance of the menarche, and accelerated secretion of the sex steroids by the ovaries results in hastening of epiphyseal closure.

In contrast to the above, if Cushing's syndrome occurs early in life and is appropriately managed by surgical ablation of the adrenals, normal growth can be anticipated in much the same manner as the growth that takes place after cessation of high doses of corticoid therapy used in children with rheumatic and/or allergic disease. The growth pattern in these children will be opposite to that of patients with the untreated

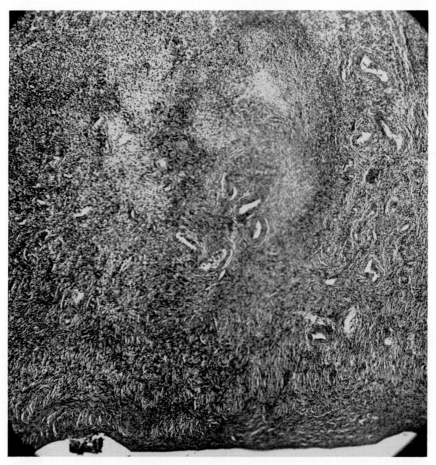

FIG. 490. *Wedge resection of an ovary from a patient with Cushing's syndrome. Fibrosis of the stroma is associated with evidence of diminished ovarian activity.*

adrenogenital syndrome in whom growth at first is greatly advanced until, with accelerated closure of the epiphyses, the over-all height of these patients becomes considerably less than that of the normal adult individual. In addition, if collapse of the vertebrae occurs (as a result of severe osteoporosis, Fig. 489) prior to puberty, these patients may never attain normal stature even when cured of their syndrome.

When Cushing's syndrome is present in a young child under the age of 12, a malignant neoplasm most likely causes the syndrome. Growth in these children is retarded, not only by the glucocorticoid secretion but also by ravages of the metastasis from the primary site.

BLOOD PRESSURE.   The blood pressure of the patient with Cushing's syndrome tends to be elevated. Nevertheless, the blood pressure in these patients in the early stages of the disease is rarely at the same level as that seen in patients with malignant hypertension. However, if the syndrome is allowed to progress, or if there is concomitant hyperaldosteronism, then there may well be significant pathologic changes in the vascular bed, such as those commonly seen in patients with long-standing or malignant hypertensive cardiovascular disease. Arteriolar disease may be very prominent in patients with Cushing's disease associated with hypertension and its sequelae.

Laboratory Findings.   HEMATOLOGIC CHANGES.   Polycythemia is seen in more than half of the patients with Cushing's syndrome. This, together with thinning of the skin, is partly responsible for the florid appearance or facial plethora. One usually sees a relative lymphopenia and eosinopenia associated with the polycythemia. In view of the specificity of the changes in corticoid excretion, the diagnostic value of hematologic findings is now of little importance because of a marked variation from one patient to another. However, it is indeed rare for any patient with Cushing's syndrome to show hematologic signs of anemia despite the marked disability they might exhibit (Figs. 491, 492). There is no evidence to prove that the patient with Cushing's syndrome shows any unusual bleeding tendency or has a deficiency of the clotting mechanism.

GLUCOSE TOLERANCE.   Patients with Cushing's syndrome characteristically show a decreased glucose tolerance.[7, 11, 15, 16, 24, 32] However, the fasting blood sugar level in these patients is usually within a normal range. Of course, there may be exceptions, as occasional patients with the disease may show definite diabetic hyperglycemic levels in their fasting blood sugar. If there is no other evident metabolic disease, a significant decrease in glucose tolerance in a patient with centripetal obesity and a normal fasting blood glucose level should suggest Cushing's syndrome.

The diagnosis is more evident if the significant decrease in glucose tolerance is not associated with abnormal glucose levels at the fourth or fifth hour of the test and if there is no evidence of liver or thyroid disease. In other words, a return to normal values after four to five

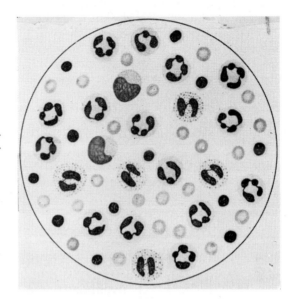

FIG. 491. Blood smear taken before corticoid therapy.

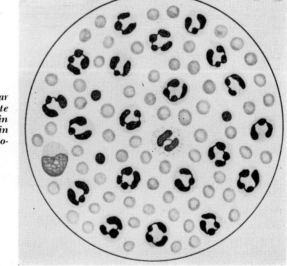

FIG. 492. Blood smear after corticoid therapy. Note the relative decrease in lymphocytes and increase in polymorphonuclear neutrophils.

hours, despite the excessive elevation of blood glucose shortly after
ingestion of the 100 Gm. glucose load, should point to the possibility of
Cushing's syndrome in a patient who had been on a high carbohydrate
diet three days prior to the test. Similar effects have been noted when
exogenous corticoids were administered.[15, 16, 24] Studies have shown
that intravenous hydrocortisone infusions did not produce a significant
elevation of fasting blood sugar during infusion despite the fact that
decreased glucose tolerance could be demonstrated by the concomitant
administration of a glucose load.[15, 16, 24]

Figure 493 shows the effects of hydrocortisone on carbohydrate
tolerance. The gray area represents the control glucose tolerance test
while the black area shows the blood sugar levels obtained during
infusion with 100 mg. of hydrocortisone in saline. The white area

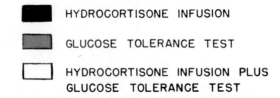

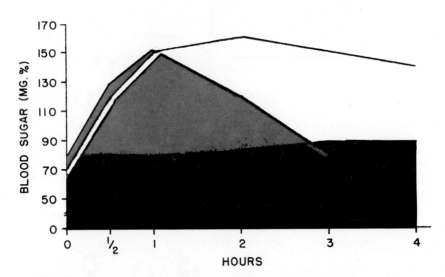

FIG. 493. Glucose tolerance test. The black curve shows the effect of hydrocortisone upon blood glucose levels. (A very minimal increase in blood sugar was
noted.) Gray depicts a normal glucose tolerance test prior to corticoid infusion.
The white area shows the effect of hydrocortisone infusion upon glucose tolerance
resulting in significant decrease in glucose tolerance.

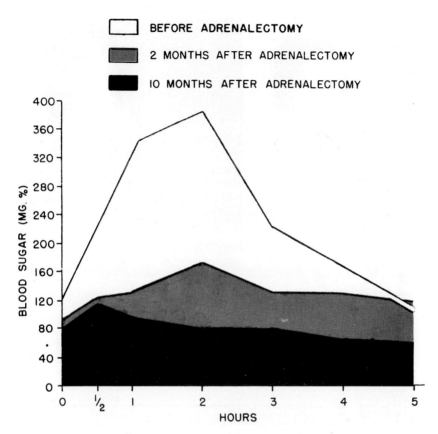

FIG. 494. *Glucose tolerance test in patient KK (Fig. 485) before and after adrenalectomy. Note the marked decrease in glucose tolerance before removal of the adrenals followed by the progressive increase in tolerance two and 10 months later.*

depicts the glucose values obtained during a glucose tolerance test performed at the time of an infusion with 100 mg. of hydrocortisone. A significant decrease in glucose tolerance was obtained. There were comparable results when glucose tolerance tests were done before and after bilateral adrenalectomy for Cushing's syndrome in the patient shown in Figs. 485, 495 and 496. Before adrenalectomy, there was a significant decrease in carbohydrate tolerance (Fig. 494). A notable increase in carbohydrate tolerance was observed (no longer a diabetic curve) two months after adrenalectomy, so that the patient's handling of a glucose load was similar to that seen in the normal patient. Glucose tolerance increased progressively until 10 months after adrenalectomy (black portion, Fig. 494) when, again, significant increase in tolerance was

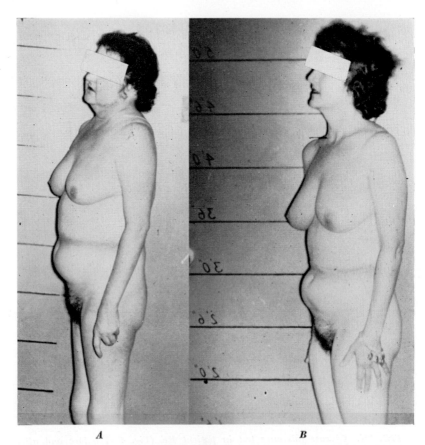

FIG. 495. *Patient KK, 34 years of age, with Cushing's syndrome due to bilateral adrenal hyperplasia, before surgery (A) and after surgery (B). Note the splendid clinical improvement which took place within 10 months after surgery. Patient lost her characteristic obesity and showed significant increase in breast size. Menstruation has taken place regularly following surgery in contrast to amenorrhea during the active phase of her disease.*

observed above that seen in the normal patient. Thus, when the source of endogenous excessive cortisone production was diminished, disturbances in carbohydrate tolerance were corrected and correlated well with the clinical improvement of the patient (Figs. 495, 496).

INSULIN TOLERANCE. While the insulin tolerance test has been an excellent diagnostic procedure in certain endocrinopathies,[10, 14, 37] its value in establishing the diagnosis of Cushing's syndrome is debatable.[9] The technique for the test is described in more detail in the section on laboratory tests; however, some facts concerned with mechanics of the insulin tolerance test will be stressed here.

The test is carried out by the intravenous administration of 0.1 unit of regular insulin per kilogram of body weight. Blood for glucose determination is obtained before the intravenous injection of insulin and then at 15, 30, 45, 60, 90, and 120 minutes after its administration. The normal curve is characterized by a 50 per cent drop in fasting blood glucose level within 20 or 30 minutes after the insulin injection (Fig. 497). This is then followed by a rapid rise of blood sugar to normal or above normal levels at the 90- and 120-minute time intervals.

The patient with Cushing's syndrome theoretically is expected to show some measure of insulin resistance because of the propensity of glucocorticoids for inducing gluconeogenesis and the supposed direct anti-insulin effects of glucocorticoids. Despite the theoretical inhibitory action of glucocorticoids upon the hypoglycemic effects of insulin, insulin resistance may be minimal or even absent in Cushing's disease.[9] Indeed, many patients with Cushing's syndrome and decreased glucose tolerance may still show normal insulin responsiveness; i.e., a normal insulin tolerance test.[9, 18, 19, 28]

It is interesting to speculate why normal insulin tolerance can be seen in the patient with Cushing's syndrome who shows a decrease in glucose tolerance when subjected to a glucose load. Experimental data from our laboratories have shown that, while exogenously administered corticoids significantly decrease glucose tolerance when the patient's carbohydrate tolerance is tested, similar doses of corticoids do not alter the

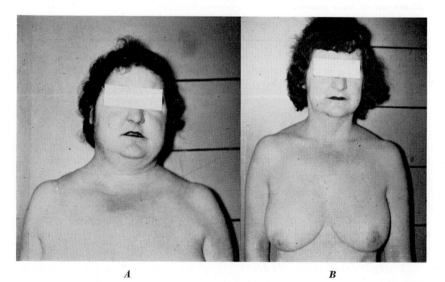

A   B

FIG. 496. Patient KK before (A) and after (B) adrenalectomy for bilateral adrenal hyperplasia. Note the definite change from a Cushing habitus to that of a normal individual.

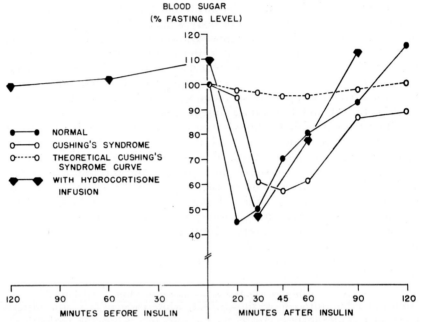

BLOOD SUGAR
(% FASTING LEVEL)

● ● NORMAL
○ ○ CUSHING'S SYNDROME
○----○ THEORETICAL CUSHING'S
        SYNDROME CURVE
◆ ◆ WITH HYDROCORTISONE
        INFUSION

120   90   60   30   20 30 45 60   90   120
MINUTES BEFORE INSULIN   MINUTES AFTER INSULIN

FIG. 497. *Insulin tolerance test. The standard insulin tolerance test is compared with that of a patient with Cushing's syndrome as well as that of a normal individual before and after hydrocortisone infusion. Note insulin responsiveness is normal in both groups.*

patient's sensitivity to intravenously administered insulin as noted in the insulin tolerance test[18, 20, 28] (Fig. 499). Indeed, the response is the same whether or not the patient receives an infusion with hydrocortisone before the performance of the insulin tolerance test. It has been suggested that corticoids might interfere with glucose utilization but they cannot alter the patient's response to exogenous insulin when there is no excessive glucose load.[18, 20, 28]

STEROID EXCRETION. *17-Ketosteroids.* The 17-ketosteroid excretion level of a patient with "pure" Cushing's syndrome is characteristically normal or below the lower range of normality. Obviously, this is not inflexible since there are patients with Cushing's syndrome who have elevated 17-ketosteroid levels, and, in some, the steroid output may be unusually high. This, however, is not the typical picture and may well represent some manifestation of a mixed adrenogenital and Cushing's syndrome or the presence of an adrenal carcinoma.

17-Hydroxysteroids (17-OH). This steroid is the pathognomonic cortical excretory product most valuable in the diagnosis of Cushing's syndrome. 17-OH may be mildly, moderately, or markedly elevated above the normal range. The diagnosis is apparent if a marked elevation is noted along with the typical clinical findings of Cushing's syndrome. However, it is frequently necessary to perform provocative tests with ACTH and/or mepyrapone, or inhibitory tests with hydrocortisone to demonstrate the presence or absence of Cushing's syndrome in those cases with indefinite clinical findings and slightly abnormal steroid excretion. Such procedures are also beneficial in demonstrating the presence or absence of neoplasm versus hyperplasia in the etiology of the disease. In case of neoplasm one must also rule out the possibility of neoplastic changes in the ovary as well as the adrenal, since at times pathologic changes in the ovary may simulate the picture occasionally seen in patients with adrenal cortical disease. The provocative and suppressive tests may also be of help in differentiating between malignant or benign neoplasms.

Specific and accurate diagnosis is necessary since, once it is definitely decided that Cushing's syndrome exists, the treatment is rather stringent and not without complications or danger. Several of the suggested procedures involved in performing the provocative ACTH test (challenge) as well as those concerned with corticoid inhibition are as follows:

1. *Adrenal Responsiveness After Corticoid Suppression.* This procedure is used to show that a specific abnormality of the adrenal cortex is present and will cause signs and symptoms of the disease.[6, 11, 34] In the performance of this test, prednisone is administered in daily doses of 20 to 30 mg. per day for seven days. Before and after the week of therapy, the patient receives a test dose of ACTH gel (40 u. intramuscularly) with 24-hour urines collected immediately after each injection. The patients with Cushing's syndrome due to adrenal hyperplasia will have a good adrenal response after both ACTH injections. In contrast, the normal patient will not have any significant increase in urinary steroids to the second ACTH injection given after the week of therapy with prednisone.

2. *ACTH Provocative Test.* If the 17-hydroxysteroids are modestly elevated, the diagnosis of Cushing's syndrome may be established by noting the patient's response to ACTH given intramuscularly or intravenously. A marked increase in 17-hydroxysteroid output (45 to 50 mg. per 24 hours or higher) in urine saved for 24 hours after 40 u. of ACTH gel or zinc ACTH administered intramuscularly is pathognomonic of the disease. ACTH may be given by infusion (25 u. intravenously in glucose-saline over a period of eight hours). Urine is collected before and during the infusion and for two eight-hour periods after the completion of the infusion. If there is a 200 per cent increase in 17-OH output after the infusion or a total excretion exceeding 45 to 50 mg. per 24 hours starting with the initiation of the infusion, then Cushing's syndrome is the most likely diagnosis. One cannot use this procedure to differentiate between neoplasia and hyperplasia except in a negative sense; i.e., patients with

significantly elevated 17-OH levels who fail to show significant and additional increases after ACTH probably have a neoplasm of the adrenal cortex. On the other hand, a marked increase in 17-OH levels after ACTH usually points to hyperplasia, although benign neoplastic lesions may also be associated with a considerable increase in 17-OH excretion.

Blood 17-OH levels may also aid in diagnosis. When intramuscular ACTH injections are used in the procedures just described, blood is drawn immediately before the injection and again three to four hours after the injection. If the infusion technique is used, blood for 17-OH is drawn before the infusion and at the end of the eight hours of infusion. Excessive increases in blood levels (over 50 mcg. per cent) of 17-OH would have the same clinical import as described for the urine studies and point towards the diagnosis of Cushing's syndrome.

More recently, Liddle has described the possible differentiation between hyperplasia and anaplastic or benign neoplasia. This involved the use of delta 1,9-alpha-fluorohydrocortisone or its 16-methylated analog, dexamethasone.[23] (Neither one of these steroids is excreted as a hydroxysteroid, nor can they be detected in the blood; thus any values obtained would represent those due to endogenous steroids and not to any of the administered compound.) A dose of 0.5 mg. of either preparation was administered every six hours for eight doses. With this method all endocrinologically normal patients had almost complete suppression of 17-hydroxycorticoid excretion.[23] Patients with Cushing's syndrome caused by hyperplasia had little change in their elevated hydroxycorticoid output. However, when these steroid doses were increased to 2 mg. every six hours for eight doses, all patients with Cushing's syndrome due to adrenal hyperplasia showed definite decrease in 17-hydroxysteroid output. On the other hand, patients with neoplasia showed no response. Thus, at low and high doses of delta 1,9-alpha-fluorohydrocortisone, one may distinguish normal adrenal function from that caused by hyperplasia as well as that caused by neoplasia. The mepyrapone test discussed in Chapter 19 can also be used in a similar manner, i.e., a pronounced increase in 17-OH excretion would occur in patients with Cushing's syndrome associated with hyperplasia, in contrast to a normal response in patients with euadrenal function.

Another point to emphasize with the use of mepyrapone is that this drug may occasionally induce a better adrenal response than that noted after exogenous ACTH. This may be explained on the basis that the ability of the adrenal to be stimulated is greater after the use of endogenous ACTH than after exogenous extracts. A poor response to ACTH was noted after the use of some of the older adrenocorticotropic preparations where it was suggested that local tissue enzymes might inactivate the parenterally administered hormone.[8, 30] It is for this reason

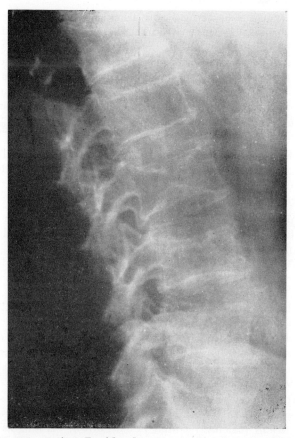

FIG. 498. Patient E with adenoma of adrenal gland which produced Cushing's syndrome. Note the marked demineralization of the
vertebrae associated with the "fish-mouthlike" changes caused by
pressure of the firm intervertebral nuclei upon the softened vertebral
bodies.

that more consistent results were obtained with intravenous ACTH as well as with highly purified preparations injected intramuscularly.[30]

Pregnanetriol. There is no evidence that pregnanetriol levels are altered in Cushing's syndrome. This steroid is diagnostically helpful only in differentiating between neoplasia or hyperplasia in patients with the adrenogenital syndrome.

BLOOD SODIUM AND POTASSIUM. Blood sodium may be either increased or normal. If there is increased aldosterone production, an increase in blood sodium and decrease in blood potassium levels may be expected. However, aldosterone levels are usually not elevated in Cushing's syndrome. Cortisone itself may occasionally induce electrolyte changes (namely, increased sodium and decreased potassium) so that occasionally significant hypokalemia may be induced with cortisone. As a rule, however, blood potassium is normal.

OTHER CHEMICAL TESTS. Lactic acid and pyruvic acid determinations are other useful chemical tests.[15] The application of these tests is limited because of a need for laboratories capable of doing these special determinations. Also, the present clinical data on these methods as diagnostic entities are meager.

Radiographic Findings. VERTEBRAL COLUMN. The skeleton of patients with long-standing Cushing's disease may show evidence of significant calcium depletion with marked osteoporosis (Figs. 498, 499). The osteoporosis in Cushing's syndrome is due primarily to the breakdown of the skeleton's protein matrix and is not due to osteomalacia (an inadequate source of calcium supply caused by faulty dietary habits or malabsorption). The loss of protein matrix of bone caused by the catabolic action of the glucocorticoid prevents adequate calcium deposition. Hence, the increased calcium excretion in urine may occur not because of excessive calcium absorption from the gut, but as a result of decreased protein matrix upon which calcium can normally be deposited. Excessive calcium is then made available for excretion.

The protein matrix of bone may be comparable to the steel framework of a skyscraper. Without the iron framework (protein matrix), mortar and bricks (calcium) cannot be laid down. As long as there is an inadequate amount of the basic supportive matrix, then there is also little foundation for calcium deposition. The result is osteoporosis. The loss of the protein matrix of the skeleton is similar to processes involving the loss of protein components of skin and muscle (Fig. 489). Osteoporosis with excessive urinary calcium loss is accompanied by considerable demineralization of the dorsal lumbar vertebrae. As a result, the intervertebral disks may become relatively firmer than the decalcified vertebrae so that the disks may compress the superior and inferior borders of the vertebrae, thereby producing a "fish-mouth" appearance of the adjacent vertebrae on x-ray examination (Figs. 498, 499).

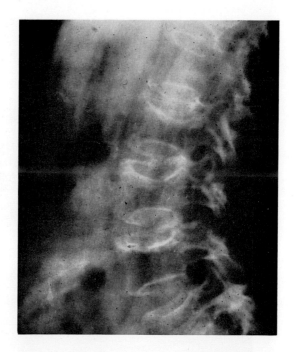

FIG. 499. Osteoporosis associated with Cushing's syndrome. Note the demineralization and "fish-mouthlike" appearance of the intervertebral spaces.

SELLA TURCICA. The sella turcica rarely is enlarged before adrenalectomy, and, when this is found, it should be considered as prime evidence of disease other than Cushing's syndrome until proved otherwise. However it should be noted, as will be discussed later, that enlargement of the sella turcica may occur in patients who have been adrenalectomized because of Cushing's syndrome. This occurs in about 10 per cent of all patients so treated.

INTRAVENOUS PYELOGRAPHY AND TOMOGRAPHY. A flat film of the abdomen or intravenous pyelography may reveal large adrenal tumors but is not valuable in small tumors or adrenal hyperplasia if there is no displacement. Perineal or presacral gas insufflation with pyelography and tomography may theoretically be more helpful in doubtful cases. However, since this technique (gas insufflation) is not without danger and even fairly large tumors are not always demonstrable (while "phantom tumors" may be seen as artifacts) these procedures have been relegated to the diagnostic limbo. If used, they may merely add points of interest, but they should not be relied on to establish a specific diagnosis.

Figure 500 shows a flat plate of the abdomen with a pyelogram in a patient with an adrenal carcinoma. There is a marked depression of the kidney evidenced by angulation of the kidney pelvis. For comparison, a normal pyelogram is presented in Figure 501. A perirenal air insufflation

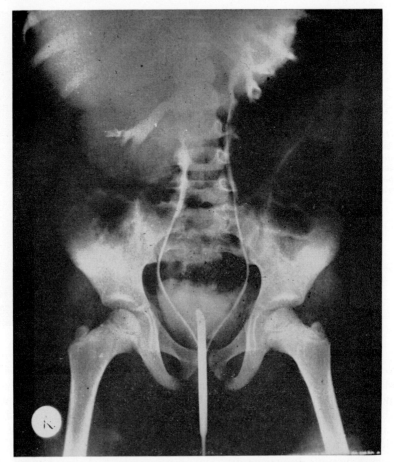

FIG. 500. *The intravenous pyelogram in a patient with a right adrenal carcinoma. Note the marked angulation of the kidney pelvis on the right side due to the suprarenal tumor.*

in a patient with an adrenal carcinoma (Fig. 502) aptly demonstrates an enlarged left adrenal mass. Left adrenal hypertrophy is also noted in Figure 503, where an adenoma was removed in a patient with marked masculinization and defeminization. On the other hand, a perirenal air insufflation shown in Figure 504 also shows unilateral adrenal enlargement. On laparotomy, no adrenal neoplasia or hypertrophy was noted. The patient with the demonstrable tumors would have been operated on regardless of x-ray findings. The patient with the "phantom tumor" did not warrant surgery but exploration was necessary after viewing the x-ray plates. It is findings such as these that have led us to question the true intrinsic value of such procedures.

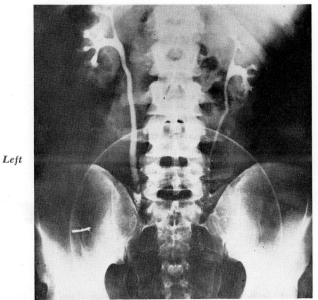

FIG. 501. Normal intravenous program. The right kidney pelvis is lower than the left as would normally be anticipated due to the overlying liver.

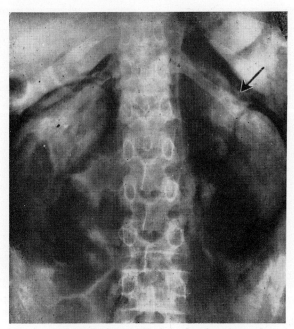

FIG. 502. A perirenal air insufflation showing left adrenal mass caused by adrenal carcinoma.

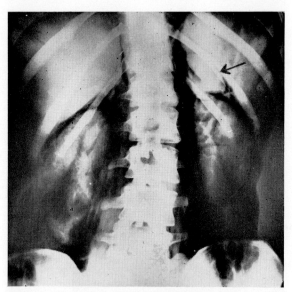

FIG. 503. A perirenal air insufflation showing left adrenal mass
due to an adenoma inducing masculinization.

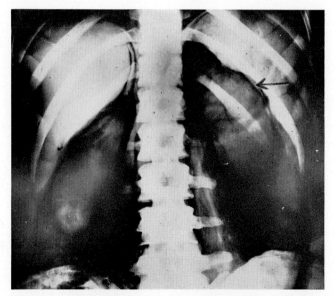

FIG. 504. A perirenal air insufflation diagnosed as a left adrenal
mass. Surgery was performed. No evidence of adrenal tumor was
noted.

TREATMENT

It is not unusual in medicine for a syndrome characterized and treated for many years by one mode of therapy to be slow to succumb to modern treatments which develop with changing concepts on the etiology of the syndrome. This is in contrast to the relatively rapid progress made in therapeutic control of other clinical entities where the physiopathology is better understood.

This divergent approach to therapy applies to two types of hyper-adrenocorticoidism—Cushing's syndrome and the adrenogenital syndrome due to adrenocortical hyperplasia. The treatment and management of Cushing's syndrome has varied according to one's concept of the disease's origin or the physiopathology responsible for its clinical manifestations. However, no universal mode of therapy receives such unanimous support as there is in the more recently recognized disturbance of adrenal function—the adrenogenital syndrome.[38-40]

Appropriate Mode of Management. In Cushing's syndrome, treatment was at first based on radiation of the pituitary gland. Later, enthusiasm arose for surgical removal of the pituitary gland, which was considered responsible for the pathologic manifestations of the disease. Surgical removal is a form of medical defeatism. Such a therapeutic approach admits our inability to medically manage the basic metabolic disturbance involved in Cushing's syndrome. With removal of the pituitary gland, normal reproductive function is completely lost.

More recently, surgery for the management of Cushing's syndrome has been directed toward the adrenal glands. At first, bilateral hemiadrenalectomy was done; now, total adrenalectomy is used to effectively control manifestations of the disease. The surgical approach in these patients may appear particularly unwise when cure of the disease by removing the offending organ creates a potentially fatal deficiency syndrome requiring appropriate replacement therapy to maintain life. If such replacement therapy is available to compensate for the necessary vital functions of the organ, surgery may be done with impunity. This application of the scalpel to eradicate the immediate or apparent cause of the disease is certainly necessary since the untreated patient would progress to a fatal outcome. In the latter instance, it appears that the physician is confronted with a dilemma whereby the organectomy may be life-saving, yet such surgery condemns the patient to a lifetime need for replacement therapy.

We have already discussed effective medical management of the adrenogenital syndrome (a form of hyperadrenocorticoidism resulting in increased androgen elaboration). The modern therapeusis of this syndrome, in contrast to surgery used in the past, is based on the epochal work of Wilkins and his co-workers. They demonstrated that a more appropriate form of therapy could be achieved by understanding the basic biochemical processes necessary for biosynthesis of the adrenal glucocorticoids in the adrenal cortex. The abnormal physiopathology of the adrenal cortex of patients with the classic adrenogenital syndrome lends itself well to medical control by the use of the glucocorticoids. This brings abnormal manifestations of this syndrome under rapid control.

In contrast, Cushing's disease has effectively resisted medical management. As a result, when the diagnosis of Cushing's syndrome is made, it becomes necessary to surgically remove the abnormally functioning adrenal glands or destroy pituitary function by radiation or excision. Correction of pathologic adrenal function is imperative since continued malfunction adversely affects the health and decreases the longevity of the patient.

Once the diagnosis of Cushing's syndrome is made, based on either clinical and/or laboratory findings, appropriate and timely therapy must be instituted. Therapy has revolved around three major avenues of approach: (1) medical management, (2) surgery, and (3) radiation.

Medical therapy is concerned with the use of the anabolic steroids including the sex steroids—estrogens, androgens, or both.

Surgical therapy usually involves bilateral total adrenalectomy in the patient with hyperplasia, or removal of the offending neoplasm if this is the cause of the disease.

Surgical hypophysectomy has been recommended by some, and in proficient hands it appears to be an excellent procedure. However, this treatment sacrifices all the other pituitary tropic hormones along with ACTH.

Radiation uses one of the following procedures:
1. Irradiation of the pituitary gland.
2. Pituitary radiation plus unilateral adrenalectomy.
3. Intranasal insertion of yttrium 90 pellets into the sella turcica.
4. Irradiation of the adrenal glands.
5. Irradiation of both the pituitary and the adrenal glands.

Medical Management.   Medical management of Cushing's syndrome was first advocated by Albright and his co-workers.[1] They showed that the use of anabolic agents, such as androgens, counteracted the protein catabolic action of the glucocorticoids and effectively diminished some of the disease's ravages.[1]

DISADVANTAGES OF MEDICAL THERAPY. Androgen therapy, of course, had arrhenomimetic effects when adequate anabolic activity was accomplished. The androgenic changes were frequently of such magnitude that female patients were prone to risk the adverse manifestations of the disease itself rather than to subject themselves to the marked virilizing stigmata associated with such treatment.

Estrogens have been used because of (1) their anabolic effect on protein structures and (2) their general ability to inhibit the pituitary tropic hormones. Since many investigators once believed that the disease was primarily of pituitary origin, it was logical to treat these patients with large estrogen doses in an attempt to ameliorate the clinical picture by significant pituitary inhibition of ACTH release. Since the disadvantages of androgens in the female are comparable to those of estrogens in the male, the feminizing effects of this steroid in the male patient are more objectionable than the disease's primary manifestations. The use of the sex steroid corresponding to the sex of the individual would certainly be more acceptable than when used in the individual of the opposite sex.

Another disadvantage of medical therapy despite its ease of administration is that complete remission is rarely if ever achieved. The chronicity of the disease itself requires medical treatment of long duration. As a result, the chronic administration of sex steroids may produce adverse clinical effects of such an extent as to be more objectionable that the undesirable features of the primary disease itself.

Potassium salts and a high protein diet may be used to supplement anabolic steroid therapy. Adding 40 to 60 mEq. of potassium per day to the diet will potentiate the anabolic effect of the androgens and minimize certain catabolic effects of the corticoids. Restricting the patient almost exclusively to a high protein diet may significantly decrease some of the clinical manifestations of hyperadrenocorticoidism.

Another disadvantage of medical therapy in Cushing's disease is that it may be administered inadvertently to patients with neoplasia rather than hyperplasia. This seems ill advised if such therapy is to be continued for a long period of time as anaplastic changes may occur and disseminate. Hence, medical management usually has been superseded by the more practical approach of either surgery and/or radiation.

Surgery.   Presently, the surgical treatment of Cushing's syndrome is the procedure of choice.[20, 29] This involves removing the adrenal glands or the offending neoplasm. This mode of therapy, of course, conflicts with the concept that the pituitary gland itself may be the primary etiologic agent of the disease. If such were the case, it seems more logical to attempt the management of Cushing's syndrome via the pituitary rather than the adrenal glands. At the present time, while the question remains open as to whether Cushing's syndrome is caused primarily by pituitary or adrenal factors, there is no doubt that the disease is primarily an expression of hyperadrenal secretion of glucocorticoids.

THE ADRENAL CORTEX IN THE ETIOLOGY OF CUSHING'S SYNDROME.   It is now well known that Cushing's syndrome may be induced by the administration of large doses of any of the glucocorticoids. In other words, when present in adequate amounts, these steroids are capable of inducing clinical manifestations of the disease with or without an intact pituitary gland.

The basophilic changes in the pituitaries in patients with Cushing's syndrome may not actually represent a positive factor in the etiology of the disease but may instead indicate a retroactive effect of the excessive glucocorticoids on the pituitary gland per se.[22] This is evidenced by the data that pituitary basophilism occurs in patients or animals given high doses of either corticoids or ACTH. Basophilism takes place when there is complete suppression of ACTH secretion by exogenously administered glucocorticoids or where there may be such intense adrenal stimulation by exogenous ACTH that the endogenously secreted corticoids would also suppress endogenous ACTH secretion. The far-advanced stage of pituitary basophilism results in cellular changes characterized by hyalinization. These morphologic alterations were described originally by Crooke, and are referred to as Crooke's cells.[7] They are seen after excessive and prolonged endogenous or exogenous corticoid effects whether or not concomitant ACTH is administered. Furthermore, it now appears that Crooke's cells are degenerative and apparently not capable of active secretion.

Surgical removal of the adrenal glands is invariably accompanied by prompt remission of the syndrome (Figs. 495, 496). It should be emphasized that, while enlargement of the adrenal gland is anticipated in most patients with Cushing's syndrome prior to adrenalectomy, some may have an adrenal gland slightly if at all enlarged. Indeed, subsequent morphologic examination of the adrenal cortex may show essentially a normal histologic picture in the adrenal cortex. Despite the normal cyto-architecture and histology, increased or abnormal function had no doubt been present because these patients with the classic syndrome showed a prompt and rapid remission of their disease after adrenalectomy.

HYPERFUNCTION OF THE ADRENAL GLAND. It would be worth while to interject here the following premises to show that circumstantial evidence may be misleading. Let us suppose that a patient with all the clinical manifestations of Cushing's syndrome has been subjected to a bilateral total adrenalectomy. Pathologic examination of the adrenal glands showed a picture not unlike that of the adrenals of a normal patient. The likelihood of the adrenalectomized patient having a dramatic remission of his Cushing's syndrome, despite the removal of normal-appearing adrenal glands, is excellent. However, if this same patient had died during the operative procedure and these normal-appearing glands were obtained at autopsy, the pathologist would have looked elsewhere for morphologic evidence of pathology to explain the patient's clinical picture of hyperadrenocorticoidism. The pituitary gland would be the most likely organ to be examined and the adenohypophysis no doubt would have contained basophilic changes characteristic of the disease. It would then have been argued that these basophilic changes were, in reality, the etiologic factor responsible for the disease since autopsy examination would not have demonstrated adequate morphologic evidence of hyperadrenocorticoidism in the adrenal. Since the histologic changes in the pituitary gland would not have been classified as retrograde effects, the pathologist would then consider the hypophysis as the primary gland in the etiology of the disease. On the basis of examination of the adrenals of many patients having adrenalectomy for Cushing's syndrome, one is compelled to accept the premise that hyperfunction of the adrenal gland may exist without demonstrable morphologic changes (Figs. 505-507). When this is the case, it is obvious why the pituitary basophilic changes, which have been noted in so many of the patients with apparently "normal" adrenal glands, bear the onus for the etiology of Cushing's disease. The prime role of the innocent-looking, though hyperfunctioning, adrenals is seen when bilateral adrenalectomy is followed by a prompt and complete remission of the syndrome.

PITUITARY ACTH SYNERGIST. Jailer and co-workers[17] presented evidence that there may be a pituitary ACTH synergist secreted from the hypophysis of patients with Cushing's syndrome. They postulated that this factor greatly augments the adrenal cortical effect of endogenous or exogenous ACTH. This substance has been found in the urine of the patients with Cushing's syndrome. When the augmenter was extracted

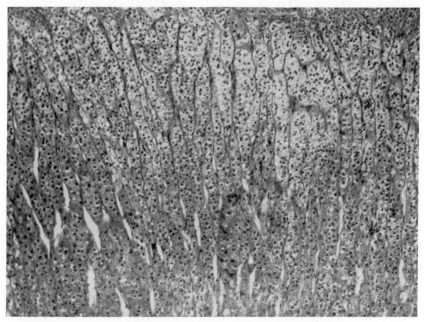

FIG. 505. *Adrenal tissue from patient KK showing normal cell structure despite the classic findings of Cushing's syndrome and the complete remission of symptoms after adrenalectomy.*

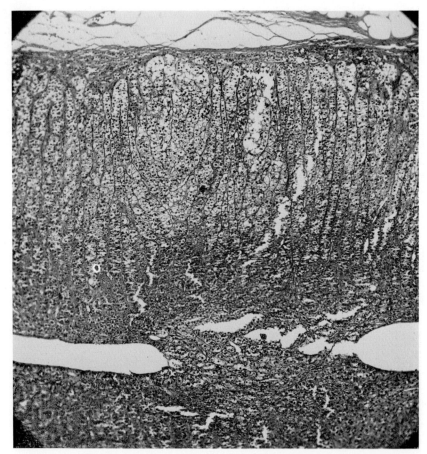

FIG. 506. *Adrenal gland removed from patient with Cushing's syndrome.*
Note the normal cell structure despite the fact that, grossly, the gland was
hyperplastic.

from the urine of these patients and assayed in hypophysectomized male
animals, it produced no notable effect on the adrenal histology or size.
However, when the same extract was administered together with ACTH,
the augmenter produced a definite synergism as evidenced by an increase
in weight of the adrenal gland over and above that achieved with ACTH
alone.[17]

A similar ACTH synergist has also been found in the urine of pregnant women. This factor, when injected without ACTH into an immature male rat, induced hypertrophy of the adrenal glands. Recently,
some doubt has been raised as to the actual presence of such an augmenter
since it became apparent that human pregnancy urine extract, via its high

gonadotropin content, had the potential of producing adrenal hyperplasia indirectly by its effect on stimulating the testes in these rats. The testicular response was then directly responsible for causing the adrenal hypertrophy. Human pregnancy extract failed to produce adrenal enlargement in female rats, nor did it have any discernible effect upon increasing adrenal weight in castrated male rats.[21]

TOTAL ADRENALECTOMY. Regardless of the possible presence or absence of a pituitary synergist, the adrenal cortex has become the prime point of attack for the surgical management of the disease. Early in the history of adrenal surgery for the treatment of Cushing's syndrome, hemilateral or bilateral partial adrenalectomy was advocated. However, it soon became obvious that partial adrenalectomy was not the desired procedure since many patients had to be reoperated on because of the recurrence of the primary syndrome in all its severity after a temporary but definite remission. There is little doubt that total, bilateral adrenalectomy is the surgical procedure of choice at the present time in patients without evidence of pituitary enlargement.

Are there any complications arising from this type of therapy or any

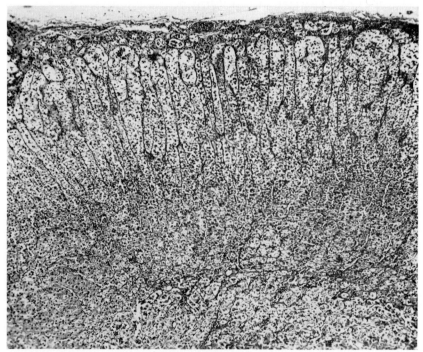

FIG. 507. The adrenal cortex of patient YS (Fig. 482). The cell structure appears normal in spite of the fact that the patient had classic Cushing's syndrome with clinical improvement following adrenalectomy.

adverse effects related to the total adrenalectomy? Obviously, the surgical procedure itself is a major risk and may result in marked morbidity or even in mortality. The risk of mortality with adrenalectomy, of course, is dependent on the skills of the surgeon and the anesthetist and on the preoperative preparation of the patient.

Our group now believes that the appropriate and most desirable surgical approach is via the abdominal route. Both adrenals can be readily visualized at the same time by this technique, and the surgeon can inspect the entire abdominal cavity (including the pelvic area) and rule out the possibility of an ovarian tumor. An ovarian tumor may be a factor in the development of Cushing's syndrome. Similarly, if the patient has an adrenal tumor, the abdominal incision readily permits inspection and palpation of both adrenal glands; it can then be determined whether one or both glands should be extirpated. If an adrenal tumor secreting glucocorticoids exists in either part of the adrenal, or replaces it entirely, the contralateral adrenal will be atrophied so that there is no need to remove this adrenal. Removal of the adrenal containing the neoplasm would leave the patient with one adrenal. Eventually, the atrophied contralateral gland could respond to the endogenous ACTH secretion which had been inhibited by the excessive glucocorticoid from the adrenal neoplasm. The patient would eventually achieve a euadrenal status. The morbidity of the abdominal method appears less than that after a bilateral dorsolumbar approach. However, the surgical procedure approaching the right adrenal from the abdomen may be technically more difficult than the lumbar incision because the liver partially obscures the field.

SURGICAL RESULTS OF ADRENALECTOMY. The results of bilateral total adrenalectomy via an abdominal incision have been very gratifying. This procedure has been instrumental in preventing errors of judgment in the removal of two adrenals when only a unilateral adrenalectomy was necessary. The abdominal exposure, for instance, would have been a wiser technique for the patient who showed only mild clinical stigmata of Cushing's syndrome due to an adrenal adenoma. The patient had exhibited a positive response to the ACTH challenge procedure. Not suspecting a neoplasm preoperatively, bilateral adrenalectomy was recommended via the dorsolumbar approach. Since simultaneous examination of both adrenals was not possible by this route, the adrenal adenoma was discovered after the nonadenomatous but atrophic gland on the contralateral side had already been removed. The atrophic adrenal is depicted in Figure 508, where one can note almost complete disorganization of the adrenal cyto-architecture. This adrenal, however, eventually would have developed into a normal gland if the one adrenal with the adenoma (Fig. 509) had been removed. Abdominal inspection of both adrenals would have uncovered the adenoma in one adrenal gland and necessitated only its removal. The atrophic gland would have recovered full function

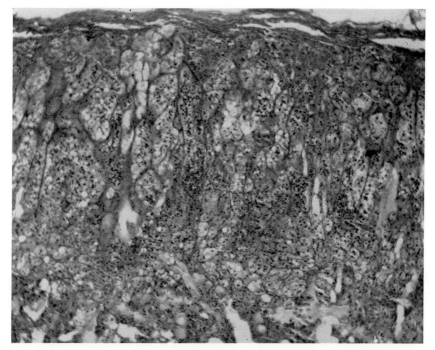

FIG. 508.   *Adrenal cortex from atrophied adrenal of patient E (Fig. 498). The patient showed marked osteoporosis and minimal clinical stigmata of Cushing's syndrome.*

and maintained the patient in a euadrenal state without the need for continuous replacement therapy with corticoids.

The clinical improvement has been gratifying and is depicted in two patients—one in Figures 495 and 496 and the other in Figure 510. The microscopic and the gross appearance of the adrenal glands of the patient shown in Figures 495 and 496 are seen in Figures 505 and 511 respectively. The combined adrenal weight in this patient was 28 mg., an enormous increase over the average adrenal weight. It is interesting to note that the patient began to menstruate regularly after surgery and showed excellent breast development (Figs. 495, 496), an indication of the resurgence of her femininity.

A more dramatic response is noted in Patient MK (Fig. 510), a grotesque-appearing female who progressively changed into an attractive feminine individual. Here too, note the progressive increase in breast size, evidence of increasing estrogenic activity. Prior to surgery, the patient, an 18-year-old female, had primary amenorrhea; since surgery, her menses have occurred regularly.

Both of these patients demonstrate the lack of specificity of end-

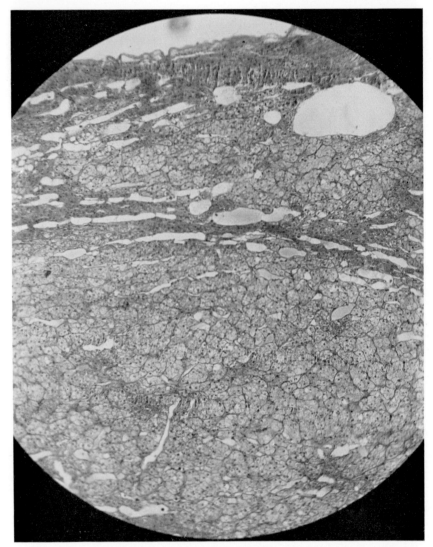

FIG. 509. *Adrenal adenoma from patient E (Fig. 498) showing the typical
adenomatous changes.*

organ hormone when the secretory product is present in high amounts.
The increased corticoid secretion in these patients was effective in inhibiting the patients' endogenous gonadotropic secretion. Removing the
hyperplastic adrenal caused normal ovarian and menstrual activity.

PRE- AND POSTOPERATIVE THERAPY. The therapeutic success of surgery on the adrenals is, of course, greatly dependent on the appropriate

pre- and postoperative care of the patient. The preparation of the patient undergoing a bilateral total adrenalectomy or unilateral removal of a neoplasm requires a sufficient amount of preoperative treatment with glucocorticoids to "cover" the patient during the surgical procedure. This prevents mild or severe adrenal crisis during and after the removal of the glands. Patients who are candidates for bilateral total adrenalectomy should be given 100 mg. of cortisone or hydrocortisone intramuscu-

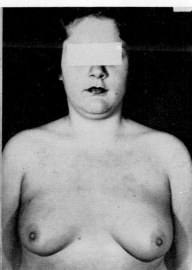

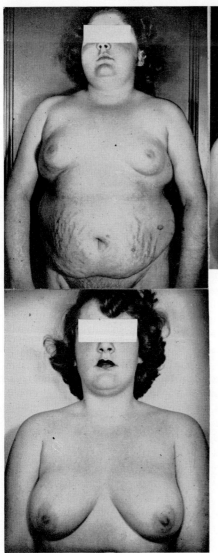

FIG. 510. Patient MK. Upper left, Before adrenalectomy. Upper right, Three months following adrenalectomy. Lower, Nine months after surgery. Note the remarkable change from a grotesque individual into an attractive woman showing excellent secondary sex development.

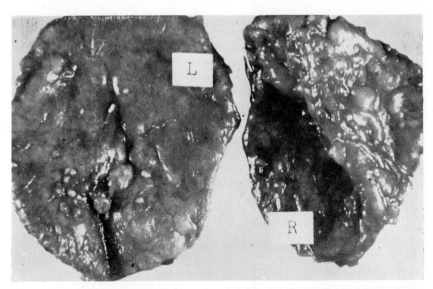

FIG. 511. *Patient KK. Gross appearance of the adrenal glands showing no evidence of adenoma formation. The combined adrenal weight was 28 mg.*

larly on the day prior to surgery, and also on the day of surgery. The corticoid is to be administered in divided doses of 50 mg. in the morning and evening of the day prior to surgery. Another 50 mg. of the corticoid is administered just preceding the admittance of the patient to the operating room if in the morning; or at 8:00 A.M. and again before surgery, if it is begun in the afternoon. At the time of surgery, an infusion containing 100 mg. of hydrocortisone hemisuccinate or 40 mg. of prednisone hemisuccinate in 500 cc. of glucose in normal saline is started. Either hemisuccinate preparation is permitted to enter by venous drip slowly enough so that the infusion is delivered throughout the entire surgical procedure. If any untoward drop of blood pressure occurs, 4 to 20 mg. of levarterenol bitartrate (Levophed) or 15 to 30 mg. of mephentermine (Wyamine) is initiated intravenously to maintain the systolic blood pressure above 100 ml. Hg. It has been suggested that phentolamine be incorporated with the levarterenol bitartrate to prevent the adverse effects that Levophed might have on producing local ischemia. These adverse results are due to profound vasoconstriction in the region of the insertion of the intravenous needle. The phentolamine will not counteract the desired systemic effects of levarterenol upon restoring vascular tone in a patient with circulatory shock.

After surgery, another 50 mg. of the hydrocortisone or cortisone is given intramuscularly, and, if the patient is passing adequate amounts of urine, 50 to 60 mEq. of potassium is administered intravenously by slow infusion. The patient should receive a total of 100 mg. of hydrocortisone or cortisone for the first 24-hour period after surgery. This is followed by 50 to 75 mg. intramuscularly on the second postoperative day, and by 50 mg. on the third day postoperatively in divided doses. On the fourth postoperative day the patient should be well enough to take steroids orally and may then be placed on 50 mg. of oral hydrocortisone or cortisone per day. The total amount is divided into four doses; each is administered at six-hour intervals. The patient's corticoid dosage is then decreased still further by the fifth or sixth postoperative day. At this time he is usually well maintained on 20 to 30 mg. of oral hydrocortisone per day, in divided doses.

9-Alpha-Fluorohydrocortisone. If, at any time during the postoperative period, the patient shows an untoward fall in blood pressure, it may be necessary to institute the mineralocorticoid 9-alpha-fluorohydrocortisone (9FF) along with the glucocorticoid. The 9FF promotes a sufficient degree of sodium retention; therefore, the patient will not develop any significant hyponatremia. However, just because the adrenalectomized individual is theoretically in need of the sodium-retaining steroid, there is no rationale for the blind or promiscuous use of 9-alpha-fluorohydrocortisone. It is used only when necessary, as evidenced by a drop in the patient's blood pressure below 100 mm. systolic and/or the presence of severe hyponatremia or hyperkalemia. In such cases, the patient may eventually be well maintained on 0.1 to 0.125 mg. of 9-alpha-fluorohydrocortisone per day or every second day. Usually, this dose restores excellent electrolyte and water equilibrium without producing a hypernatremic state. If the salt-retaining steroid is used in the above dosage, it is not necessary to restrict the potassium intake or encourage a high salt diet.

HYPERPIGMENTATION. A serious complication noted in patients totally adrenalectomized for Cushing's syndrome has been described[13, 26, 27, 31, 32] Actually, this complication does not involve any of the signs or symptoms anticipated as a result of the surgical procedure itself and has been associated with the development of a pronounced increase in pigmentation despite adequate glucocorticoid replacement therapy. Changes in the sella turcica have been described and are associated with a significant and progressive enlargement of the pituitary gland.[28] The reason for these postoperative changes is not known. The appearance of this "postadrenalectomy syndrome" again raises the question as to the site of primary origin (pituitary versus adrenal) of the disease. It may be that the relatively few patients (approximately 10 per cent) who develop these findings do so because of a pituitary adenoma which was present prior to adrenalectomy, and that, once this pituitary is released from the suppressing effects of the excessive endogenous adrenal steroids, it increases its activity and thereby provides the impetus for hypertrophy and hyperplasia or even for neoplasia with an anaplastic propensity.

The physiologic doses of corticoids used as maintenance therapy are not capable of inhibiting the surge of increased pituitary activity and growth. The accompanying increase in pigmentation may be a manifestation of this uncontrolled pituitary secretion. Certainly, it is a clinical warning of the presence or beginning of pituitary neoplastic activity. It has been reported that the adenomas may progress to an adenocarcinoma. If a patient has had a total adrenalectomy and is on adequate adrenal replacement therapy but despite this begins to show a marked increase in pigmentation accompanied by some decrease in the visual fields, an enlarging pituitary neoplasm is possible and appropriate therapy must be started. The enlargement of the sella turcica may vary from minimal to excessive. When significant erosion of the clinoid processes is noted, there is usually a commensurate encroachment upon the visual fields.

Most of the cases reported, including those with an adenoma or carcinoma, were maintained on the usual doses of corticoids. It must be emphasized, however, that the postadrenalectomy syndrome has been seen only in patients who have had Cushing's syndrome. It has not been reported in patients where adrenalectomy was done for reasons other than Cushing's syndrome. It has never appeared in a patient with Addison's disease. Therefore, it may be stated categorically that the continued use of corticoids in the absence of the adrenal glands is not a prerequisite for the development of this syndrome. In any event, when the postadrenalectomy syndrome develops, it then becomes necessary to subject the patient to other methods of control involving either radiation of the sella or removal of the enlarging neoplasm of the adenohypophysis.

Enlargement of the sella turcica has occurred in only one of our patients subjected to an adrenalectomy because of Cushing's syndrome. She had been well maintained on corticoid replacement therapy with no adverse effects for two to three years, when she suddenly developed increasing pigmentation (Fig. 429). At that time, there was some suspicious enlargement of the sella turcica as compared to her preadrenalectomy skull x-ray pictures. Soon after, the patient developed a sudden acute episode of left ophthalmoplegia, with diplopia and marked restriction of the visual fields in this eye plus moderate diminution of fields in the right eye. Some hypesthesia was evident on the left side of the face. Carotid angiograms demonstrated some deviation of the path of the left middle cerebral artery, probably due to an expanding intrasellar neoplasm. Accordingly, neurosurgical intervention was advised. However, before the final preparations for intracranial exploration could be completed, sudden and rapid spontaneous improvement in visual fields and in the ophthalmoplegia occurred. Surgery was deferred and pituitary irradiation suggested. Before radiation was initiated, however, almost complete restoration of the visual fields was noted. This eventually progressed to normal by the time the course of radiation therapy had been completed. The ptosed eyelid also had recovered full function after radiation therapy. Since that time, there has been no recurrence of diplopia and skin pigmentation has returned to normal. The question now arises, "Were the patient's symptoms, physical findings, and the deviation of the left middle cerebral artery caused by a vascular compression resulting from an aneurysm or was there a pituitary neoplasm?" Regardless of the etiology, the radiation of the sella turcica resulted in complete subsidence of the patient's hyperpigmentation.

ADVANTAGE OF ADRENALECTOMY. The surgical ablation of the adrenals for the treatment of Cushing's disease has one decided advantage over pituitary ablation by either radiation or surgery.[24] In the adrenalectomized patients, normal pituitary activity of other tropic modalities will continue. In other words, these patients show no evidence of disturbances in thyrotropic or gonadotropic function. Hence, the adrenalectomized patient would still be capable of reproductive function and would not require gonadal or thyroid replacement therapy. This would not be true for individuals treated by pituitary extirpation or radiation. The maintenance of the panhypopituitary patient, while not particularly difficult with the endocrinologist's modern armamentarium, is certainly more complex and expensive than the therapy of the adrenalectomized patient. In addition, total adrenalectomy will usually produce permanent remission in all patients except those developing the postadrenalectomy syndrome. This is not true for patients treated with radiation therapy alone. Obviously, if an increased number of cases of hyperpigmentation associated with sellar enlargement and impairment of the visual fields occur following adrenalectomy, then one would be forced to reconsider the pituitary gland rather than the adrenals in the treatment of Cushing's syndrome. Clues should be sought for the diagnosis of hypophyseal hypertrophy and accentuated pigmentation. On the basis of our present experience, we would be less inclined to do a bilateral adrenalectomy and would direct our therapy toward the pituitary gland if the patient shows evidence of enlargement of the sella turcica and/or increased melanin deposition.

Radiation Therapy. The management of Cushing's disease by pituitary irradiation has, of course, been used since attention was first centered on the pituitary gland when Cushing reported that pituitary basophilism is probably a factor in the etiology of the syndrome. There are two major approaches for radiation of the pituitary gland.

PITUITARY IRRADIATION. Pituitary irradiation alone has been the procedure of choice of many radiologists and has been subscribed to by those who believe that the origin of the disease lies in the pituitary it-self.[8, 35] Therapy has involved the administration of 4000 to 6000 r. directed toward the pituitary gland.

Adverse Effects. In the past, there was always the possibility that radiation could induce some adverse effects on brain structure adjacent to the hypophysis. However, such undesirable possibilities are now kept to a minimum by the competent modern radiotherapist through improved instruments for concentrating the rays and through his greater skill in directing the destructive radiation beam.

Sosman's early recommendation for the use of a total dose of 1700 r. administered over a six- to 10-day interval has proved to be of limited value. This dosage produces permanent remission in only a minority of patients.

Some authorities believe that radiation is innocuous. They advocate its use initially, and, if no improvement occurs, then bilateral adrenalec-tomy can be done. Unfortunately, there has been a significant rate of recurrence of Cushing's syndrome in patients who had a temporary re-mission after radiation therapy. These exacerbations may occur less with a more intensive course of therapy, but then the risk of destroying the other modalities of pituitary function becomes greater and occasionally a permanent hypopituitary state is induced. Thus, while radiation of the pituitary gland in doses which are not destructive to all pituitary function may yield only temporary remission, more effective treatment may result in permanent remission but may also be accompanied by alteration or diminution in other modalities of pituitary tropic activity.

Other adverse effects of radiation, albeit minimal, are the permanent alopecia and the persistent hyperemia and telangiectasia it induces at the skin sites of penetration of the x-ray. No doubt the patients effectively treated by pituitary irradiation would not be expected to develop the hyperpigmentation and sellar enlargement noted in some individuals undergoing a bilateral total adrenalectomy. All these factors must be weighed carefully before selecting radiation or other therapy for the management of the Cushing patient.

PITUITARY IRRADIATION AND UNILATERAL ADRENALECTOMY. Some au-thorities recommend the use of pituitary irradiation plus unilateral adre-nalectomy.[33] The logic of such an approach lies in the fact that patients receiving this treatment do not require adrenal cortical replacement therapy as do those after bilateral adrenalectomy. Such treatment is said to be effective because radiation of the pituitary is of such magnitude that it diminishes excessive ACTH release and thereby prevents compen-satory hypertrophy of the contralateral intact adrenal gland. Our experi-ence with this procedure is nil; however, Soffer and his group in their extensive use of this method are convinced that it is the procedure of choice. Approximately 60 per cent of their patients treated this way have shown complete clinical remission. In the event of a recurrence of their syndrome these patients must then be subjected to a second surgical procedure to remove the intact adrenal gland. Since there is always the possibility of repeated surgery, it would appear that if one were to radiate the pituitary gland, radiation should be done first without a unilateral adrenalectomy. If the disease occurs after a remission—or if a remission fails to occur—a total bilateral adrenalectomy could then be done. The patient would be spared a second surgical procedure.

INSERTION OF YTTRIUM 90. Irradiation of the pituitary gland by the insertion of yttrium 90 is an effective and comparatively nontraumatic method used in the treatment of Cushing's syndrome. Radon seeds and colloidal gold also have been used for the same purpose. Apparently, this therapeutic approach has been successful in managing certain patients with Cushing's disease. These patients retain some modalities of pituitary activity other than those referable to the adrenal cortex. Thus, if adrenal-ectomy seems contraindicated, the use of transnasal implantation of radioactive material into the sella turcica is a procedure that warrants further exploration, particularly because of ease of administration. In addition, the entire technique in the hands of the expert is relatively innocuous. Complications from this type of therapy are reported to be minimal. Erosion through the sphenoidal sinus with the possibility of infection and encephalitis, however, must always be kept in mind.

Iatrogenic Hyperadrenocorticoidism. Iatrogenic hyperadrenocorticoid-ism of the Cushing type must also be considered in a general discussion of Cushing's syndrome. The prevalent use of high doses of the different corticoids in treating a variety of inflammatory and neoplastic disorders may induce the typical clinical changes of Cushing's syndrome. These changes include: buffalo obesity, facial plethora, striae, weakness, etc. In these patients, obviously, the withdrawal or diminution of the dose of corticoid decreases the extent, either totally or partially, of the iatrogenic hyperadrenocorticoidism. Since it may be necessary to main-tain the patient on large doses of the corticoids to preserve life, the physician must decide whether to permit the primary disease to run rampant or to create another disease by virtue of the therapy itself. This quandary may be minimized if one realizes that sometimes only a slight decrease of corticoid dosage may be necessary to reverse some of the adverse effects due to medication, while still maintaining the desired clinical effect of holding in abeyance the ravages of the primary disease for which the patient is being treated.

DIETARY CONTROL. *High Protein Intake.* Many of the undesirable effects of induced Cushing's disease secondary to large doses of corticoids may be avoided if the patient follows certain dietary restrictions which should include a high protein diet, almost to the exclusion of carbohy-drates. At the same time, increased potassium supplementation of the diet is advisable. These recommendations may be helpful in diminishing the clinical features of hyperadrenocorticoidism while still permitting the patient to be maintained on the effective dose of corticoids necessary to hold his primary disease in abeyance.

Potassium Supplementation. Potassium supplementation should be given in the amount of 80 to 120 mEq. per day. This is well tolerated in the liquid form, potassium gluconate, available as an elixir (Kaon Elixir), of which four to six tablespoons per day provide adequate potassium supplementation. Each tablespoon supplies 20 mEq. of elemental potassium.

Conclusions. Therapy for Cushing's syndrome is still dependent on a relatively archaic method—ablation of the metabolically malfunctioning organ. Perhaps, as in the adrenogenital syndrome, the basic physiology of the disturbances noted in Cushing's syndrome will eventually be understood, and then one may provide a more logical and less drastic therapeutic approach to this disease, initially described by Cushing and made famous by the elegant metabolic studies of Albright and his co-workers.

Pulmonary Carcinoma and Cushing's Syndrome. In the past few years an increasing number of patients have been noted to have both pulmonary carcinoma and Cushing's syndrome.[2, 3, 5, 25, 36] As a rule, the majority of the carcinomas found were of the oat-cell type, i.e., small cells. Interestingly enough, a predominance of females has been noted when the two diseases occur simultaneously. This is in contrast to the uncomplicated bronchial carcinoma which is seen much more frequently in males. At the present time, 29 cases of Cushing's syndrome associated with bronchogenic carcinoma have been recorded. A significant number of patients with this syndrome fail to show an accentuation of the characteristic clinical stigmata usually seen in patients with Cushing's syndrome. The absence of the full-blown Cushing's syndrome might be explained, in part, by the virulent nature of the pulmonary disease so that, when the two occur together, death may take place before full manifestation of Cushing's syndrome is possible. In addition, since the bronchogenic carcinoma is associated with weight loss in itself, some of the clinical characteristics of Cushing's disease might be obscured. A frequent and unexplained finding in many of these patients has been a hypokalemic alkalosis.[3]

The manifestations of the clinical picture and some of the chemical findings of Cushing's syndrome may be due to secretion of ACTH by the tumor cells of the anaplastic pulmonary lesion. Since the elevated glucocorticoid level of many of these patients is not suppressed with adequate doses of dexamethasone, it appears that the main source of the increased ACTH secretion is not the pituitary, but rather the pulmonary neoplasm.

There are other tumors that may be found in a patient with a clinical picture of Cushing's syndrome. These include neoplasms of the thymus, liver and pancreas. While seen less often than the pulmonary anaplastic lesions, they are next in frequency to the bronchogenic carcinomas. Neoplasms of the thyroid, ovary and testes have also been associated with Cushing's disease. The reason for simultaneous presence of a neoplastic growth and Cushing's syndrome is not known. One can theorize—and this is only conjecture—that if neoplasms are caused by a "virus-like substance," the increased elaboration of glucocorticoids in the Cushing patient may accentuate the spread of such neoplasms due to a breakdown of the normal body mechanism protecting the patient against spread of such a neoplasm.

References

1. ALBRIGHT, F., PARSON, W., AND BLOOMBERG, E.: Cushing's syndrome interpreted as hyperadrenocorticoidism leading to hyperglyconeogenesis: Results of treatment with testosterone propionate. J. Clin. Endocr. 1:375-384, 1941.

2. ALLOTT, E. N., AND SKELTON, M. O.: Increased adrenocortical activity associated with malignant disease. Lancet 2:278-283, 1960.

3. BAGSHAWE, K. D.: Hypokalaemia, carcinoma, and Cushing's syndrome. Lancet 2: 284-287, 1960.

4. BLODGETT, F. M., BURGIN, L., IEZZONI, D., GRIBETZ, D., AND TALBOT, N. B.: Effects of prolonged cortisone therapy on the statural growth, skeletal maturation and metabolic status of children. New Engl. J. Med. 254:636-641, 1956.

5. CHRISTY, N. P.: Adrenocorticotrophic activity in the plasma of patients with Cushing's syndrome associated with pulmonary neoplasms. Lancet 1:85-86, 1961.

6. CHRISTY, N. P., WALLACE, E. Z., AND JAILER, J. W.: Comparative effects of prednisone and of cortisone in suppressing the response of the adrenal cortex to exogenous adrenocorticotropin. J. Clin. Endocr. 16:1059-1074, 1958.

7. CROOKE, A. C.: A change in the basophil cells of the pituitary gland common to conditions which exhibit the syndrome attributed to basophil adenoma. J. Path. Bact. 41:339-349, 1935.

8. DOHAN, F. C., RAVENTOS, A., BOUCOT, N., AND ROSE, E.: Roentgen therapy in Cushing's syndrome without adrenocortical tumor. J. Clin. Endocr. 17:8-32, 1957.

9. FABRYKANT, M., JACKSON, R. S., AND ASHE, B.: Cushing's syndrome: Failure to demonstrate diminished peripheral glucose uptake and insulin resistance. Metabolism 6:116-126, 1957.

10. FRASER, R. W., ALBRIGHT, F., AND SMITH, P. H.: The value of glucose tolerance test, insulin tolerance test and glucose-insulin tolerance test in diagnosis of endocrine disorders of glucose metabolism. J. Clin. Endocr. 1:297-306, 1941.

11. GELLER, J., ALVAREZ, A. S., GUTMAN, A., DEFREITAS, A., GABRILOVE, J. L., AND SOFFER, L. J.: The effect of prednisone on adrenal responsiveness to corticotropins in normal subjects and in patients with treated and untreated Cushing's syndrome. J. Clin. Endocr. 18:409-416, 1958.

12. GESCHWIND, I. I., AND LI, C. H.: Inactivation of adrenocorticotropic hormones in vitro by tissues. Endocrinology 50:226-233, 1952.

13. GLENN, F., KARL, R. C., AND HORWITH, M.: The surgical treatment of Cushing's syndrome. Ann. Surg. 148:365-374, 1958.

14. GREENBLATT, R. B., AND KUPPERMAN, H. S.: Diagnostic value of the glucose tolerance and insulin tolerance tests in endocrine disorders. Southern Med. J. 40:737-744, 1947.

15. HENNEMAN, D. H., AND BUNKER, J. P.: The pattern of intermediary carbohydrate metabolism in Cushing's syndrome. Amer. J. Med. 23:34-45, 1957.

16. IANNACCONE, A., GABRILOVE, J. L., SOHVAL, A. R., AND SOFFER, L. J.: The ovaries in Cushing's syndrome. New Engl. J. Med. 261:775-780, 1959.

17. JAILER, J. W., LONGSON, D., AND CHRISTY, N. P.: Cushing's syndrome—an adrenal or pituitary disease? J. Clin. Endocr. 16:1276-1280, 1956.

18. KUPPERMAN, H. S.: Extrapancreatic factors in diabetes mellitus. Postgrad. Med. 20:151-159, 1956.

19. KUPPERMAN, H. S., BERNSTEIN, A., FORBES, A., COPE, O., AND ALBRIGHT, F.: Remission in Cushing's syndrome after bilateral hemiadrenalectomy. J. Clin. Endocr. 13:154-164, 1953.

20. KUPPERMAN, H. S., PERSKY, M., LINSK, J., ISAACS, M., AND ROSENBLUTH, M.: The paradoxical effect of intravenous hydrocortisone upon carbohydrate metabolism. Ann. N. Y. Acad. Sci. 61:494-501, 1955.

21. LANMAN, J. T.: The adrenal fetal zone: its occurrence in primates and a possible relationship to chorionic gonadotropin. Endocrinology 61:684-691, 1957.

22. LAQUER, G. L.: Cytological changes in human hypophyses after cortisone and ACTH treatment. Science 112:429-430, 1950.

23. LIDDLE, G.: Tests of pituitary-adrenal suppressibility in diagnosis of Cushing's syndrome. J. Clin. Endocr. 20:1539-1560, 1960.

24. LUFT, R., OLIVECRONA, H., IKKOS, D., AND HERNBERG, C. A.: Treatment of Cushing's disease by pituitary surgery. Report of two cases. Acta Endocr. (Kbh) 24:1-7, 1957.

25. MEADOR, C. K., LIDDLE, G. W., ISLAND, D. P., NICHOLSON, W. E., LUCAS, C. P., NUCKTON, J. G., AND LUETSCHER, J. A.: Cause of Cushing's syndrome in patients with tumors arising from "nonendocrine" tissue. J. Clin. Endocr. 22:693-703, 1962.

26. MONTGOMERY, D. A. D., AND WELBOURNE, R. B.: Cushing's syndrome: a review. Quart. Rev. Surg. Obstet. Gynec. 16:201-215, 1959.

27. MONTGOMERY, D. A. D., WELBOURNE, R. B., McCAUGHEY, W. T. E., AND GLEADHILL, C. A.: Pituitary tumours manifested after adrenalectomy for Cushing's syndrome. Lancet 2:707-710, 1959.

28. PERSKY, M., LINSK, J., ISAACS, M., JENKINS, J. P., ROSENBLUTH, M., KUPPERMAN, H. S.: Acute effects of intravenous hydrocortisone on glucose and insulin tolerances, and levels of serum and urinary inorganic phosphorus. J. Clin. Endocr. 15:1247-1256, 1955.

29. PRIESTLEY, J. T., SPRAGUE, R. G., WALTERS, W., AND SALASSA, R. M.: Subtotal adrenalectomy for Cushing's syndrome: Preliminary report of 29 cases. Ann. Surg. 134:464-475, Sept. 1951.

30. RENOLD, A. E., JENKINS, D., FORSHAM, P. H., AND THORN, G. W.: The use of intravenous ACTH: A study in quantitative adrenocortical stimulation. J. Clin. Endocr. 12:763-797, 1957.

31. SALASSA, R. M., KEARNS, T. P., KERNOHAN, J. W., SPRAGUE, R. G., AND MacCARTHY, C. S.: Pituitary tumors in patients with Cushing's syndrome. J. Clin. Endocr. 19:1523-1539, 1959.

32. SIEBENMANN, R. E.: Invasiv wachsendes, vorwiegend basophiles adenom des hypophysenvorder lappens bei Cushing-rezidiv nach subtotaler adrenektomie.

Schweizerische Zeitschrift für Allgemeine Pathologie und Bakteriologie 18:1189, 1955.

33. SOFFER, L. J., EISENBERG, J., IANNACCONE, A., AND GABRILOVE, J. L.: Cushing's syndrome. Ciba Foundation Colloquia on Endocrinology Vol. VIII—The human adrenal cortex. Little Brown and Co., Boston, 1955, p. 487.

34. SOFFER, L. J., GELLER, J., AND GABRILOVE, J. L.: Response of the plasma 17-hydroxy-corticosteroid level to gel-ACTH in tumorous and non-tumorous Cushing's syndrome. J. Clin. Endocr. 17:878-883, 1957.

35. SOSMAN, M. C.: Cushing's disease—pituitary basophilism. The Caldwell Lecture: 1947. Amer. J. Roentgenol. 62:1-32, 1949.

36. THOMPSON, G. S., HORWICH, L., AND DAVIS, J. C.: Carcinoma of bronchus and Cushing's syndrome. Lancet 2:534-536, 1962.

37. WETCHLER, B. B., AND KUPPERMAN, H. S.: The importance of the glucose tolerance and insulin tolerance tests in obstetrics and gynecology. Bull. Mgt. Hague Mat. Hosp. 9:111-116, 1956.

38. WILKINS, L.: The diagnosis of the adrenogenital syndrome and its treatment with cortisone. J. Pediat. 41:860-874, 1952.

39. WILKINS, L., LEWIS, R. A., KLEIN, R., GARDNER, L. I., CRIGLER, J. F., JR., ROSEMBERG, E., AND MIGEON, C. J.: Treatment of congenital adrenal hyperplasia with cortisone. J. Clin. Endocr. 11:1-25, 1951.

40. WILKINS, L., LEWIS, R. A., KLEIN, R., AND ROSEMBERG, E.: The suppression of androgen secretion by cortisone in a case of congenital adrenal hyperplasia. Bull. Johns Hopkins Hosp. 36:249-252, 1950.

chapter 22

Hyperaldosteronism is one of those rare diseases that piques the imagination but occurs so infrequently that most clinicians and endocrinologists rarely have the opportunity to see a patient with the classical disease. The cases reported in the literature and the known cases total less than 200 in number. However, before elaborating upon the various clinical signs and symptoms, it would be well to review some of the factors and mechanisms involved in aldosterone secretion and regulation.

ALDOSTERONE SECRETION

Site of Secretion. The site of aldosterone secretion or storage appears to be in the zona glomerulosa. Two groups of investigators, Giroud, Stachenko and Piletta,[24] with separate *in vitro* incubation of the glomerulosa and inner zones of rat and beef adrenal glands, and Ayres and associates[3] with incubation of ox-adrenal-capsule strippings composed mainly of zona glomerulosa tissue, have shown that in the test animals employed the zona glomerulosa is the major site of aldosterone production. Bloch and co-workers[8] found sodium-retaining activity in extracts from adrenal tissue of human fetuses from the ninth to twenty-first weeks of gestation. They hypothesized, and it has since been confirmed by Farrell,[17] that adrenal androgens are synthesized in the reticular zone, glucocorticoids in the fascicular zone, and mineralocorticoids (aldosterone) in the glomerular zone, the outer layer of the adrenal cortex.

Hyperadrenal
Corticoidism – III.
Hyperaldosteronism and
Mechanism of
Aldosterone Secretion

Regulating Mechanism. While there is little question concerning the site of aldosterone secretion, much investigation is still being carried on to clarify the mechanisms regulating the secretion of this steroid.

ROLE OF ACTH. There is considerable evidence pointing to the role of adrenocorticotropin (ACTH) in aldosterone homeostasis (Fig. 512A). ACTH can enhance aldosterone secretion from the adrenal, albeit this stimulation, comparatively speaking, is much less than the increase in corticoid secretion during the same stimulation.[2, 13, 17, 23, 30, 32, 34]

HYPOPHYSECTOMY AND ALDOSTERONE SECRETION. Despite hypophysectomy, aldosterone is secreted by the adrenals in amounts which will maintain normal electrolyte metabolism[2, 13, 34] Deane and Greep,[15] in 1946, studied the adrenals of hypophysectomized rats and concluded that the zona glomerulosa remained the same size or actually increased in width following hypophysectomy. They also demonstrated that the secretory activity of the zona glomerulosa is maintained at an almost normal level following removal of the pituitary gland, as evidenced by cytologic criteria. In addition, fat-staining techniques have adequately demonstrated the presence of ketosteroid precursors in this layer. These findings support those described above and substantiate the belief that the glomerulosa layer primarily secretes mineralocorticoids. It appears that the rate of secretion of these steroids is not markedly changed following hypophysectomy. More recently, the post-hypophysectomy output of al-

793

dosterone has been found to be 50 to 60 per cent of the pre-extirpation level, whereas the glucocorticoid secretion drops down to 10 per cent of the prehypophysectomy level.[32] Furthermore, a normal zona glomerulosa has been found in the adrenals of hypophysectomized human beings at autopsy.

The above citations confirm the clinical observation that while hypophysectomized human beings may show evidence of pathologic alteration of carbohydrate and protein metabolism, they maintain relatively normal electrolyte balance without hypophyseal assistance.

Extracellular Fluid and Aldosterone Secretion. Bartter and others[4, 28] have shown that some changes in extracellular fluid volume may exert a strong influence over aldosterone secretion (Fig. 512A). The effect of fluid volume on aldosterone release can be shown to be independent of total body sodium or of serum sodium concentration and increase in glomerular filtration rate (GFR). Secondly, when body fluids are diminished without sodium deprivation, by withdrawal of water, aldosterone excre-

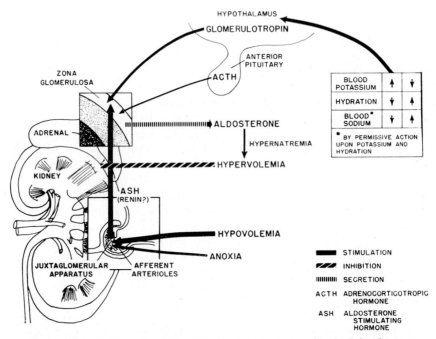

FIG. 512A. *A diagrammatic presentation of the factors involved in the secretion of aldosterone. Note the direct influence of the juxtaglomerular apparatus upon the zona glomerulosa. Both anoxia and hypervolemia influence the response of the juxtaglomerular apparatus and affect its tropic action upon the zona glomerulosa. The secretion of glomerulotropin by the hypothalamus is influenced by the sodium, potassium, and water levels of the body.*

tion rises despite increasing serum sodium concentration and decreasing GFR.[7] The way in which volume change affects aldosterone secretion is not definitely known.

INTRAVASCULAR VOLUME CHANGES. Although the above studies on intravascular volume are convincing, work by other investigators casts some doubt on their validity. Expansion of the intravascular volume at the expense of interstitial fluid by infused hyperoncotic albumin paradoxically resulted in sodium retention.[25, 36] Infusion of iso-oncotic albumin, which expanded intravascular volume without change in interstitial volume, did not bring about the expected naturesis. Indeed, in some cases, there was a fall in sodium excretion. Although variations in sodium excretion are not equated with changes in aldosterone levels, these experiments at least suggest cautious appraisal of the evidence that changes in intravascular volume alone are the effective stimuli for the secretion of aldosterone. It should be pointed out that an alteration in intravascular volume will affect the renal excretion of sodium without altering aldosterone secretion. Therefore, variations in serum and urine sodium concentrations are not sufficient to cause changes in aldosterone secretion. Finally, Farrell points out that the effects of body water are best seen when the subject is depleted of sodium beforehand. He also noted that changes in aldosterone secretion in dehydration studies were within the normal variation.[17, 18]

It must be emphasized that sodium change, independent of intravascular volume, may, under certain conditions, also control aldosterone secretory rates. The work presented concerning volume control does not mitigate against this possibility.

Central Nervous System Factor. Bartter's group[5, 6] has attempted to delineate the afferent pathways through which the central nervous system senses the alterations in intravascular volume (Fig. 512B). Mills and associates[29] found that section of the cervical vagus nerves prevented the return of an acutely elevated aldosterone secretion to normal levels, Bartter[6] showed that constriction of the thyrocarotid arterial junction was followed by an increased aldosterone secretion, and, conversely, that denervation of this area prevented an increased secretion of aldosterone. However, again, it should be pointed out that disagreement is rampant. Davis[13, 37] denervated the entire cervical carotid arterial system, including the carotid sinus and thyrocarotid arterial junction, and failed to influence the high rate of aldosterone secretion, the sodium retention, and the formation of ascitic fluid in dogs with thoracic caval constriction.

Right Atrium. Farrell and associates[1] have attempted to show that the right atrium contained receptors regulating aldosterone secretion. However, Davis[13] has also presented convincing evidence which, he feels, provides little support for this hypothesis.

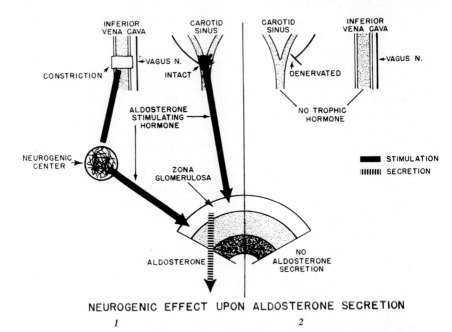

NEUROGENIC EFFECT UPON ALDOSTERONE SECRETION

1   *2*

FIG. 512B. *Neurogenic factors controlling aldosterone secretion. 1, Note that the aldosterone-stimulating centers in the vena cava and carotid sinus respond to alteration in intravascular pressure. These pressure changes are induced by variation in blood volume. The pressure centers in the vena cava, indirectly via the neurogenic center, and directly from the carotid sinus, release the stimuli influencing aldosterone secretion. When these centers are denervated (2), there is no stimulus for aldosterone secretion.*

Influence of Potassium.   When potassium is removed from the diet, aldosterone secretion, if originally elevated, is consistently lowered. When large loads of potassium are administered, aldosterone secretion is increased. Deane and co-workers[16] observed hypertrophy of the zona glomerulosa to follow potassium administration, and atrophy to follow potassium deprivation in the rat. Laragh[27] has reported increases in urinary aldosterone levels following potassium administration in man and in the dog. However, the question of the effect of potassium administration on aldosterone production is still not completely settled. Potassium depletion does not prevent secretion of aldosterone and efficient sodium conservation in response to sodium deprivation. Rosnagle and Farrell[33] were unable to detect increases in the aldosterone level in adrenal venous blood following potassium infusions. Thus, a direct effect of potassium on the adrenal gland is not yet proved. However, it may well be that potassium influences aldosterone secretion only indirectly, either by effecting release of glomerulotropin or by altering the activity of the juxtaglomerular apparatus.[14, 22, 26, 35]

Diencephalon. In 1956, Rauschkolb and Farrell[31] suggested that the diencephalon contains a center for control of aldosterone secretion (Fig. 512B). They found that decerebration and removal of tissue anterior to the midbrain was followed by a marked reduction in aldosterone output, whereas decortication was without effect. Midbrain lesions, which extended into the rostral pons, induced a significant increase in aldosterone output, suggesting the existence of an inhibitory area. Farrell concluded that the diencephalon controlled the secretion of a humeral tropic factor which in turn stimulated aldosterone secretion by a direct stimulatory effect on the zona glomerulosa.[20] This center received stimulatory and inhibitory influences from peripheral receptors, and could be influenced by other parts of the brain stem. He presented the theory purely as a working hypothes's.[19, 20, 31] It has been criticized by Davis[13] and by Daily and Ganong.[12] The latter authors reported that the only hypothalamic lesions which influenced aldosterone production were those occurring in the median eminence. Recent observations on "adreno-glomerulotropin" by Farrell[19, 20] confirmed his earlier beliefs that lipid extracts of the pineal selectively stimulate aldosterone secretion. Farrell also prepared synthetically a substance which has been shown to have many of the properties of the pineal extract. This synthetic product was capable of stimulating aldosterone secretion. The fact that the decapitated dogs were still capable of responding to stress with an increased aldosterone output does not negate the pineal or hypothalamic concept of Farrell, but again merely indicates that there are a number of different mechanisms regulating aldosterone secretion other than those emanating from the hypothalamus.

PRIMARY HYPERALDOSTERONISM

Primary hyperaldosteronism, first described by Conn,[9, 10] was evoked when Conn considered the symptomatology of the disease as well as the biochemical alteration and correlated these findings and observations with excess secretion of a mineralocorticoid.

The signs and symptoms of hyperaldosteronism are primarily due to hypokalemia. The associated muscle weakness due to excessive potassium loss had been noted prior to Conn's description of the syndrome but was invariably associated with acidosis instead of alkalosis. The low body potassium accompanied by acidosis as seen in renal tubular acidosis was ascribed to the potassium loss via the kidney and urine, and was considered to be an attempt by the body to compensate for the failure of the kidney to form and secrete ammonia. The alkalosis seen with hyperaldosteronism was also observed in the past, but, prior to Conn's description, was not correlated with increased mineralocorticoid excretion or production.

Clinical and Laboratory Findings.   The following signs and symptoms are noted in hyperaldosteronism:

Urinary

Polyuria and associated polydipsia
Nocturia
Albuminuria
Decreased glomerular filtration
Vacuolar nephropathy
Alkaline urine
Low urine specific gravity

Muscular

Weakness
Periodic paralysis
Flaccid paralysis
Tetany
Positive Chvostek's sign
Positive Trousseau's sign
Necrosis of muscle tissue
Muscle cramps

Central nervous system

Headaches
Paresthesia
Amblyopia

Cardiovascular

Hypertension
Cardiac enlargement
Absence of edema (usually but not always)
Alkalosis
Hypokalemia (below 3 mEq.)
Hypernatremia

Incidence.   The disease may be divided into two types:

1. Congenital (three times more common in men than women), and usually associated with hyperplasia.

2. Acquired—neoplastic (more common in women than men), and seen in 70 to 80 per cent of all patients with hyperaldosteronism.

Most of the patients are between the ages of 30 to 45 years, although there have been reports of the syndrome in patients as young as nine and as old as 63 years.

Diagnosis. The diagnosis is based upon the basic triad: benign hypertension, polyuria, and hypokalemia. An interesting point about the low serum potassium is that the patient with hyperaldosteronism continues to secrete large amounts of potassium despite the hypokalemia. Thus, a high potassium clearance with low serum potassium is characteristic of the syndrome.

SPECIFIC TESTS. Increased aldosterone excretion and secretion may be noted. However, marked elevation of excretion of aldosterone occurs in patients with malignant hypertension.

CONFIRMATORY TESTS. Plasma volume is increased at least 25 to 50 per cent more than anticipated.

A prompt rise of the serum potassium occurs following the administration of 300 mg. of spironolactone (Aldactone) t.i.d. to q.i.d. for three to four days. A rise of the low serum potassium to normal at the end of the third day would support the diagnosis of hyperaldosteronism. More recently, by the use of micronized spironolactone, smaller doses in the range of 75 mg. t.i.d. to q.i.d. may be used with good results.

Treatment. The treatment of primary hyperaldosteronism consists of surgical extirpation of the adenoma, if present, or complete adrenalectomy in those patients with adrenocortical hyperplasia.

SECONDARY HYPERALDOSTERONISM

Much more commonly seen are the patients with secondary hyperaldosteronism associated with edematous states, particularly the nephrotic syndrome, hepatic cirrhosis, and congestive heart failure. While edema is not commonly seen in primary hyperaldosteronism, its presence does not necessarily rule out the syndrome. This is particularly true of patients with adrenal tumors.[11, 21] The signs and symptoms of secondary hyperaldosteronism are very similar to those seen in the primary disease. Therapy is directed at the secondary nature of the disease and is usually not surgery. An important point is that the use of diuretics may cause secondary hyperaldosteronism. This is due to the decrease in extracellular fluid volume which stimulates aldosterone secretion despite the concomitant decrease in serum potassium.

The role of aldosterone in hypertension and congestive heart failure is a subject of enormous magnitude. Both digitalis and aldosterone act similarly in that each steroid is capable of releasing intracellular potassium into the extracellular spaces (Fig. 513). Since these two steroids are similar in their action upon intracellular metabolism, it may well be that they compete with one another for the tissue substrata. It also is conceivable that aldosterone may enhance the effect of digitalis through its role in potassium depletion. This may be particularly so since digitalis may act upon cardiac muscle to promote a potassium depletion and

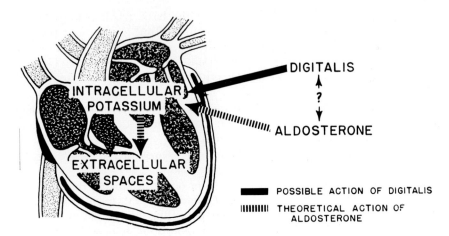

FIG. 513. *Relationships of digitalis and aldosterone. Both are important in releasing intracellular potassium into the extracellular spaces.*

thereby achieve a more profound digitalis effect in a patient with high potassium levels. However, since further discussion on this topic would be out of the realm of endocrinology, nothing more will be said on the action of these two steroids.

References

1. ANDERSON, C. H., McCALLY, M., AND FARRELL, G. L.: The effects of atrial stretch on aldosterone secretion. Endocrinology 64:202-207, 1959.

2. AUGUST, J. T., NELSON, D. H., AND THORN, G. W.: Aldosterone. New Engl. J. Med. 259:917-923, 1958.

3. AYRES, P. J., HECHTER, O., SABA, N., SIMPSON, S. A., AND TAIT, J. F.: Intermediates in biosynthesis of aldosterone by capsule strippings of ox adrenal gland. Biochem. J. (Proc. Biochem. Soc.) 65:22, 1956.

4. BARTTER, F. C.: The role of aldosterone in normal homeostasis and in certain disease states. Metabolism 5:369-383, 1956.

5. BARTTER, F. C., MILLS, I. H., BIGLIERI, E. G., AND DELEA, C.: Studies on the control and physiologic action of aldosterone. Rec. Progr. Hormone Res. 15:311-335, 1959.

6. BARTTER, F. C., MILLS, I. H., AND GANN, D. S.: Increase in aldosterone secretion by carotid artery constriction and its prevention by thyro-carotid arterial junction denervation. J. Clin. Invest. 39:1330-1336, 1960.

7. BIGLIERI, E. G., AND FORSHAM, P. H.: Studies on the expanded extracellular fluid and the responses to various stimuli in primary aldosteronism. Amer. J. Med. 30:564-576, 1961.

8. BLOCH, E., BENIRSCHKE, K., AND ROSEMBERG, E.: C_{19} steroids, 17β-hydroxycorticosterone and sodium retaining factor in human fetal adrenal glands. Endocrinology 58:626-633, 1956.

9. Conn, J. W.: Presidential address: Part I, Painting background. Part II, Primary aldosteronism, a new clinical syndrome. J. Lab. Clin. Med. 45:3-17, 1955.

10. Conn, J. W.: Evolution of primary aldosteronism as a highly specific clinical entity. J.A.M.A. 172:1650-1653, 1960.

11. Cortes, F., Shuman, C. R., and Channick, B. J.: Primary aldosteronism, observations on 2 cases. Amer. J. Med. Sci. 239:324-337, 1960.

12. Daily, W. J. R., and Ganong, W. F.: The effect of ventral hypothalamic lesions on sodium and potassium metabolism in the dog. Endocrinology 62:442-454, 1958.

13. Davis, J. O.: Mechanisms of salt and water retention in congestive heart failure. The importance of aldosterone. Amer. J. Med. 29:486-507, 1960.

14. Davis, J. O., Carpenter, C. C. J., Ayers, C. R., Holman, J. E., and Bahn, R. C.: Evidence for secretion of an aldosterone-stimulating hormone by the kidney. J. Clin. Invest. 40:684-696, 1961.

15. Deane, H. W., and Greep, R. O.: A morphological and histochemical study of the rat's adrenal cortex after hypophysectomy with comments on the liver. Amer. J. Anat. 79:117-145, 1946.

16. Deane, H. W., Shaw, J. H., and Greep, R. O.: The effect of altered sodium or potassium intake on width and cytochemistry of the zona glomerulosa of the rat's adrenal gland. Endocrinology 43:133-153, 1948.

17. Farrell, G. L.: Regulation of aldosterone secretion. Physiol. Rev. 38:709-724, 1958.

18. Farrell, G. L.: The physiological factors which influence the secretion of aldosterone. Recent Progr. Hormone Res. 15:275-297, 1959.

19. Farrell, G. L.: Recent observations on adrenoglomerulotropin. Endocr. Soc. Abst. page 15, 1961.

20. Farrell, G. L., Pratt, A. D., Jr., and Mellinger, J. F.: Adrenoglomerulotropism: a diencephalic factor specific for aldosterone secretion. In Currie, A. F., Symington, T., and Grant, J. K.: The Human Adrenal Cortex. The Williams & Wilkins Company, Baltimore, 1962, pp. 196-203.

21. Fine, D., Meiselas, L. E., Colsky, J., and Oxenhorn, S.: Primary aldosteronism: Report of a case and discussion of the pathogenesis. New Engl. J. Med. 256:147-152, 1957.

22. Ganong, W. F., Milrow, P. J., and Cera, G. G.: Effect of angiotensin and ACTH on adrenocortical secretion in hypophysectomized, nephrectomized dogs. Endocr. Soc. Abst. page 14, 1961.

23. Genest, J.: Angiotensin, aldosterone and human arterial hypertension. Canad. Med. Assn. J. 84:403-419, 1961.

24. Giroud, C. J. P., Stachenko, J., and Piletta, P.: In vitro studies of the functional zonation of the adrenal cortex and of the production of aldosterone. In Muller, A., and O'Connor, C.: Aldosterone. Little, Brown and Company, 1958, pp. 56-72.

25. Goodyer, A. V. N., Peterson, E. R., and Relman, A. S.: Some effects of albumin infusions on renal function and electrolyte excretion in normal man. J. Appl. Physiol. 1:671-682, 1949.

26. Hartcroft, P. M., Newmark, L. N., and Pitcock, J. A.: Relationship of renal juxtaglomerular cells to sodium intake, adrenal cortex and hypertension. In Moyer, J. H. (ed.): Hypertension. W. B. Saunders Co., Philadelphia, 1959, pp. 24-30.

27. Laragh, J. H., and Stoerk, H. C.: A study of the mechanism of secretion of the sodium retaining hormone (aldosterone). J. Clin. Invest. 36:383-392, 1957.

28. LIDDLE, G. W., DUNCAN, L. E., JR., AND BARTTER, F. C.: Dual mechanism regulating adrenocortical function in man. Amer. J. Med. 21:380-386, 1956.

29. MILLS, I. H., CASPER, A., AND BARTTER, F. C.: On the role of the vagus in the control of aldosterone secretion. Science 128:1140-1141, 1958.

30. MULLER, A. F., RIONDEL, A. M., AND MANNING, E. L.: Effect of corticotrophin on secretion of aldosterone. Lancet 2:1021-1024, 1956.

31. RAUSCHKOLB, E. W., AND FARRELL, G. L.: Evidence for diencephalic regulation of aldosterone secretion. Endocrinology 59:526-531, 1956.

32. RAUSCHKOLB, E. W., FARRELL, G. L., AND KOLETSKY, S.: Aldosterone secretion after hypophysectomy. Amer. J. Physiol. 184:55-58, 1956.

33. ROSNAGLE, R. S., AND FARRELL, G. L.: Alterations in electrolyte intake and adrenal steroid secretion. Amer. J. Physiol. 187:7-10, 1956.

34. ROSS, E. J., VAN'T HOFF, W., CRABBÉ, J., AND THORN, G. W.: Aldosterone excretion in hypopituitarism after hypophysectomy in man. Amer. J. Med. 28:229-238, 1960.

35. TOBIAN, L.: Interrelationship of electrolytes, juxtaglomerular cells and hypertension. Physiol. Rev. 40:280-312, 1960.

36. WELT, L. G., AND ORLOFF, J.: The effects of an increase in plasma volume on the metabolism and excretion of water and electrolytes by normal subjects. J. Clin. Invest. 30:751-761, 1951.

37. YANKOPOULOS, N. A., DAVIS, J. O., KLIMAN, B., PETERSON, R. E., AND CASPER, A.: Evidence that a humeral agent stimulates the adrenal cortex to secrete aldosterone, in experimental secondary hyperaldosteronism. J. Clin. Invest. 38:1278-1289, 1959.